'The publication of this volume of papers from the Klein archive, together with critical discussion by notable Klein scholars, is a most exciting event. Every chapter is of interest, not only for its historical significance, but also because Klein's clinical and theoretical thinking is further explored in the excellent commentaries and related to later developments in psychoanalysis. I recommend it most warmly. It forms an essential and impressive part of the array of recent books about Klein which attest to the continuing fertility of her legacy.'

Margaret Rustin, Honorary Consultant Child Psychotherapist,
Tavistock and Portman NHS Foundation Trust,
co-author of *Reading Klein*

'This volume adds significantly to our understanding of Melanie Klein, her thinking and her internal world. We see her as a child, powerless to prevent the losses inflicted on her family; longing for knowledge and for the power to reduce suffering. We learn of Klein's early defiance, a hint of the powerful thinker whose radical ideas were later to spark fierce debate across the psychoanalytic world. We are shown too, a softer, more vulnerable and less certain Klein. Melanie Klein's humanity shines out of the chapters in this book.'

Penelope Garvey, Training Analyst British Psychoanalytical Society

ESSENTIAL READINGS FROM THE MELANIE KLEIN ARCHIVES

Essential Readings from the Melanie Klein Archives: Original Papers and Critical Reflections brings together a selection of previously unpublished material by Melanie Klein, one of the key architects of child psychoanalysis, and sets it in the context of the contemporary understanding of her work, with contributions by a range of leading Klein scholars.

The book contains lectures, letters, notes and an autobiography by Klein, as well as key pieces of analysis on Klein's work from major Kleinian analysts, with contributions from Claudia Frank, R.D. Hinshelwood, Jane Milton and Maria Rhode based on wide-ranging research into Klein's archive. Bringing the work of Claudia Frank to an English audience for the first time, there is also a new chapter by Maria Rhode featuring further case material on Klein's famous young patient 'Dick', the subject of Klein's 1930 paper on symbolism, which is discussed in relation to current ideas about the autistic spectrum. This material fleshes out our understanding of Klein's thinking, shines new light on the major features of her work, and the influences on the analyst herself.

Melanie Klein was a pioneering and sometimes controversial figure within psychoanalysis, whose new approach to child analysis and new understanding of our inner world were revolutionary. Her large archive (now available online) contains papers and drafts of papers, notes for lectures and seminars and a vast amount of case material, all of which is of scientific interest. *Essential Readings from the Melanie Klein Archives* will be of great interest to Klein scholars, as well as to researchers and readers in the wider history and development of psychoanalysis.

Dr Jane Milton is a psychiatrist and a training analyst of the British Psychoanalytical Society. Having worked as a consultant psychiatrist at Kings College Hospital and the Tavistock Clinic, she is now in full-time psychoanalytic practice. She is archivist for the Melanie Klein Trust and has published books and papers on various psychoanalytic topics.

ESSENTIAL READINGS FROM THE MELANIE KLEIN ARCHIVES

Original Papers and Critical Reflections

Edited by Jane Milton

Routledge
Taylor & Francis Group
LONDON AND NEW YORK

First published 2020
by Routledge
2 Park Square, Milton Park, Abingdon, Oxon OX14 4RN

and by Routledge
52 Vanderbilt Avenue, New York, NY 10017

Routledge is an imprint of the Taylor & Francis Group, an informa business

British Library Cataloguing-in-Publication Data
A catalogue record for this book is available from the British Library

Library of Congress Cataloging-in-Publication Data
A catalog record has been requested for this book

ISBN: 978-0-367-33789-6 (hbk)
ISBN: 978-0-367-33790-2 (pbk)
ISBN: 978-0-429-32198-6 (ebk)

Typeset in Bembo
by Integra Software Services Pvt. Ltd.

CONTENTS

ACKNOWLEDGEMENTS

I first acknowledge my gratitude to the Melanie Klein Trust for appointing me as archivist, giving me the privilege of working with this fascinating material. The trustees, who retain copyright, have given permission to publish all the material presented here. I am particularly grateful for the support of John Steiner who agreed to write the Foreword. The help of colleagues from the Trust website www.melanie-klein-trust.org.uk/ has been appreciated, particularly Anne Amos, Eleanor Sawbridge-Burton and Caroline Graty.

Claudia Frank owns copyright for her three chapters (6, 7 and 8) and has given permission for translation and publication. We would like to acknowledge the journals in which the material appeared:

Psyche-Zeitschrift Fur Psychoanalyse Und Ihre Anwendungen published Frank, C. (2003) 'Zu Melanie Kleins zeitgenössischer Bezugnahme auf Hitler und den Zweiten Weltkrieg in ihren Behandlungen'. *Psyche-Z Psychoanal*, 57: 708–728 (Chapter 6).

Luzifer-Amor: Zeitschrift zur Geschichte der Psychoanalyse published two of Frank's articles. The first is 'Angstberuhigung "Zu Melanie Kleins unveröffentlichtem Beitrag". On reassurance' (Chapter 7).

The second is '"Ist es ein Tier im Inneren?" Melanie Kleins unpubliziertes "Don Juan Paper"' (1939). In *Luzifer-Amor*, 41: 120–140 (Chapter 8).

Psychoanalysis and History gave kind permission for publication of two articles: Hinshelwood, R. (2006) 'Melanie Klein and repression: An examination of some unpublished notes of 1934'. *Psychoanalysis and History*, 8: 5–42 (Chapter 9).

Hinshelwood, R. (2008) 'Melanie and Klein and countertransference: A note on some archival material'. *Psychoanalysis and History*, 10: 95–113 (Chapter 10).

The International Journal of Psychoanalysis gave kind permission for two articles. The first is Hinshelwood, R.D. (1997) 'The elusive concept of "internal objects" (1934–1943). Its role in the formation of The Klein Group'. *Int. J. Psychoanal.*, 78: 877–897 (Chapter 11). The second is Milton, J. (2018) 'From the Melanie archive: Klein's further thoughts on loneliness'. *Int. J. Psychoanal.*, 99 (4): 929–946 (Chapter 12).

I am indebted to the Estate of W.R. Bion for allowing me to publish two letters written to Klein by Wilfred Bion, and to the Elliott Jaques Trust for allowing me to publish the letter to Klein from Elliott Jaques. All three of these letters appear in Chapter 12.

My gratitude goes to Christopher Hilton and Christy Henshaw of the Wellcome Library, who with colleagues made digitization of the Klein Archives possible. Christy's determination and energy in giving priority to digitization of the work of female scholars like Klein was particularly timely and helpful for me.

I want to thank Sophie Leighton for her excellent translations of Claudia Frank's three papers into English. Helga Skogstad also kindly worked with me during the process of choosing and translating the papers.

Particular thanks to my friend Mary Piercy for her skill in deciphering some of the eccentricities of the Archives, and for her quick and efficient typing, sorting of references and other invaluable contributions during the writing of the book.

FOREWORD

In the five years since her appointment as Archivist to the Melanie Klein Trust, Jane Milton has made this rich source of psychoanalytic thinking much more widely known especially through her regular blogs on the Melanie Klein Trust website. Now she has brought out this fascinating and important book which is much more than a contribution to history: it is highly relevant to contemporary analytic theory and practice and will be welcomed by a wide range of readers.

The first part of the book consists of four lectures given between 1936 and 1939 to a lay audience, which expound Klein's basic findings in simple but uncompromising terms. We see accounts of the play technique, the role of the unconscious, the place of sadness and loss in children and a discussion of the thorny question of what psychoanalysis can offer a child in difficulty. Most of the ideas have become incorporated in Klein's later work but these remain excellent summaries and are a pleasure to read. They indicate that some of her theories were well established in the 1930s and have not been greatly modified in later work.

The remainder of the book consists of papers by Claudia Frank, Bob Hinshelwood, Maria Rhode and Jane Milton herself who have worked in the Archives and discuss and explain material they have found there. The reader needs help to put the material in context and this is ably provided by the scholarship of these authors.

Readers will find their own favourites among these chapters and I will only mention a few that I found particularly interesting. One was the discovery by Claudia Frank of several sections in which Klein comments on the threat from Nazi Germany which entered and influenced the phantasy life of her patients. This seems to contradict the view that Klein ignored the external environment. She found that some patients identified with the Nazi violence and feared that an internal Hitler figure had done terrible damage. I was surprised to find that Klein also addressed the need to deal with real external threats and that unconscious phantasy can interfere with our capacity to do this. She described how splitting is necessary if we are to turn our hatred against external sources of evil and direct our love to the protection of good objects. A breakdown of splitting as a result of phantasies of destructiveness can therefore have a paralysing effect on our ability to defeat external dangers. Splitting helps us to trust our capacity to love and enables us to hate our enemies with full strength and to oppose what is felt to be evil in the external world.

Hinshelwood's discussion of Klein's comments on countertransference was also very interesting. While she clearly had reservations about the use of countertransference it is clear that she accepted that the analyst was profoundly influenced by the patient especially in the case of psychotic patients who use violent splitting and projection into the analyst. When they cannot handle the negativity the analyst may defend himself against such intrusions by reinforcing the positive transference. Elsewhere in her lectures in technique she described the opposite possibility when we over-emphasize the negative transference and fail to recognize the love beneath the hatred.

Jane Milton's discussion of Klein's paper 'On the Sense of Loneliness', which was published posthumously in 1963, makes use of the various versions and additions which she was collecting to use in a book on the subject. The original paper is moving and probably influenced by her own loneliness near the end of her life but it is clearly unfinished and leaves us curious to understand the essence of loneliness. Klein linked loneliness to a longing to regain an idealized early relationship to the mother, perhaps especially a pre-verbal one. She also emphasized the importance of integration and suggested that we feel lonely when separated from parts of ourselves when these have been split off and projected. In a surprising comment she suggests that an understanding of our bi-sexuality was important in loneliness I think because she felt that a good relation between male and female elements is vital for a sense of completeness. Jane Milton sensitively discusses the additional material and even though it does not answer the fundamental questions it does provide important context including the way Klein listened to her colleagues and pupils, especially Bion, Jaques, Segal and Rosenfeld.

For me the chapter on Klein's patient Dick by Maria Rhode raises important questions about the use of part-object language in our work with disturbed patients. I remember the problems Dick had with symbols when he saw some pencil shavings on Klein's lap and said 'Poor Mrs Klein', but I had forgotten that she believed that his concrete thinking enabled her to speak in part-object terms referring particularly to the body. For example in her play she spoke to him about a 'Daddy-train' and a 'Dick-train' and when he made it roll to the window and said 'Station' she explained: 'The station is mummy; Dick is going into mummy.' When he shut himself in a space between the doors saying 'dark' she explained to him: 'It is dark inside mummy.' Later she interpreted that Dick wanted to cut faeces out of mummy's tummy.

Klein was concerned with attacks on the mother's body and the babies, faeces and father's penis that it contained, and we are familiar with these concepts as unconscious phantasies. However in recent times we have tended to avoid interpreting directly to the patient in these terms and Maria Rhode's account makes me wonder if we have lost something in the process and might try to reassess this aspect of our technique.

Other readers may focus on different themes and there is plenty to stimulate interest and thought. Jane Milton's editorial overviews are extremely useful and much of Klein's unpublished material is stimulating and provocative. It is clear that a great deal of rich material remains to be studied that will provide fertile areas of exploration for years to come.

by John Steiner

CONTRIBUTORS

Professor Claudia Frank is a medical doctor and IPA psychoanalyst in private practice in Stuttgart. She is a training analyst of the Deutsche Psychoanalytische Vereinigung, and has served as chair of their training committee. From 1980–2001 she held a chair at the Department for Psychoanalysis, Psychotherapy and Psychosomatics at the University of Tübingen. She has published widely about the technique, theory, history and applications of psychoanalysis. Her 1999 book (translated into English in 2009) *Melanie Klein in Berlin: Her First Psychoanalyses of Children* was a major contribution to Klein archival studies. She is currently co-Editor of *Jahrbuch der Psychoanalyse.*

Professor Robert D. Hinshelwood is a Fellow of the British Psychoanalytical Society, and a Fellow of the Royal College of Psychiatrists. He was Director of the Cassel Hospital and is now Professor Emeritus at the University of Essex. He has a long interest in the history of psychoanalysis, and is a founder of the Journal *Psychoanalysis and History*. He has published many books and articles in the psychoanalytic field.

Dr Jane Milton is a psychiatrist and a training analyst of the British Psychoanalytical Society. Having worked as a consultant psychiatrist at Kings College Hospital and the Tavistock Clinic she is now in full-time psychoanalytic practice. She is archivist for the Melanie Klein trust and has published books and papers on various psychoanalytic topics. She has particular interest in the development of psychoanalysis in Ukraine.

Professor Maria Rhode is Emeritus Professor of Child Psychotherapy at the Tavistock Clinic and University of East London, and Clinical Associate of the British Psycho-Analytical Society. She trained as a Kleinian child psychotherapist at the Tavistock, where she formerly co-convened the autism workshop and now sees toddlers at risk of autism. She is co-editor of *Psychotic States in Children* (with Margaret Rustin and Alex and Hélène Dubinsky); of *The Many Faces of Asperger's Syndrome* (with Trudy Klauber); and of *Invisible Boundaries: Psychosis and Autism in Children and Adolescents* (with Didier Houzel).

EDITOR'S INTRODUCTION

The Melanie Klein Archives

In this book I aim to show the reader some of the riches of the Melanie Klein Archives. Owned by the Wellcome Library but with copyright retained by the Melanie Klein Trust, the Archives are a fascinating source of unpublished material from the pen of this major figure in the history of psychoanalysis.

Melanie Klein (1882–1960) knew that her ideas were important and was concerned that they should survive her. They were subject to huge controversy in her lifetime, especially after Freud and other Viennese refugees arrived in London just before the Second World War. At this point she was in danger of expulsion from the British Society and had to fight to show that her ideas were as rooted in Freud's as were those of Anna Freud and others. A whole section of the Klein Archives is concerned with the Controversial Discussions where this debate took place. I think that Klein's fear for the survival of her ideas must be part of the reason she kept so much material and ensured its preservation.

The Melanie Klein Trust, to whom Klein bequeathed her papers, is a charity set up near the end of Klein's life, with the aim of preserving and disseminating her legacy. After Klein's death the Archives were stored in the home of her close colleague Hanna Segal. In 1984 the Trust donated them to the Medical Archives Centre of the Wellcome Library, where the fragile material could be preserved and made available to scholars.

Besides family letters and photographs, Klein left diaries, drafts and full versions of papers both published and unpublished, teaching material, ideas for papers, and so on. The dearth of professional letters suggests that Klein destroyed these. She did however keep an enormous amount of case material. Of the 29 boxes of papers (each consisting of several hundred sheets), 12 are of clinical notes; it is clear that Klein, unlike Freud, thought that her unpublished notes were worth preserving, and there is evidence that she had been intending to use at least some of them in future publications. Klein tended to date her clinical notes, but most of her notes on theory and technique are, frustratingly, often undated.

The material is catalogued in five sections as follows:

A Personal and biographical, 1879–1982;
B Case material;
C Manuscripts;
D Notes;
E Controversy within the British Psycho-Analytical Society, 1939–1944;
F Family Papers.

The earlier papers, before Klein's arrival in London in 1926, are in German and some of them are written in 'Deutschschrift'; the Klein Trust has had the help of Ines Schlenker in deciphering the handwriting and Sophie Leighton in translation from German into English. However the later material is in English. Some material is handwritten by Klein; much material is in typescript, often with corrections in Klein's handwriting.

At first scholars were able to consult the original documents in the Wellcome Library reading room. Over the years, in attempts to maintain access without deterioration, they were microfiched, and later some of them were copied on to CDs. Finally, in early 2018, through collaboration between the Trust and the Wellcome, the process of full digitization was completed. The papers are now available to the general public online, through the Wellcome Library. A few child files remain under restricted access until the 2030s.

To view a digital file through the Wellcome Library catalogue (https://wellcomelibrary.org), the code digklein is used, followed by the file catalogue number. For example to view the additional loneliness notes described in Chapter 13 the entry would be digklein C.29. When the file name appears, clicking 'view online' will then open it.

Researching the Archives

Immersion in the Archives shows one how Klein never thought of theory independently of practice – a theoretical passage will quickly flow into a set of session notes, and vice versa. Often one finds scribbled in Klein's hand on a piece of material 'for book on (subject) X' or 'to illustrate Y'. She seems alive with ideas until the last, and full of plans for further publications, still at the height of her powers when she died aged 78.

Over the years my predecessor as archivist, Elizabeth Spillius, who described herself as becoming a complete Archives addict, researched the Archives, supported others in doing so, and published material herself (see Spillius, 2007 and Spillius et al., 2011). Since succeeding her in 2014 I have tried to continue this work. I try to discover what has already been researched and published. I work closely with the team who run the Trust website, an excellent source of information and news about Klein and post-Kleinian developments. I write a blog post every few months, which can be found via the website, where I bring out small but interesting nuggets that I have discovered in the Archives. As an example I will give my first blog post from 2016.

This short vignette comes from archive file PP/KLE/D.16, itself part of a larger collection D. 1–17, referred to in the Archives catalogue as 'Techniques Notes'. D.16 is a large, miscellaneous bundle of lecture and seminar notes, bits of theory and bits of clinical material. A small number of pages within the file are dated between 1940 and 1943, suggesting that this extract also belongs to around that time. I have found no mention of this patient in Klein's published work. It consists of one and a half pages of typed material, appearing in the digital archive on D.16, images 57 and 58.

Defences in infancy

A very important defence, linked up with turning away from the object, is turning away from the satisfaction itself. Instance: Patient, 50 years old, in whom we discovered that all her life she had no need for liquids and drank extremely little. The doctor disapproved of this lack of liquid. In her youth she was proud that she needed so little liquid, and on expeditions could give up her share to others. This never struck her as strange. The material in this particular context definitely pointed to the early relation to the breast – that she did not need the breast and milk, and got compensation from that. That was very important in a number of ways in her make-up. We found that liquid was equated to fluidity in mental ways and attitudes, and her rigidity, which she was aware of as a strong limitation, was connected with 'solid' ways, e.g. putting everything in its place. This could be worked out in many ways in her mental life, 'solid' ways, everything worked out carefully: obsessional ways and rigidity of mind. Later, when came up again, showed how it influenced her social intercourse with people. She had not been able to ponder leisurely over a talk with people. She felt that other people could so much more easily return a smile, and converse easily, and so on. Again connection with the rejection of liquid came in, quite clearly in connection with her mother, who actually despised caressing names, thought too big gifts to friends unnecessary, and had an attitude of restricting tenderness and easy ways. From there we got back again to the earlier rejection of liquid and could link this up with the lack of tenderness, caressing, conversing, in her babyhood. This patient had noticed the rigid ways of her mother in connection with younger brothers and sisters, of whom there were many, and she had definite memory about these ways of her mother in connection with these babies. Also memory that her mother refused to feed the youngest baby. It was quite obvious that the mother actually had this attitude. My point is the link between easy, friendly, loving sexual intercourse and early relation at the breast. Interesting point that in spite of these ways of the mother some of the brothers and sisters developed entirely different attitudes from those of the patient.

Although I cannot know about all the work that has been done in the Archives I will mention a few scholars besides Elizabeth Spillius who have already devoted much time to them. Pearl King and Riccardo Steiner (King & Steiner,

1992) made use of section E in their important book about the Controversial Discussions. Phyllis Grosskurth (1986) consulted archival material for her biography of Klein. Claudia Frank was one of the first scholars to study the Klein Archives in depth and did extensive research on them in the 1990s. She writes in German but some of her work is available in translation, for example her research on Klein's early work in Berlin (Frank, 2009). Three of her papers originally published in German have been translated for this volume. Some of Robert Hinshelwood's considerable archival research appears here also. Michal Shapira (2013) and Sue Sherwin-White (2017) have all made substantial use of the Archives in their books. John Steiner's (2017) publication of Klein's lectures and seminars on adult technique was a major contribution.

Contents of this book

Part 1 of this book, 'In Klein's own words', publishes for the first time four of Klein's lay lectures given between 1936 and 1939, her autobiography of 1959 and one important letter from 1955. The lay lectures were written for conferences on Education and Child Guidance and are very readable and engaging. Klein's academic papers can sometimes feel indigestible, but she perhaps felt freer writing for a lay audience.

Chapter 1, 'The need for psychoanalysis in certain types of difficult children', appears in archive PP/KLE/C.49. It was written for a conference of the National Education Fellowship held in Cheltenham in the summer of 1936. The NEF was a movement between the wars connecting lay enthusiasts for educational reform with major figures in the developing disciplines of psychology and education.

Klein states her respect for the good educator with some psychological understanding, who shows belief in the child's good intentions, in order to strengthen these. However, she explains that she has in mind children whose feelings of love and kindness are so deeply buried that it is impossible to detect them. She gives the example of 12-year-old John, who has lost his mother. He is greatly inhibited and can neither trust nor take anything in from others, including his teachers. He fears closeness, is over-pleasing and at times deceitful, and is prone to fits of violence and cruelty towards other children. In Klein's view John's tendency to excess aggression has led to fears of his destructiveness towards the good object and retaliation in kind; the loss of his mother had confirmed his worst fears about the results of his destructiveness.

Klein shows how careful analytic work with John enabled him to resume learning at school, make good contact with others, and to develop a real fondness for a few other people. Only by analysis of their aggressive impulses and resultant anxieties can the analyst uncover the feelings of guilt arising from these impulses and gain access to buried feelings of love. Klein's stress on uncovering love buried under hate is stressed also in Klein's recently published lectures on technique (Steiner, 2017).

The material of Klein's lecture in Chapter 2, 'On play', is to be found in archive file C.50. It was given at the Child Guidance Inter-Clinic conference of Great Britain 1937. I explain in this chapter the context of the relatively new Child Guidance movement, and I also give the backgrounds of the discussants taking part in this workshop.

Chapter 3, 'The importance of the unconscious mind for the whole personality', and Chapter 4, 'Sadness and loss in the emotional life of the young child', both contain lectures given at the London Institute of Education in May 1939. They were part of the Joseph Payne lecture series, the overall topic of which was 'Psychoanalysis and Normal Development'. All the material of these two chapters is to be found in archive C.51.

Chapter 5, 'Autobiography and reflections', contains two items. The first is a recently unearthed letter that will in due course be placed in the Wellcome archive. It was written in 1955 and I find it moving in the way it expresses how at last Klein is beginning to believe that her ideas will survive her. This is followed by Klein's autobiography of 1959, found unexpectedly in Money-Kyrle's archives at the Wellcome by Robert Hinshelwood. The autobiography appears, in an earlier, more fragmentary form, in Klein's archive file A.52. This was published with explanatory notes by Janet Sayers and John Forrester in 2013. The version found in the Money-Kyrle archives is nearer to completion. It had, as Hinshelwood shows, been sent to Money-Kyrle with a view to its being included in Klein's collected works, but in the event was not and, being the only copy at the time, was lost to view for many years.

Part 2 of this book, 'Studies from the Melanie Klein Archives', is devoted to research done on parts of the archives by Claudia Frank, R.D. Hinshelwood and Maria Rhode and myself. Of the eight chapters, versions of seven have previously been published in journals, but three of those only in German, translated here for the Klein Trust by Sophie Leighton. The final chapter, 13, was kindly written by Professor Maria Rhode especially for the book and is a study of Klein's further notes on 'Dick'. Maria was given special access to this closed file, and has carefully preserved confidentiality. Dick was the 4-year-old child who formed the basis of Klein's seminal 1930 paper 'The importance of symbol-formation in the development of the ego' (Klein, 1975[1930]). Here Klein writes about some early sessions with Dick, a very disturbed child who by modern diagnostic criteria would be considered on the autistic spectrum. It turns out that Klein continued to work with Dick, on and off, into young adulthood, keeping copious notes on the work; she may have intended to write further about him.

Maria Rhode is a specialist on the study and treatment of autism from a psychoanalytic perspective. She has drawn careful attention both to Dick's clearly autistic features, and also to his more ordinary capacities, and not least to the surprisingly positive and rapid way he responded to a psychoanalytic approach. Rhode is interested in how Klein, inevitably of her time, and before the diagnosis and understanding of autism even existed, was sensitive to the fact that there was something more, and different, about Dick. For example many years before Frances Tustin was to understand about the autistic child's fear of 'pouring out' through holes in the skin, Rhode shows how Klein intuited something about this and tried to describe it, even though she as yet had no theory in which to frame her observations.

The three newly translated chapters by Claudia Frank are a result of her painstaking work in the Archives in the 1990s. Chapter 6 is entitled 'Melanie Klein's contemporaneous references to Hitler and the Second World War in her therapeutic sessions'. Claudia shows how, contrary to a commonly held prejudice, Klein by no means concentrated on internal to the exclusion of external reality. Here she is shown working with her adult and child patients during the war, and skilfully analysing the complex interaction between external and internal worlds, particularly in relation to destructiveness and reparation. The 'Hitler inside us' or 'the war inside' are evocative concepts also used by Michal Shapira (2013) independently using some of the same material but looking from a sociological perspective.

Chapter 7, 'An unpublished contribution of Melanie Klein on reassurance' (from file C.67), Claudia shows to be a contribution to a piece of research on psychoanalytic technique conducted by Edward Glover in the British psychoanalytic society in the1930s. She discusses the paper against the background of discussions conducted in London at that time, which included contributions from Klein's psychoanalyst daughter Melitta Schmideberg and from James Strachey. Although Klein consistently considered 'correct interpretation' to be most effective means of reassurance, she occasionally also accepted a non-interpreting approach. In this respect the paper presented here goes further than any of her published writings.

Klein's unpublished Don Juan paper, as Claudia Frank's meticulous research shows, was written in 1939, although she may have written a brief summary of her thoughts in 1934, after seeing a performance of a play by Obey about this character. The relevant archival material, in file C.91, is discussed in Chapter 8. Claudia describes how the character of Don Juan has been portrayed by many writers, going back to the early seventeenth century. The Don Juan of Obey's play is a more tormented and tragic character than the better known Don Giovanni of Mozart's opera. In this venture into applied psychoanalysis, Klein links his state with defences against primitive depressive anxieties, linked to oral destructive and devouring impulses. To illustrate her theme, Klein brings clinical material from the treatment of a 5-year-old boy, also mentioning an adult case.

Professor R.D. Hinshelwood contributes three chapters, all of which have previously appeared in journals. They have all been modified slightly to make them more suitable as book chapters. In Chapter 9, 'Melanie Klein and repression: An examination of some unpublished notes of 1934', Bob points out that Klein rarely uses the term 'repression' in her published works, referring early on at least as much to 'splitting of the object' and later to 'splitting of the ego' together with 'projective identification'. He was thus struck to find 15 pages of notes in archive file B.89 entitled 'Early Repression Mechanism'. In this chapter he researches this material from a historical perspective, seeking to discover how Klein's preference for the term 'splitting' had come into being.

Hinshelwood argues that Klein originally intended in these Notes to set early defences (evacuation/destruction) in relation to classical repression. However, he shows how these 15 pages of Notes provide insight into the very process of invention, evidencing how Klein reworks the physical sequence of the pages at least once, with certain pages re-ordered and interpolated as Klein re-orders her thinking about early and late defence mechanisms.

In Chapter 10, 'Melanie Klein and countertransference', Bob explores Klein's relationship to the concept of countertransference, hardly mentioned in her published work. From 1950 onwards a number of analysts revised the view of countertransference simply as an obstruction, suggesting that it can sometimes give us vital information about our patients. Among these was not only Paula Heimann, who was later to become estranged from Klein, but also colleagues to whom she remained closely associated, like Rosenfeld, Bion and Money-Kyrle. She must thus have been able at least to tolerate such views in her followers.

In this chapter, in addition, Hinshelwood publishes five pages from the archive file D. 29. This contains two sets of notes on countertransference in response to a paper given by Bion to a symposium on The Psychology of Schizophrenia at the IPA Congress of 1953, held in London. Hinshelwood shows that Klein does in fact confirm a view of countertransference as a possible product of the patient's projective processes, as of course later Kleinians have fully exploited. Hinshelwood sees her as taking an intermediate position between that of Freud and that of her followers who were beginning to use the concept clinically. He feels that this position was one which allowed her followers freedom in developing the notion and use of countertransference, in spite of her relative scepticism.

In Hinshelwood's Chapter 11, 'The elusive concept of "internal objects"', he uses three archive files, C.68, C. 92 and D.16, to trace a debate about the concept of 'internal objects' which took place between 1934 and 1943, a time when a group of analysts was forming around Melanie Klein. The debate is set within a complex of personal, group and organizational dynamics, which the paper starts to unravel. Hinshelwood uses Bion's notion of 'group schism' to show how opposed groups of analysts formed to support members against severe anxieties at this time. These anxieties were the fact of war and possible invasion, the Nazi destruction of psychoanalysis on mainland Europe, and the death of Freud shortly after his refugee friends and followers arrived in the British society.

Hinshelwood shows how between 1935 and 1942 'internal objects' were the subject of frequent scientific meetings and at the centre of debate. To protect Klein's views an informal study group was set up by 1939 called the 'Internal Objects Group'. Today 'internal objects' are not a subject of great contention in the British society, though they are still conceptualized in somewhat different ways, with some classical colleagues preferring to use the differently shaded term 'internal representation', and others not using the concept much at all.

My own Chapter 12, 'Klein's further thoughts on loneliness', arose out of a study of archive files C.27, C.28 and C.29. All are connected to Klein's final, posthumously published paper 'On the sense of loneliness'. I discovered that four differing versions of the paper, prepared for spoken presentations to different audiences, were written between 1958 and 1960. There is evidence from Klein's copious additional notes that she intended to write a monograph addressing loneliness from a psychoanalytic point of view. Previously unpublished letters to Klein from Wilfred Bion and Elliot Jaques and extracts from Klein's own notes are included, organized under a number of headings. I find the material moving and I suggest that some of the themes Klein was working on may have had particular relevance for her personally in what turned out to be the very last months of her life.

References

Frank, C. (2009). *Melanie Klein in Berlin: Her first psychoanalyses of children*, ed. E. Spillius. London: Routledge. Translated by Sophie Leighton.

Grosskurth, P. (1986). *Melanie Klein: Her world and her work*. London: Knopf.

King, P. and Steiner, R. (eds) (1992). *The Freud–Klein controversies 1941–45*. London: Routledge.

Klein, M. (1975[1930]). The importance of symbol formation in the development of the ego. In *Love, guilt and reparation and other works. 1921–1945: The writings of Melanie Klein volume 1*. London: Hogarth.

Sayers, J. and Forrester, J. (2011). The autobiography of Melanie Klein. *Psychoanalysis and History, 15*(2), 127–163.

Shapira, Michal (2013). *The war inside: Psychoanalysis, total war and the making of the democratic self in post war Britain*. Cambridge: Cambridge University Press.

Sherwin-White, S. (2017). *Melanie Klein revisited: Pioneer and revolutionary in the psychoanalysis of children*. London: Karnac.

Spillius, Elizabeth (2007). *Encounters with Melanie Klein: Selected papers of Elizabeth Spillius*. Edited by P. Roth and R. Rusbridger. London: Routledge.

Spillius, E., Milton, J., Garvey, P., Couve, C. and Steiner, D. (2011). *The new dictionary of Kleinian thought*. London: Routledge.

Steiner, John (ed.) (2017). *Lectures on technique by Melanie Klein*. London: Routledge.

The digitized Melanie Klein Archives can be accessed via the Wellcome Library (https://wellcomelibrary.org).

PART 1

In Klein's own words

1

THE NEED FOR PSYCHOANALYSIS IN CERTAIN TYPES OF DIFFICULT CHILDREN

Melanie Klein (edited by Jane Milton)

Introduction

Melanie Klein gave this lecture at a conference of the National Education Fellowship (NEF) held in Cheltenham in 1936. The NEF was a movement connecting lay enthusiasts for educational reform with major figures in the developing disciplines of psychology and education, such as Carl Gustav Jung, Jean Piaget and John Dewey. The conference theme was the educational foundations of freedom and a free community, and it was to be the last before the onset of the Second World War. Brehony (2004) notes that, unlike the NEF conferences of the 1920s, amongst 50 listed contributors there was little sign of psychoanalysis in the discussions other than contributions from Melanie Klein and Susan Isaacs. Klein's manuscript, hitherto unpublished, is to be found in Wellcome Library archive file PP/KLE/C.49 and is available to view online. Klein's typescript is heavily corrected in her own handwriting. Klein's style, as with others of her lay lectures, is clear and approachable, with detailed clinical illustration. She focuses here on the interaction between environment and the inner life of phantasy, particularly aggressive phantasy, in causing severe disturbance, which she says responds only to psychoanalytic intervention. Her main case illustration is a boy of 12 whose lack of trust and inability to get close to others in a loving relationship are linked to fears of the damage he does in phantasy through his aggression.

The lecture: The need for psychoanalysis in certain types of difficult children

In my contribution to this Symposium I want to consider the special question of those difficult children with whom various modes of psychotherapy or other measures, such as favourable changes of environment, educational influences, giving the child opportunities for play and for suitable occupation, do not achieve their purpose. Such methods, beneficial as we know they may be in some cases, fail or do not achieve lasting results with children whose difficulties are very deeply rooted.

In considering the causes of severe emotional difficulties in children, one would, broadly speaking, say that they arise from two sources. Unfavourable circumstances, especially in the very early days, have a lastingly bad effect upon the child's mind. The other source is his own aggressive impulses, which give rise to fear and feelings of guilt in his mind, since to begin with they are directed against the very people on whom he is dependent and of whom he is most fond – first of all his mother.

Even where circumstances are favourable, the child's impulses and phantasies of a frightening nature, which necessarily develop in his mind and which are bound up with his instinctual life, may give rise to severe psychological difficulties. Again, however unfavourable the environment may be, one cannot attribute psychological disturbances exclusively to it since the child's own impulses and phantasies play a fundamental part in the effect such experiences will have upon his mind. This explains why environmental influences and changes do not always and necessarily do away with the child's difficulties. If his difficulties are due more to deep unconscious conflicts than to the external pressure of circumstances, he will not be accessible to any method which cannot go down to the sources of these difficulties. That is why certain types of disturbances can be relieved only by the specialized technique of psycho-analysis, which is able to penetrate to the unconscious causes of the child's conflicts.

From among the variety of types of difficult children who do not respond to education and other methods and with whom I think only psycho-analysis can be effective, I am choosing today as an example the case of a child who seems to illustrate my thesis clearly. Children of the type which I am singling out here, when offered friendliness, seem unable to accept it, and are incapable of real affection. They are usually extremely distrustful, though they may disguise this. They are uneducable in the true sense of the word, for though they sometimes make an apparent adaptation, they are driven to this mainly by fears and the wish to escape punishment, or in order to get certain advantages.

A boy, let us call him John, aged twelve, came to be psycho-analysed on account of inhibition in learning and character difficulties. He came from a poor and simple but intelligent family. The general impression he gave was that of a diffident and shy child, who avoided looking one in the eyes; but at the same time apt to be overbearing and inclined to fits of violence and cruelty towards other children. Though John was very keen to get on with his teachers and peers he did not manage to do so, and was definitely uncompanionable and unpopular. He was prone to lying and stealing and was generally unreliable, and did not show affection for anyone. Though hypocritical in some ways – for instance, deceitful if he got into trouble – he was not inclined to simulate affection but tended to withdraw from people and not to confide in them.

In analysis it appeared that John had no belief in anybody's kindness or reliability; least of all did he trust his own good feelings, and that was the reason for his deep mistrust of others. His adaptation, as far as he achieved this, was mainly determined by fears, and the wish to avoid trouble or to get something out of it. Another important motive for his attempts at adaptation was his obsessional fear of being thought to be different from other children, and his anxiety of being laughed at and humiliated, which led him to avoid being conspicuous. He was incapable of real affection, and friendliness seldom stirred any response in him. This development had been greatly influenced by the death of John's mother which had occurred some years earlier. He had been very fond of her and also of his sisters but his relation to them gradually became less satisfactory after his mother's death, and he seemed to lose his affection for them. John's relation to his father was never really affectionate, though he was careful not to get into trouble with him.

Psycho-analysis brought out the fact that the death of his mother had not been the fundamental cause of his unfavourable development, though it made things infinitely worse. Fits of violence of a definitely asocial or even criminal type which occurred during the psycho-analytic hours were found to go back to situations in his early babyhood. Actually when a baby, he once had a quite dangerous fit of violent rage because the bottle, being too hot, had to be taken away again after he had already seen it. Intense greed, and in connection with this, very strong destructive impulses against his mother as a result of any dissatisfaction or frustration had given rise to great anxiety of having injured her – or rather, of going on injuring her whenever hate flared up. An unbearable conflict was thus created which determined his whole later development; the same person whom he deeply loved was the one who was most exposed to his hate, because she was the one from whom he most wanted gratifications. This greedy love was also the source of his intense jealousy, since he could not stand anybody else enjoying her love or attention.

It is a characteristic of the infant's mind that aggressive phantasies, which go with destructive impulses, are felt to be a real danger to the object of them, and give rise to feelings of guilt. The strength of aggression no doubt varies with individuals, and another important variable factor is the child's ability to stand his anxieties and feelings of guilt.

If the child is not altogether overcome by them, these anxieties and feelings of guilt quite early give rise to the wish to make good and they will thus be greatly modified in the course of the development, with the help of a favourable environment. But if this deep struggle between destructive impulses and feelings of love and constructive tendencies has not for one reason or another come to a more or less satisfactory solution in the first few years of life, it influences all later relationships. In psycho-analysis however (and this is one of the means by which fundamental changes are brought about) conflicting feelings and impulses of various kinds – love, hate, distrust, guilt, fears, and so on – are revived in connection with the analyst, on whom they become temporarily focussed, and can thus be submitted to analysis.

To return to John: his aggressive impulses and his fears had been extremely strong to begin with, but had become modified to a certain extent later on. When his mother's death occurred however, this was felt by him to be a confirmation of his fear that his strong sadistic tendencies had been effective. As a result, his feelings of guilt increased enormously, and his trust in his own good feelings and in his constructive tendencies decreased. Moreover, he felt that he could get no more goodness in the world, since in his mind he had destroyed the source of all goodness.

During his analysis, feelings of love and confidence in the analyst came to the fore, alternating with violent hate and distrust; but he strongly denied both to himself and to the analyst these growing feelings of love.

One day in analysis John told me a little French rhyme about a kitten that played with grandmother's ball of wool and tangled it. Grandmother got cross, and the kitten in a cowardly way ran off; but soon came back because he knew very well that grandmother was really very kind and patient. John then suddenly realized that in his mind the good grandmother stood for the analyst, who had been so patient with him. But this spontaneous realization of his friendly feelings towards me was soon followed by an outburst of violence in which he threw his knife (a blunt one) at me and just missed me. He then told me that he would not have minded if he had hit me, and actually he did not show any feelings of sorrow or concern. Later in the same hour in which he had made this attack on me he told me that there were two things that I must never say. These were 'being fond' and 'kill'.

His violent reaction can be explained in the following way. His becoming aware of love and gratitude towards me had had the effect of making him feel all the more that the loved mother, whom I represented to him at the time, was also the one whom he wanted to injure, because at the same time as he loved her, he hated her, first for not gratifying his very strong and greedy desires and then because fear lest she would retaliate for his aggressive intentions. [Such a fear] gives rise to increased hate, anxiety and distrust of the person whom the child is attacking in phantasy.

When he became aware that he loved me, his fears that he would destroy me – as in his phantasy he had destroyed his mother – were aroused. This fear led him to test, by his attack, whether he was actually dangerous to me and also whether I would retaliate. The old conflict between love and hate and the fear for the safety of the loved one had reappeared in full strength, and was overwhelming. Feeling that he was possessed of uncontrollable greed, incapable of bearing frustrations and unable to control his murderous tendencies, he could not bear to realize that he loved a person whom at the same time he felt in danger of destroying.

To illustrate this further: John used to bring sweets with him, which he saved especially for this purpose and ate during the psycho-analytic sessions. He did this partly to be able to control his outbursts of violence against me. Once, when he had set burning a great amount of paper in my room, he said afterwards, 'This would not have happened had I had sweets with me.' He had then already come to understand that if he avoided frustrations, he could better control his aggressive impulses.

In the past, he had buried his love because he could not cope with the conflict between love and hate, for greed and jealousy were overwhelmingly strong in him. Since he could not trust himself to love anybody without endangering that person, he had therefore had to shut himself off from friendly influences. Along with this, his constructive tendencies and his belief in them became inhibited.

As I have pointed out before, very early in development, feelings of guilt as a result of aggressive impulses towards the loved object give rise to wishes to repair the damage which has been done in phantasy. These wishes to restore and to make good are at the bottom of all constructive tendencies, and influence all later creative and productive activities, and also learning and intellectual development.

John was so overwhelmed by the dangerousness of his destructive tendencies that he could not trust in his constructive ones. The fact that his tendencies to make reparation could not develop and his distrust of everybody and everything, were responsible for his incapacity to take in knowledge, for his general intellectual inhibition, and for all his other difficulties.

When the analysis touched the unconscious reasons for these difficulties, his violence gradually diminished and his capacity to learn and to be a companion, greatly improved. He became able to make good contact with others, developed real fondness for a few people and his whole general attitude altered favourably.

I want to stress two important facts, first that there is a connection between aggressive impulses and constructive tendencies; the link developing early in life between the love felt for and therefore guilt towards the object which has been injured in phantasy and therefore the guilt experienced at its injury. The second point is that this early connection may be broken off if fears and the feelings of guilt are too overwhelming.

If, in the infant's mind, a balance cannot be kept between love and hate, between aggressive impulses and efforts to make reparation – then feelings of love and all that these imply may become entirely buried.

Good educators, being led by true psychological understanding have, of course, always known that to show trust and belief in the child's good intentions, even where these can hardly be detected, is sometimes a good way of bringing them to the fore and strengthening them. But as we also know, even these means do very often fail. If feelings of love and kindness are so deeply buried that for all practical purposes they do not exist, it is futile to appeal to them.

Moreover, in the type of case I have referred to, any approach of the kind – anything which might be felt as appealing to the child's good feelings – may even increase his anxieties and suspicions. For in the depths of his mind he feels that he cannot be trusted, because of his uncontrollable aggressive impulses, and that it is safer for others and also for himself if people are on their guard against him.

With a child of this type it is only by analysing his aggressive impulses and phantasies and the various anxieties to which they give rise that the psycho-analyst uncovers the feelings of guilt arising out of these impulses, and then also gains access to the buried feelings of love.

The conclusion presents itself that the specialized treatment of psycho-analysis, carried out by properly trained psycho-analysts should be made available as an adjunct to education for those children for whom it is indispensable. It is true that there are many difficulties in the way of the general application of psycho-analytic treatment. It often takes some length of time, and it can only be given individually – to one child at a time and for several periods a week.

There are, however, cases in which a shorter course of psycho-analytic treatment can produce very far-reaching results which are unobtainable by any other method. We must also remember that much time, effort and money are now being spent on attempting to stabilize and educate children who cannot, as I have tried to show, benefit by such methods. The fact that we are not yet in a position to apply this treatment more generally should not allow us to lose sight of the fact that in some cases, which are more numerous than is yet realized, mental health and education are only possible if psycho-analytic treatment is given.

We must

[Here the first part of the document stops. Clearly Klein intended to say something further in this, her conclusion to the lecture, but the pages are now missing. However there is an additional note taking the form of some clinical material, typed in a slightly different format. We do not know whether or not Klein spoke from these notes in her lecture.]

Clinical material

There had been very difficult days in connection with the preparation for the exam. When he heard that he could not come and see me on Saturdays, which he wished to do, because this time would be left for the exam, this obviously frightened him very much and he at once turned very aggressive against me. There had again been hours when he would not go out of the waiting room and I had to go out as soon as he started to throw his Yo-Yo at me in a rather dangerous way. The Yo-Yo now took the place of the hard balls he used to throw at me, also standing for an internal object which he could control and which could come back to him. In these treatment sessions, he was reading in an obsessional way, eating greedily lots of sweets and sometimes allowing me a few minutes' explanation before he left me, already in the doorway. It was important for him to polish his shoes with boot polish, which he had brought to me and kept in my house because he felt that at school they did his shoes badly.

He had started to make a great mess in the waiting room. He threw papers from the sweets about, spitting out sweets at me or on the floor, and sometimes he mentioned that they are awful. When he had said this he pulled a sliding piece of wood from the desk and kicked it over and over again. Repeatedly, he had played with fire in a rather dangerous way, bringing fireworks into my room, which made an awful smoke, and once he found a box of matches. He started to burn the wallpaper so that I had in both cases to use force to take these things away. It had not the effect of frightening him away the next day but obviously was a reassurance that in such violent situations I could control him. He had taken to defecation in the bathroom, but denied every time that he had defecated. Once when he had spent some long time there he said that he had made fireworks. Another time that he had just looked at his chocolates and tried to find out which was better. When I interpreted more and more the burning quality of his dangerous faeces, identified with the chocolate, which was also meant to be the bad penis, the bit of the desk, and that there was a vicious circle by which everything was poison because his own burning poisoning faeces burnt him and the whole house, and that this would get back into him again as my speech got into him and that was why I could only speak when he allowed it, and then only a little. He felt relieved, but at the end of the hour hit me with the newspaper, which was folded up in a long piece. Before he left me I pointed out that this long bit of paper was in his mind the same thing as the wood from the desk, and that he felt driven or controlled by this phantom penis (his own expression for somebody who appears suddenly and goes). The next day he wanted to see my newspaper.

After all these interpretations which I had repeatedly given he asked why I did not have chrysanthemums in my garden and won't they grow, and told me that they grow until December. Complains that I don't have them.

The day before Guy Fawkes Day he did not come, a thing which was quite unusual. Though he is often late, he most rarely stays away. The next day he came feeling rather sorry for not having come, very friendly, and said he did not feel like coming. I interpret that his staying away was to save me, because he was so afraid of again having to test on me whether his faeces will prove burning and destructive to me, and thus he needs to discover by setting fire to things in my house.

[The next page is headed 2a and Klein has written 'insert on page 2' (the previous page of the manuscript). I suggest that it was intended to follow the words in the second paragraph 'tried to find what was better'. The next sentence 'when I interpreted more and more' would then have been condensed.]

2a

He took the boot polish down and smeared it in the waiting room, and threw bits at me and out into the hall. Then being concerned whether I could clean it and not wanting to go until he saw that I took a brush and washed it, he said, 'You see you can clean it.' I interpreted about burning faeces, connected chocolate, boot polish, which was supposed to be good in one way and to clean him, but got mixed up with bad faeces because his wish to keep the good faeces apart from the bad burning ones inside him and inside me never succeeded. I interpreted the two excuses he gave for defecation. One that it was fireworks, the other that he was looking at chocolate to see which he could eat. All this connection with burning faeces, boot polish and chocolate, things thrown at me and attacking me, together with other aggression, were things which seemed so important in resolving his anxieties

[Page 3 of the manuscript then appears to follow on from the end of the page before: 'set fire to things in my house'.]

He then showed me silver coins which he had with him from his collection, and he was very friendly and asked me to watch with him the fireworks going on in the neighbouring gardens. Also asked me did I want to do work with him, because I was not saying anything. I pointed out to him that this was the first time he had been friendly without any reaction of anxiety or hate; that he had left me with being sorry that I have no chrysanthemums growing in my garden. It was meant to be babies which should grow undisturbed in me, and that was why he had not come the next day, which was connected with Guy Fawkes Day. He finds it most difficult to realize that he is fond of me and wants to save me from his destructive tendencies; that he has often to be more destructive to prove that he does not care. Also is so frightened that I am destroyed, since he got what he thought was proof that she was destroyed by the death of his mother. That he is in despair of putting me right. Parting from me in a few weeks' time increases this anxiety, and so does the exam, but for all these reasons he denies that he is sorry to leave me, that he is fond of me and that he is most worried about doing harm.

This was the first time he could listen to such an interpretation without any reaction of hate or anxiety. We went on looking at the fireworks and it was only towards the end of the hour that he again showed me all his coins, silver coins, and I interpreted this as a much more hopeful feeling that he has not got burning and poisoning faeces, but quite good ones – the silver coins – and that also I could see that while he so often before had asked me not to look at him or at his book, etc, hiding away from me, now he was showing me something. At the end of the hour, he asked me for two pence to go back by bus to school, saying that otherwise he would have to leave me early, and he did not want to do this. He knows that we had arranged that I should not lend him money because this caused trouble, but feels that he would bring it back. Towards the end of the hour he again gets angry and tears at newspaper. I interpret that leaving me always arouses his hate even if it is not my fault that he goes.

The next morning, the first thing he does is to give me the coppers [Klein had clearly decided to give him the money in spite of her doubts about doing so!], having brought especially bright new ones, and shows me a full box of cigarette cards which he was going to sort out in my room, not objecting in the least to interpretations which were all on the line of his greater hope about his inside and the good things inside; and while he was sorting out these, after the interpretation, he asked me, 'Do you think I will have time to finish?' I interpret this not only as his wish to put these cards in order before he goes home, but also the question whether I could finish his analysis before he goes for the holidays. He showed me that the cards represent people and all sorts of things, but pointed out some animals in brown. He doesn't like them, but just keeps them with the collection.

I interpret on the line of contents of body, people inside him, and his hate of the two brown people and faeces, which he could not help having; but he obviously feels less worried about them, because they are less in quantity than the good things. [Margin note here – 'need to show him boundary between me and not me is often vague in the unconscious'.] I had also interpreted that the anxiety of the exam connected with the phantom penis and the dangerous me, who seemed to become so dangerous when he had attacked me. (Obviously frightened – had to go towards end of hall before he left, and not say a word while he was going out.) Interpret on the line of internal examiners – Father and Mother – united, and also that his anxiety about learning and not knowing things was connected with what he felt to be this mixed mess inside him. In the last two days he also mentioned that he thought that he knows things already for school, and spoke of the date of the exam without special worry, also saying on those two days he would have to miss time with me.

When anxiety was so acute and sometimes I could only put in a few interpretations at the end, I was often restricted to ten words.

The difference between his reaction to interpretation of his loving the object and his concern and distress and his reaction some weeks ago is all the more striking because then he still reacted in a very violent way. He had mentioned after having. . ..[Klein's marking] doing a lot of things for him, that he had got from the man where he buys sweets and who sometimes let him have a little more, that he had given him more change than he should have done. I interpret that this rather good man stands for me and that he thinks he does exhaust my patience and my time, and also that he cheats me, because he so often insists on staying longer (putting it carefully). He did not deny this, and wanted to go up into the playroom out of the waiting room, which was sign of lessening anxiety, but that was the day when he started to burn the wallpaper and then to throw burning matches at me, so that I used force to take the matches away from him. This time no reaction of aggression or of hate followed this. That he is in distress of separating from the good object. Quite obvious that this parting now has less pain because his belief in his own destructiveness, the bad penis, and therefore also in my being destroyed, is lessened.

Reference

Brehony, K.J. (2004). A new education for a new era: the contribution of the conferences of the New Education Fellowship to the disciplinary field of education 1921–1938, *Paedagogica Historica*, *40*, *5–6*, 733–755, DOI: 10.1080/0030923042000293742

2

ON PLAY

Melanie Klein (edited by Jane Milton)

Introduction

In this chapter, set within its wider context, is a lecture that Klein gave in London in January 1937. She was taking part in the third, biennial Child Guidance Inter-Clinic Conference of Great Britain. This material is found in Wellcome Library archive PP/KLE/C.50, available online. C.50 contains the Proceedings of the conference, which covered diverse social, educational and therapeutic topics ranging from remedial teaching to juvenile court procedure. Klein gave her lecture during a session entitled 'Discussion on Play'. It is published here for the first time, followed by some comments from Joan Riviere on Klein's manuscript, presumably made in advance of the conference, and which Klein may have incorporated into her talk. The Proceedings contain a summary of the discussion of Klein's paper, probably compiled by Susan Isaacs.

Child Guidance was a relatively new and promising movement. It originated in the United States after the end of the First World War, was at first funded philanthropically, and then adopted by Education Boards and finally the British National Health Service. Teams consisted of psychiatrists, psychologists and social workers, with child psychotherapists later becoming an important addition. In the preface to the Proceedings (C.50 images 5–6) it is noted that invitations were issued to all professional workers in child guidance clinics in England, Scotland and Wales and to other people having specialized knowledge of the subject. The 258 delegates who attended included representatives of 45 clinics or centres. They also included members of Government Departments, of University staffs, and Medical Officers of Health and Directors of Education, from areas especially active in child guidance work.

Chairing the Discussion on Play on the first afternoon of this two-day conference was Dr C.L.C. Burns, with speakers listed as Mrs Melanie Klein, Dr M. Lowenfeld,

Miss G. Chesters and Dr Susan Isaacs. Dr Margaret Lowenfeld was a paediatrician who became a pioneer child psychiatrist and psychotherapist. Like Klein she recognized the importance of play both in child development and in enabling the child to communicate what could not be put into words. In the late 1920s Lowenfeld established one of the first Child Guidance Clinics in Britain, in Notting Hill, London. A hallmark of Lowenfeld's work was the use of the sand tray, alongside small toys; this popularized the sand tray approach to play therapy. Her approach differed from Klein's, in that it was not based on psychoanalysis, about which she clearly had some suspicion.

Dr C.L.C. Burns was a child psychiatrist who wrote on the psychology of young offenders. He spent time in the Children's Department of the Tavistock Clinic in its early days, then became Director of the Birmingham Child Guidance Clinic. Miss G. Chesters cannot be identified but from her remarks in this discussion clearly worked with children individually and in groups, perhaps in a nursery setting. Dr Susan Isaacs was an educationist, psychologist and finally a psychoanalyst who became a close colleague of Klein. She directed the Malting House School in Cambridge, an educational research project inspired by Klein, where children were encouraged to express their phantasy life.

The lecture

Play

[Klein's typescript of her lecture is found in C.50, images 105–143. Her original page numbering has been inserted in square brackets so as to make sense of comments by a colleague, probably Joan Riviere, at the end.]

[Page 1] The value of play as a means of education has long been known, and in this connection we think of Froebel, whose teachings profoundly influenced educational methods. In recent years the importance of children's play from the therapeutic point of view has been widely recognised. This is largely due to the discoveries of psycho-analysis. The study by this method of the depths of the child's mind has led to the discovery that play is the means by which the unconscious as well as the conscious mind of the child finds fullest expression, and that it is by means of play that children can be cured of even grave mental disorders.

The methodical development of the play technique of psycho-analysis goes back to the years round about 1920. Repeated observations in the analysis of small children, some of whom spoke very little, convinced me that children reveal even more of their unconscious thoughts and feelings as well as of their [page 2] experiences in play than do grown-ups by verbal associations. I found that the children's play could be analysed in the same way as the dreams of adults, and that by interpretations of the details of play, step by step anxieties grew less; imagination became more free, and play more varied. In order to explain the way in which relief is obtained through play analysis I must first shortly recapitulate some of the fundamentals of psycho-analysis.

Fears and conflicts develop in the child's mind not only for external but also for internal reasons. His aggressive phantasies are directed against the same persons whom he loves most. If his mother satisfies his needs he loves her; if she doesn't satisfy them he hates her and attacks her in phantasy. That is where the deepest conflict in human minds has its origin. It is a characteristic of the young mind that the child should feel that his hating impulses have real effects. Hence fears of various kinds and feelings of guilt set in. Fears of the parents as dangerous and retaliating figures and anxiety [page 3] lest the loved persons should be injured and destroyed by his aggressive wishes, remain active in his unconscious mind. The wish to repair what has been injured in phantasy also arises very soon and is an important factor in all sublimations and in the development of social conscience.

Aggressive and erotic phantasies, the desire to repair and to make amends, all these impulses and phantasies are a motive force in play activities and find expression through them. Play is a bridge between reality and phantasy and in this respect is most important for the relief of anxiety and tension, as well as for the pleasure and the happiness which it brings to the child. The child's phantasies are put to a reality test in his play.

[Here Klein has included an extra page (C.50 image 108) noting that it should be inserted on page 3. Some faint marks on her copy suggest that the insertion is intended at this point. It reads as follows:

> Insert p 3
>
> Here I refer to mutual play, with other children and with adults, and also to solitary play, for as well as having facilities for free play with others, it is important that the child should be given opportunity to play by himself and to develop his phantasies alone. Mutual play and solitary play have different influences on the child's mental life, but both are of the greatest value for his development.]

In a game, for instance, a child shoots a lion. But although it is lions he wants to shoot in conscious feeling and thinking, the lions are but the distorted picture of these phantastic parents felt to be dangerous who the child fears will eat him up because he wanted to eat them up in his aggressive phantasy. These phantastic beings are thus the products of his own [page 4] aggression and fears; but they cannot in the depths of his unconscious mind be entirely separated from the real parents, since it was these whom he attacked in his phantasy. The aggressive wishes and the hate are here displaced from the parents on to the lion. This is the way in which fears of wild animals and fears of other animals and beings develop, which are so well known to us as phobias.

The boy who in play shoots the lion is, however, not only expressing his aggression; he is also gaining much reassurance of various kinds. Through this play he gets a proof that nothing has actually happened, that he is not really attacked by the lion (father), nor has he in fact killed him. That is to say, he obtains a proof that his aggressive desires are not omnipotent, and that the dangerous parents, who in his unconscious mind are represented by the lion, are not so dangerous as he feared. Moreover, if his mother, let us say, or somebody else who stands for her, falls in with such a game, this is a further and most important proof that a good mother exists, that she does not [page 5] mind his aggression which is, in the deep unconscious, ultimately directed against her.

Much could be said about the manifold unconscious motives and drives which underlie play activities, but I am restricting myself here to emphasizing the liberation of erotic and aggressive phantasies, the expression of restitutive phantasies and the reassurances of all kinds gained by testing in play and thus seeing whether the various unconscious fears are justified or not in reality. But these reality tests imply also the cooperation of the child's conscious mind and his intellectual interests and powers. At the same time as he is dealing with his unconscious conflicts he is also mastering his experiences – past and present – solving some of his conscious problems and thus adapting himself to the demands of reality as a whole.

Freud discovered that erotic and aggressive feelings, thoughts and phantasies become repressed because they are felt to be bad by one part of the mind, which he termed the 'super-ego'. These impulses, feelings and phantasies are not put out of action [page 6] by repression. They remain active in the unconscious mind, and the effect they produce can be most beneficial or most harmful. It is well known that imagination and the free play of phantasy are connected with intuition and creative powers. The roots of imagination and phantasy life are, however, in the unconscious mind, and they are closely connected with phantasies and impulses both of an aggressive and of a restitutive nature. For even the very young child strives – and this is also partially unconscious – to make good for the injuries done in phantasy to people. If the unconscious phantasies and impulses are not too deeply repressed they act as a continuous stimulus to the child's activities and interests, and first and foremost to his play. They are, to a certain extent, liberated as well as worked over in play and in other activities. Constructive interests and good relations to people lessen the intensity of the unconscious conflicts; for satisfactory activities and happy relationships relieve the sense of guilt largely derived from internal sources. Mental stability and wealth of personality depend largely on a [page 7] good interplay between the unconscious and the conscious mind – between the individual's phantasy life and his relation to reality. If, however, the repressions are too powerful, unconscious conflicts will remain too strong, and there will be a constant clash in the unconscious and between the conscious and the unconscious mind. The results of this are mental difficulties and inhibitions of all kinds.

From this follows that emotional development cannot be separated from intellectual. Unconscious conflicts inhibit intellectual growth, and anything which helps to relieve mental stress will also promote intellectual development. It is a grave mistake to try to influence intellectual growth at the expense of phantasy life. Maria Montessori though she saw the value of the child's expressing his constructive tendencies in practical matters and in this way has favourably influenced educational methods, has entirely failed to understand the part which the phantasy life plays in the child's personality. In her recent [page 8] lecture at the Institute of Medical Psychology, speaking about what she calls the 'phenomenon' of the 'repetition of the exercise', she especially referred to one child of three and a half years who was 'doing an exercise which consisted in taking a set of cylinders of graded dimensions out of their holes in a stand into which they fitted with absolute exactness, and fitting each into its place again'. We gather from Montessori's description that the deep absorption which this child exhibited in carrying out this exercise – forty-two times as Montessori reported – was concentration on this function, from which the child derived such benefit that she seemed completely changed after the performance. In Montessori's words, 'Something had awakened deep down in the child's being.' This may well be true; but psycho-analytic work leads to conclusions as to the nature of the inner process very different from those Montessori arrived at. The drive to repeat the function over and over again is characteristic of a certain tendency to obsessional trends which are very common in the [page 9] stage between three and five years of age, in which, as Montessori tells us, this phenomenon of 'repetition of the exercise' can mostly be observed. It is shown in many forms of play, even where not such precise apparatus is put at the child's disposal as the Montessori material, which lends itself so well both to precision and to acquiring skill in the exercise itself. Anyone who observes children of this age and even earlier (and I dare say this has always been observed since mankind existed) can see that if a child has no other toy – or even if he has – he may go on for a long time playing with such a thing as a tin with buttons in it, taking the buttons out and putting them back, or taking off the lid of the tin and putting it on again. A normal child will do this kind of exercise especially if the material given is interesting and affords him opportunities for an intellectual achievement, for instance, such material as a jigsaw puzzle. Moreover, the children Montessori speaks about were very poor, some of whom might not have had a toy before; [page 10] and she also mentions the fact that she could not achieve the same results with rich children. We hear, however, from her that these poor children, who were so interested in the special Montessori material, did not care for dolls. But this observation can surely not be generalized.

We all know what great happiness the majority of children, and especially poor children who are lacking in toys, experience when given a doll or a Teddy bear or other toys – how fond they may grow of these toys and how they will still cherish them when the toys are old and worn out.

As to the absorption shown by the child whom Montessori mentions, psycho-analytic experience leads us to conclude that along with such activities go conscious and unconscious phantasies which find part expression in the activity. No doubt there are present also such things as pleasure in carrying out the function, intellectual satisfaction in the skill needed to carry out the exercise, etc; but the phantasy part is entirely overlooked by Montessori. In some Montessori classes the children are [page 11] not allowed to play with the material in the way they often would like to do. In other classes the children actually play with this material in a fanciful way, for example, they may pretend cylinders are people or engines, and so on. For the child plays even if he is not meant to do so. Poor children who have no toys may use a scrap of paper or a rag as a toy; for their phantasy-life – fortunately – cannot be stopped.

Montessori's neglect of the phantasy-life and the unconscious processes in the child's mind leads her to over-emphasize intellectual achievement and explains why she should think that toys are unimportant. She says: 'Toys – at least the common kind of toys – lend themselves to no exact form of exercise, no real purpose. The complex activities requiring exercise if development is to be normal are not able to function through toys . . . The playthings have merely external value, and the only feeling they call forth is that of possession.' And again, 'The children had merely been given toys and had never had the chance to occupy themselves with things having use and meaning.' To my [page 12] mind there are few things more pathetic than that there should exist children who have never had a toy to play with.

A toy can signify many different things to the child, as is easily observed. No nurse or mother who has watched with interest a child going to bed with his Teddy bear or his doll would doubt that he finds comfort and reassurance and pleasure in its company because it is felt to be a friend, or perhaps a baby, and stands for a protective and friendly being. In playing with her doll a little girl can satisfy in phantasy her longing for a baby of her own, which, as ordinary observation shows, is very strong in girls and will often be expressed quite openly by some of them at a certain age. This frustrated wish, and all the conflicts which go with this frustrated wish – the wish to be like mother, to be in her place, to have children, to have Daddy as a husband, and so on – all these are not only given expression, but at the same time the child's conflicts are mitigated and partly relieved and comfort is gained through her play with her doll. [Page 13] The value of toys, in giving pleasure and comfort and developing feelings of love and affection and thus also influencing the child's relations to people – that is to say, the value of toys for the emotional development of the child – cannot be over-rated.

Montessori's theory as to the nature of the benefit which the child derives from the absorption in the 'repetition of the exercise' would lead to the conception that it is the lack of concentration, the lack of precision, which is at the root of unfavourable mental development, and that the child blossoms out if the teacher puts it in a position in which it can exercise this function in a good way. Psycho-analytic experience shows, however, that it is the other way round. Very painstaking efforts are sometimes made to do away with intellectual inhibitions with the hope that this would also improve the child's mental stability, but analytic experience shows that such attempts are being made from the wrong end. There are no doubt some severe cases in which especially skilled teachers are able to bring about [page 14] considerable improvement in learning, which is beneficial for the child all round. But this method will not be successful in very many cases, and even so it will only relieve special symptoms and not cure the child altogether.

I have mentioned before that unconscious phantasies provide an important stimulus for the development of interests and activities of all kinds, and that the over-strong repression of phantasies leads to the inhibition of activities, and first of all to the inhibition of play. In this connection, I will mention one of the many instances of the kind which I take from the analysis of a German boy of seven years of age. (I quoted this case in a paper [editor's note: this refers to Klein (1985 [1923]) 'The Role of the School in the Libidinal Development of the Child'].)

Instead of the German double 's', he always wrote only one, – apparently by mistake – until a phantasy, discovered in analysis, afforded the explanation. The one 's' was himself, the other his father. They were to embark together on a motor boat, for the pen was also a boat, the copy-book a lake. The 's' that was himself got into the boat that belonged to the [page 15] other 's' and sailed away in it quickly upon the lake. This was the reason why he did not write the two 's's together; the boat and the pen stood for the male genital, the copy book, i.e. the lake, stood for his mother. In phantasy he was taking away father's genital and having intercourse with his mother by going upon the lake. His frequent use of an ordinary German 's' in place of a long one proved to be determined by the fact that the part of the long 's' that was thus left out was for him 'as though one were to take away a person's nose'. This mistake proved to be determined by castration-wishes against his father and disappeared after this interpretation. The same child had a marked inhibition in doing division sums, all explanations proving unavailing, for he understood them quite well, but always did his examples wrong. He told me once that in doing division he had first of all to bring down the figure that he still required; he climbed up, seized it by the arm and pulled it down. It seemed to him as if his mother stood on a stone thirteen yards high and someone came and caught her by the arm so that they tore it out [page 16] and divided her. Shortly beforehand, however, he had phantasied about a woman in the circus who is sawn in pieces, and then nevertheless comes to life again, and now he asked me whether this were possible. The repeated interpretations of these phantasies, both in the case of the writing and of the sums, completely removed the inhibitions. I must add that these phantasies which were connected with his writing and his arithmetic also played a great part in his play. By removing the inhibition of these phantasies, first of all his play became more free. Generally speaking, inhibitions in play in many cases precede inhibitions in learning, for the very reason that the same type of phantasies play a part in both. These phantasies had been inhibited because they were linked up with wishes of a kind which the child's conscience disapproved of.

Our experience has shown that the repression of these phantasies because of their forbidden content – forbidden by inner forces, by the super-ego – is apt to inhibit the activity that goes along with these phantasies. The proof for this is [page 17] that, together with the liberation of these phantasies by means of the analytic work, the activity becomes possible, and gradually improves. The analyst may often have the gratification, after a period of analysis of a child, of hearing from the mother or from the teacher that the child is now so much better at his reading and takes great pleasure in it; or has so much improved in doing his sums. (This applies to older as well as to younger children.) If the inhibition is lessened, the child then becomes capable of profiting by educational methods. The pleasure which he now derives from these activities, the gratification of achieving something, becomes now an additional factor in his mental stability. He may now spend much time and effort in making figures and numbers as precisely as possible: and here use is made of certain obsessional tendencies which, as I said before, are characteristic of the child between three or four and about eleven years of age. These trends need not be in any way pathological, if they are not too strong. They are connected with the tendencies to order and tidiness and intellectual curiosity [page 18] and interests which are part of the normal development. In the early ages, let us say between three and five years, children express these tendencies predominantly in play and in everyday occupations. But increasingly these trends play a part in the ways the child acquires knowledge and is busy perfecting intellectual activities, school work, and so on, to the satisfaction of his teachers. The child derives much gratification in satisfying these tendencies in the way I have described, and it is as important for him to give expression to them as to express his phantasy life. But as I said before, intellectual activities and the phantasy-life cannot be judged separately. Where unconscious difficulties are over-strong, intellectual activities become inhibited, and this inhibition again affects the child's intellectual development.

In play, the actual life of the child – with all his experiences, great and small, everyday and unusual – finds expression. But also, his past experiences from the earliest days onwards are [page 19] represented. Thus the child's play is a bridge between phantasy and reality, because he gives expression to both, side by side, and because he can represent in play the interplay between experiences, past and present, and his phantasy life. For the child's phantasies, from the earliest stage of development onwards, influence his perception of reality, and on the other hand, his experiences influence his phantasies, and thus there is a constant interplay between real experiences and phantasies.

I want to illustrate this by a very ordinary hour of play analysis with a child who can be called quite normal, since his neurotic anxieties, which had never been of a very abnormal type, had at this stage of analysis already been almost resolved. The analysis is not far from its completion. In the session before the one I am going to describe, the child, aged five years nine months – let us call him Tony – had shown some anxiety on account of an accident which his elder brother had had, his foot having been hurt by a cupboard which he had pulled down on himself. Tony had even produced a slight accident in my room, managing to [page 20] slip, so that the stool which he was holding with one hand fell a little on him. Then he had remarked that it hadn't been so bad as his brother's accident. At the beginning of the next day's session, which I want to deal with, Tony looked happy and excited. He told me that the doctor had seen his brother's foot and said it was not injured inside, but only bruised. The relationship to this brother had been very difficult in the past, the brother having at times been very unpleasant to Tony. Tony then started to jump about in the room, saying that he was mad. Then he suggested that I should be the audience and that he was the clown at the circus. (He had been with his brother to the circus a few days before, and it was after this performance that his brother was playing the clown and had the accident.) Tony decided that I was to be a Granny and wanted me to have company. He put all the small cushions which I have in my playroom – five in number – beside me representing children, and I had to carry on a conversation with them. Then he [page 21] brought a flannel, asking me to make it into a shape, and that was to be 'Father Gran', adding 'You should have a husband.' Then he got angry with the 'Father Gran', saying he had missed so much of the clown's performance, and suddenly took him, threw him up to the ceiling, and said that I was to cry and call out instead of Father Gran. After Father Gran had fallen back on the floor, he brought him back to me, put him on the table and asked me to cheer him up. When I asked what had happened to him, had he hurt himself, Tony got rather worried and said he didn't know, adding, 'I don't think he is very ill. He just has three hundred scratches.' One of the babies was supposed to have made a noise and Tony proceeded to treat him in the same way as he did Father Gran, he threw him up to the ceiling. I had again to indicate the baby's crying, and then he brought him back to me, suggesting that I should cheer him up and put him to sleep. Tony again said, with a rather worried look, that he was probably not seriously hurt, then added, 'We don't [page 22] know, we shall see. Probably he is only bruised' (repeating thus the experience of his brother's accident). Later on he wanted me to look after the child, to see whether he was still sleeping, and said, 'He has woken up and is crying' (obviously pleased that he was not dead). Saying this, he threw this tiny cushion against my breast and was most astonished to find that it stayed there for a little while, and said, 'Now you are giving him the breast.' He seemed quite pleased. Then Tony decided that Father Gran should look after all the children and that I should also be a clown. I had to make all sorts of movements which he indicated, then to dance to his music (that is, his singing). Next he wanted us to dance holding hands, and then suggested that we should lie down on the floor. He put one leg of the table in between my feet, caressed my head, and suggested that he would jump over me – which I declined. When I asked him while we were performing, 'what about Father Gran and the children?' he said 'Never mind them. You [page 23] stay here.'

During this hour, I had given Tony various interpretations. I referred to his jealousy of his brother, which was quite strong, and which was expressed in his behaviour towards the cushion baby. (In this way he changed his older brother into a child younger than himself. He had expressed his wish to me before that he would like to be the elder of the two.) In this connection I interpreted to him that he had often had death wishes against his brother because of jealousy and also because the brother had often treated him badly. He was quite aware of these death wishes, but not aware how sorry and frightened he had been because of the accident. I told him also that he would like to have his Granny with him, as he had had her just recently on his holidays. In this relation the children (cushions) represented himself and the whole family. The five cushions expressed his wish that his mother should have more babies, partly because his jealousy of possible children and his aggressive wishes against these unborn children had led him [page 24] to fear that he had prevented the babies from arriving. (Two days before, we had had a talk in which Tony had very strongly enquired into all the details of child-birth and sexual intercourse, putting together various details, which he had known unconsciously and partly consciously, but which had now come fully to consciousness, and about which he wanted to clear his mind as a definite piece of conscious knowledge. He had then asked me why his mother had not more children, and also said that women should have 50,000 children, and that he was going to have fifty children, a wish he had repeatedly expressed before.) I now reminded him of this previous talk, and interpreted that he also wanted me to have five children. A further interpretation which I gave him was when he was tossing Father Gran in the air and injuring him. I reminded him that, as analysis had shown before in full detail, he had often been jealous of his father and wished him to die, because he wanted to have mother to himself, have sexual intercourse with her and give her babies. I told him that he had expressed his death wishes against his [page 25] father in the way he had treated 'Father Gran', and that Father Gran and Granny were standing for Daddy and Mummy. (That is also why he used the name 'Father Gran'.) I went on to say that he had represented Daddy and Mummy through Granny and Father Gran because it was less painful to him, and because his grandfather was actually dead. I also explained to him that in his longing to have his grandfather alive he had brought him back to life in the play. Another interpretation was that the whole treatment of baby and Father Gran linked up with the accident to his brother, his feelings of guilt in connection with this, and also his fear that something similar could happen to him. That is why he played he was a clown in my room, as his brother had done when the accident happened, thus showing that he could bring it to a better end. His jumping about and his dancing was also to show that he could use his feet and was all right. I explained also that his dancing with me and our lying on the floor represented sexual intercourse with me, and that we had gone away together and [page 26] left behind father and the children, referring all this back to his wishes in connection with his father and mother.

Much has been expressed in this one hour which I cannot refer to in more detail. But I should still like to stress how in this hour actual experiences had stirred phantasies and feelings of guilt in relation with present and past experiences, and had also stirred or brought to the fore phantasies of quite an early kind. His present-day interests and ambitions were also very clearly expressed.

Here we see his wish to be a man, a father, to have children, but also to be skilful, his ambitions to be admired as a clown. Again, everyday experience and activities come in. His dancing lessons which he had recently started were a stimulus for showing his cleverness in dancing. In making me dance and showing me the movements while he made the music to it, he had put himself into the position of the dancing teacher and me into the one of the child.

[Page 27] One could easily describe the happenings of this analytic hour in a very simple way. The child played that he was a clown, I was his audience; he wanted me to have the whole family with me, then decided that I should play with him, and in between showed a certain amount of aggression towards Father Gran and one of the babies. This is quite an ordinary game, and you may say that there is no need whatever to suggest that there are unconscious phantasies and motives underlying it. But looking at it from the conscious point of view, one cannot, of course, discover the unconscious content; this can only be done by means of the psycho-analytic method. Furthermore, this one hour is taken out of the whole context of the analysis; and this unconscious content and all the associations and interpretations which I mentioned can only be understood in connection with the whole of the analysis. Material of the kind I mentioned had appeared before, and had been interpreted. The interpretations I gave in this hour were [page 28] based on those I had given before. As regards the need to look for the unconscious content, I would say that it is most essential to do so in cases where the disturbance of the child is grave, and that it is very helpful also in less severe cases.

Here we come to the differences between non-analytic play therapy and the play technique of psycho-analysis. Comparing first the processes which underlie play analysis and non-analytic play therapy, I feel that I touch on a topic which would deserve a paper in itself, while I shall have time to say only a few sentences about it.

I have mentioned repeatedly how important in psycho-analysis is the resolution of anxiety. In non-analytic play therapy also, if the inhibited child begins to play, and the less inhibited child is developing his play more and more, no doubt some anxiety is being relieved by the therapist. The anxiety relieved in play therapy however must necessarily be much more superficial than that resolved in psycho-analysis. In [page 29] the former case the relief is produced by the very fact that the play therapist has become to the child a good helping figure, and this counteracts anxieties in the child, and thus phantasies can come up. The child now plays more freely, and a good circle is set going, with all the beneficial effects which play brings.

I have just said that the play therapist is felt by the child to be a friendly and encouraging person. Here she makes use of what has been termed positive transference. In psycho-analysis however – and that is an important difference – the analyst makes use both of the positive and of the negative transference. That is to say, all the hate as well as the love which the individual has felt from his earliest days onwards, and which has been partly repressed, are transferred on to the analyst. All the bad phantasy figures which have existed in the patient's mind – I remind you of the lion, which as I suggested stood for the distorted picture of the parents who were felt to be dangerous – all these bad phantasy figures, and [page 30] also the good ones, become related to the person of the analyst and thus brought to consciousness. By means of this and by the patient's understanding of how his anxieties of these bad figures came about in the past, these figures now lose some of their power over the mind, and this goes along with a diminution or resolution of fundamental and deep anxieties. The success of an analysis and the permanence of its results depend largely on the fact that the analyst works both with the negative and with the positive transference. Because he works with the negative transference he releases anxieties of a strength which can only be dealt with by the specified technique of analysis. To illustrate this by an everyday experience of the child analyst: I may discover in a child's mind, while he is in my playroom, that the strong anxiety he produces is due to his phantasy that I, the analyst, am an awful witch who is going to cut him in pieces. Through my interpretation I resolve this special anxiety, the child begins to play happily, and I may then become a nice fairy to [mislabelled 30, duplicated this page number] him. This would mean that through my interpretation I have been able to resolve the negative transference, and that has resulted in the positive transference coming up.

To contrast this with the attitude of the non-analytic play therapist: I want to make clear that the play therapist can and shall make use of the positive transference in the same way as the successful educator does. She cannot make use of the negative transference and should not try to get in direct touch with the unconscious. Of course she cannot prevent anxiety – sometimes very acute anxiety – or distrust and dislike of her coming up in the child. If this happens she can only use the friendly means at her disposal. I stressed the word 'direct' touch with the unconscious because the indirect touch with the unconscious is there all along. That is indeed just what brings about the good understanding between her and the child. But she should not attempt interpretations, since she is not able to cope with the [page labelled 31] anxiety which may thus be released. Let us go back to the instance of the analytic hour with Tony, and think of an interpretation which the play therapist might be tempted to give in the case of a child playing a game of the kind. We will suppose that her interpretation links on to the aggressive behaviour of the child towards Father Gran and the baby. The amount of anxiety stirred by touching upon the anxieties and feelings of guilt connecting with the death wishes of Tony against his brother, his father, his grandfather and the unborn baby, might be overpowering. And there would be no means of relieving these anxieties and his feelings of guilt. In the non-analytic play therapy, and this is the conclusion from what I have said so far, fundamental processes in the unconscious remain unaltered, though they are temporarily influenced. Only one part, and a more superficial part, of his unconscious impulses and phantasies finds expression.

Taking again the instance of the 'lion game': as I said before, the child will not know whom he wants to shoot if he [page labelled 32] shoots the lions;

nevertheless a great mental relief is obtained by one part of the phantasy being liberated – namely his aggressive wishes against the lions and his anxiety of them. Buried in his unconscious remains the fact that he actually wants to shoot his parents. He also gains great relief and reassurance against the anxiety of the phantastic parents – though he does not know that it is they of whom he is afraid – by the friendly and cooperative attitude of the play therapist. Since in his positive transference he transfers to her predominantly his feelings of love towards his mother, she gives him, in the setting of the play, the proof that a good mother exists and not only a lion-mother, and that this good mother understands and forgives his aggressive wishes against her and against father expressed in the play.

Corresponding to the more limited means at her disposal, the results of the play therapist are necessarily more limited than those of the psycho-analyst. It is more likely that the play therapist will be able to relieve one symptom or some [page labelled 33] symptoms than to effect full mental stability and a change in the whole of the personality. She may also not be able to cure graver cases, and she may have to give up cases in which the anxiety or the play inhibition is too strong. But she may achieve very beneficial results in a large number of milder cases. There are many mentally unstable children who have suffered badly from lack of understanding. With such children, the fact that they come in nearer contact with an understanding and friendly person who, in a specially favourable setting, provides them with the opportunity to play might make all the difference in their lives. Even children who have not altogether been lacking in love and understanding, and nevertheless become neurotic, may be helped to a certain extent by play therapy.

As in every work which is concerned with human relationships, the personality of the play therapist and her attitude is a very important factor for the success of the therapy. A friendly, passive, and really understanding attitude is felt [page labelled 34] by the unconscious mind of the child. His unconscious mind knows that he is allowed to bring out phantasies which he might not be able to act out in the presence of a less understanding person, or of his own mother even if he loves her. I think the often-used word 'detached' is here very much in place. The play therapist needs to have a real and friendly interest in the child, but at the same time she should be willing to wait for whatever the child's mind brings forth. Though she may encourage his phantasies, she should not be over-anxious for him to express them; and, moreover, she should not aim at his giving expression to special sets of phantasies. If she has a really understanding attitude towards his aggressive tendencies, he will feel that. But if she is too much interested in the expression of this part of his phantasies she might stir more aggression, and by this, more anxiety than she could resolve. On the other hand, she should not try to induce him too much to express his constructive tendencies. I think much of the success of the play therapist [page labelled 35] will depend on her inner willingness to follow what the child's mind is trying to express, and then she will probably be able to keep the balance between play of an aggressive and of a constructive nature, and thus enable the child to find the mental relief which play can afford.

I have tried to convey to you in this paper the meaning of play and its value for therapy. I cannot finish, however, without stressing the importance of play in ordinary life for the favourable development and for the happiness of the normal child, from the earliest days until he grows up. First of all there is the happy play between the mother and her baby. This not only helps to establish a good relationship between them but is the beginning of what could be called a prophylactic therapy. For play – mutual as well as solitary – is a means of gradually stabilizing the child's mind, building up his happy relationships to people, contributing towards the wealth of his personality – in fact, furthering his all-round development.

[Page labelled 36] Much is to be hoped from the growing understanding of what play can do for the normal and for the mentally unstable child, which finds expression in the increasing facilities for play therapy in different parts of the country.

Commentary on draft of lecture by Joan Riviere

In C.50 Images 144–145 someone other than Klein, almost certainly from the handwriting Joan Riviere (personal communication Marion Bower, see also Bower, 2019), has given two pages of handwritten comments as follows:

> Clinic Lecture p. 7, line 5
>
> Constant clash in the unconscious and between – I don't think the constant clash in the unconscious will be clear to most people. The clash between conscious and unconscious will be grasped as a conflict between 2 kinds of wishes but not so easy to see the clash between 2 elements having – so it will be thought – the same qualities or character (or relative to superego/conscience/Ego).
>
> p. 9 box and beans rather than tin and buttons if really ever since mankind existed.
>
> p. 16, 2 lines from end – Super-ego. This is a more technical term than appears in the earlier part of the book.
>
> p. 28 The main difference between the play technique of psychoanalysis and the non-analytic play treatment lies in the modes of resolving or dealing with anxiety. The rest of your paragraph needs more elucidation; it is not clear and sounds dogmatic.
>
> Clinic Lecture p. 30 [here it seems as if the commentator is referring to the repeated page 30] Does the reader really know what the negative transference is? Its repetition does not much inform him; can't line 2 be recast so as to say what is going on in his mind rather than what it is technically called?

p. 31 I find this page unconvincing. You do not say what the non-analytical therapist would *do*; its vagueness suggests that we do not know and are out to attack the procedure with such concepts as that only the more superficial parts are reached.

Then on p. 32 it does not seem that you explain the analytic therapy sufficiently. It isn't pure shooting but erotically intentioned and erotically satisfying shooting that is going on. It is a shooting that is saturated with *meaning*.

p. 33 it is *more likely* (p. 32) that the non-analytical therapist will do this rather than that – such unsupported statements sound like polemics: the evidence is not adduced.

Summary of the discussion on play

This summary is published in the proceedings C.50, images 26–32. As is it written from the point of view of someone knowledgeable about psychoanalysis with an understanding of Klein's views, it was probably Susan Isaacs, who was also on the panel.

Dr Lowenfeld stated that since she had no experience or knowledge of psycho-analytic play and equally found herself unable to accept Mrs Klein's description of non-analytic play – although it must be done extempore and without preparation – she would attempt to give an outline of her own conception of play and therapy based on play.

She did not like the words 'unconscious thought', because they were a contradiction in terms. Much thought was non-cognitive, but she believed it to be in a sense conscious, but the consciousness of a different order to that of cognition. Children's thought, up to the age of the control of speech, as an instrument of expression, was of this nature. It was three dimensional in quality, entirely subjective in aspect, and was best expressed in play, and particularly play with certain specified pieces of apparatus. She argued for an approach to this problem, which should be on all fours with the approach to other forms of psychological problems; that is, the experimental approach, in which objective evidence remained of observations carried out, which could be examined apart from the child, in which repeat experiments could be made and results checked: and touched briefly upon the method used at the Institute of Child Psychology, where such proceedings were carried out. She stated that she herself believed and hoped in another place to be able to show that Spearman's neogenetic laws could, with certain crucial modifications, be shown to hold in this region of the mind also.

As regards the negative transference, she could not agree with the statement of the previous speaker, that this could only be handled with safety in a psycho-analytic atmosphere, owing to the anxiety aroused. Negative effect of the strongest possible kind was a daily commonplace of the method of handling used in the Institute of Child Psychology, and the dire results of non-interpretation on psycho-analytic lines, suggested by the last speaker, had not been found to occur. Dr Lowenfeld agreed with the last speaker as to the seriousness of negative emotion in children, and stated that her endeavour and that of her co-workers was to transfer this emotion on to the material of the play-room, in connection with which it was worked through. In the ICP and in private, every effort was made to minimise personal transference relation and turn it on to the material instead. In general, this attempt proved successful and children were able to work out safely in this way their negative effects, however intense.

Her procedure in the treatment of a child had two aspects. (1) To provide material for the adequate expression, and working through of the ideas and experiences of the child's primary system of ideas and experiences, which was of a nature suitable for the expression of these ideas. (2) To help him to bridge the gap between his two-dimensional, logical, cognitive side and the subjective phantastic primary side.

She pointed out how even in the best adjusted adult human beings, this cannot be altogether successful as no adult, but a great poet, however conscious of them he may be, finds means for the successful verbalisation of his profoundest and most dynamic emotions.

Miss Chesters followed Dr Lowenfeld and spoke on group play. Just as behaviour in general tends towards the maintenance of equilibrium, so the function of spontaneous play appears to be the relief of tension and the restoration of balance. With most of the children referred to a clinic these self-balancing processes have broken down. Many children have little opportunity for adequate provision of satisfactory conditions for play. From a practical point of view this involves the consideration of the playroom situation with its social and material provision.

To deal first with the playroom situation. Initiative in play and conversation is left to the child, the role of the worker being that of an interested, understanding adult companion. The child's play is met without criticism, while expressions of feeling extraneous to the situation as created by him are refrained from. While he finds in the worker a real source of confident friendly feeling, her behaviour must not be such as will intrude upon the expression of his phantasies, and he must be able to use her as a representative figure, just as he can use a box as a ship, a cradle, a motor-car or just a box.

Socially, most of the children are still at the stage of needing to monopolise the adult, and view their contemporaries as troublesome rivals. Their problem is the modification without dislocation of feeling of this infantile attitude. Consequently, the child is met as he demands while any showing of more social feeling is encouraged, and ultimately, as his anxiety is relieved, he becomes able to relinquish his monopolising behaviour, and to form co-operative relationships with his fellows.

Further, the child needs intellectual support from the worker. He has many questions which his contemporaries are no better able to answer than he is himself, and it is for the worker to give him understanding of the general subject to which they are related.

The material to be provided must be of a kind which can give the child the means of expressing and solving his problems, but not such as must be used in too specific a way. Amongst the essential materials are found to be water, sand, dough and plasticine. In playing with them the child can deal with a great number of problems. They are capable of a great variety of representation, while allowing both for messing and constructive play. They relieve the child of fear of his own destructiveness, for what is made can be destroyed and made again, without the child's feeling that he has done irreparable damage. Such materials also provide him with a ready link between his phantasy and reality play, for as his more primitive feeling finds relief, he becomes progressively interested in the possibilities of the material itself. Washing and scrubbing materials, feeding bottles and tea sets, small vessels, rubber tubing, boats, trays and shovels are necessary for such play. Further necessary material is an empty cupboard or clothes' basket for tucking-in games; painting and drawing materials; matches, small pieces of paper and a big tin for making fires; and dressing-up clothes. Useful supplementary material is found to be small figures of animals and people, dolls and a dolls' house, bricks, toy trains and cars, and hammer toys.

To conclude. Play in small groups and under conditions such as have been described can give relief to the children less severely ill than those to whom the available individual treatment must be given, and can make possible for them the progressive restoration of balance functioning normally in happier children.

Mr Dickson, of Notre Dame Child Guidance Clinic, Glasgow, stated his method of encouraging the child to work through his emotional problems and to work towards an adjustment to his contemporaries. In the playroom at Notre Dame Clinic, there are a doll's house 9 by 12 ft and a fixed rail lay-out. Such material can be used by the child on its own, and also, is of such a nature that it tends to bring children together. He held that in a child guidance clinic interpretation to the child, only desirable in 10 per cent of cases, should be left to the psychiatrist. The one worker in a playroom should be a 'sympathetic adult', not a 'playmate'.

Dr Danzinger, of the Parents' Association Institute, described yet another aspect of play, i.e. play in relation to the child's development.

Toy materials may be used in order to diagnose the child's stage of development. The word material mentioned by Dr Lowenfeld may be used in order to study the amount of planning the child puts into his 'task', and to discover if retardation is due to intellectual or emotional causes.

Thus the type of play a child produces is of great importance in assessing his stage of development.

Dr Susan Isaacs summed up what had been a most interesting discussion. She first brought out the points on which all were agreed: the prophylactic value of play at all ages; the diagnostic value of play from emotional and intellectual standpoints; the therapeutic value of play. She mentioned, however, that Mrs Klein and Dr Lowenfeld display important differences of theory and of practice concerning play therapy. She pointed out that Mrs Klein was the first to show how the child could express his feelings towards the analyst and other people by his use of toys and play material. She agreed with Dr Lowenfeld that the child can be helped to express emotions, feelings and thoughts which have never been articulated, stating that the analyst also works with this level but regards unconscious fantasy as the most important. She stated also that no technique can rule out an emotional relationship with the therapist entirely.

'Analysts may be said to prefer to help one or a few of the mother's children very thoroughly, whilst child guidance workers prefer to do something for every member of the mother's family,' said Dr Isaacs. Some prefer a wide survey, some, detailed work. There was room for both, and each was indebted to the other. Special reference was then made to the great debt we all owe to Mrs Klein, and to the fundamentally important work she had done in the exploration of the child's unconscious.

The meeting passed the resolution:

> That this meeting recognises the great importance of play therapy in all types of child guidance work, and recommends the provision of trained play therapists as part of the staff clinics.

References

Bower, M. (2019). *The life and work of Joan Riviere: Freud, Klein and female sexuality*. London: Routledge.

Klein, M. (1985 [1923]). The role of the school in the libidinal development of the child. Chapter 3 in *Love, guilt and reparation and other works. The writings of Melanie Klein vol 1*. London: Hogarth.

3

THE IMPORTANCE OF THE UNCONSCIOUS MIND FOR THE WHOLE PERSONALITY

Melanie Klein (edited by Jane Milton)

Introduction

This previously unpublished lecture is to be found in the Melanie Klein Archives at the Wellcome Library in file PP/KLE/C.51 and can be viewed online. Like the material in Chapter 4 that follows, it was given at the London Institute of Education in May 1939 as part of a series known as the Joseph Payne lectures, the overall topic of which was 'Psychoanalysis and Normal Development'. Like Klein's other lay lectures it is clearly and compellingly written, showing her passion for her subject, and full of illustrative examples from the everyday life of infants.

The lecture

The importance of the unconscious mind for the whole personality

Professor Clarke, Ladies and Gentlemen,

I would like to say that it gives me very much pleasure to have the opportunity of speaking in the Institute of Education on Psycho-Analysis, which has been my work for a great number of years.

I am particularly glad to be able to speak on the relation between Psycho-Analysis and Normal Development, since it is not generally realized that psycho-analytic studies have an important bearing on the ordinary development of the ordinary child.

Every advance in education has been arrived at by an increase in our knowledge of human nature. Great educationalists have always been good psychologists, for they had an intuitive understanding of the child's mind long before the science of psychology had been systematically developed. For instance, Froebel intuitively understood the vital importance of play for the child's development, and our present psychological knowledge confirms his view and has much to add to it. We now not only appreciate the value of play, but also fully understand those unconscious mental processes which make play an imperative need of the child.

The close connection between psychology and education is so evident that I need not enlarge on it. I am speaking to you as a psychologist, and my purpose in these lectures is to present a picture of personality as seen through the facts revealed by the work of psycho-analysis. I shall give you a short account of those deep fundamental emotions in the child which influence all his later interests, lead to their development and fulfilment, or to their inhibition and loss.

In this first lecture, I wish to deal with 'The Importance of the Unconscious Mind for the Whole Personality'. I will then go on in my second lecture to discuss 'The Development of Interests and their Inhibition', and in my third will deal with 'The Problems of Adolescence' in particular.

Certain discoveries of the workings of the mind made by Sigmund Freud, from the year 1896 onwards, have been developed by him and his collaborators into a body of knowledge which has not only fundamentally changed psychotherapy but profoundly influenced all sciences dealing with the human mind. The psychological knowledge gained first of all through the study of mentally ill people proved in course of time to be the key to the understanding of the normal personality also; for in the process of studying mental disturbances, Freud came to understand the structure of the mind in general and its normal functioning. In considering here the normal personality, I would like you to bear in mind that normality is not a rigid and narrow set of qualities. Within the range of the normal there lies an infinite variety of states of mind, modes of behaviour and qualities of temperament.

Early in his work Freud found in the treatment of patients that psychological symptoms were relieved when certain thoughts, feelings and early memories, hitherto unknown to the patient, were brought to light. Freud discovered that if the patient allowed himself to express his thoughts and feelings freely as they came to him, an unconscious meaning could be detected, going beyond the meaning which the patient had expressed in so many words. In following this method of free association further, Freud came to understand that there exists a part of the mind which is quite unconscious, and is yet most powerful in its effects. Certain thoughts and feelings are kept under repression, banished to a less accessible part of the mind, as it were; and yet they exert a strong and sometimes disturbing and harmful influence on the whole personality. Freud found that when these repressed thoughts and impulses were brought to light by his method and thus submitted to the full consciousness and judgement of the individual, their unfavourable effect ceased, and mental disturbances were thus relieved. Further studies showed that repression is a normal, inevitable and useful mechanism, and that only an excess of it, and certain conditions under which it is experienced, make it harmful in its effects.

The precise method of free association allowed Freud not only to gain access to the unconscious part of the mind, but to understand more and more of the way in which it works.

At this point I would like to say one or two words about the question of evidence. I am very much aware how dogmatic many of the statements I make must necessarily appear to those who have no acquaintance with the evidence upon which they are based, and in the time at my disposal it is impossible for me to remedy these defects. It has to be remembered that we are dealing with the unconscious mind, and that the description 'unconscious' is meant with complete seriousness. Certain phantasies, wishes and feelings remain truly unconscious in the full sense of the word, and any untrained observer who hears of them without having got to know them in his own mind may feel that they are strange and unlikely – actually that they are untrue.

The psycho-analytic technique requires a long and highly specialized training. The student has to learn to appreciate the unconscious meaning of the actual words and gestures, tones of voice, memories and thoughts of the patient. His perception is gradually educated to see also the way in which all the various things which the patient states and feels and remembers are related to each other. Psycho-analysis is above everything else an empirical study, and there are many ways in which we gain proofs or correction of our views, but these tests and means of verification would take me far too long to describe to you. Confirmation of the working of the unconscious mind can also be gained in such sciences as anthropology, mythology and folk lore, since the primitive modes of thinking characteristic of the unconscious mind appear very clearly in primitive medicine, magic, ritual, etc. Again, we can verify some of the psycho-analytic conclusions by observing the play, talk and behaviour of the young child, in whom unconscious phantasies manifest themselves more readily and directly than they do in adults. Many of the things which the child says appear so strange to us because of the nature of the unconscious, which strikes our conscious minds as bizarre or even grotesque.

To demonstrate the principle of free association I will give you an instance of a first interview with a fifteen-year-old patient of my own. I had asked him to speak as freely as he could about whatever went through his mind. At his request, I had given him an explanation of the purpose of the treatment, and had mentioned that by means of psycho-analysis I might find the unconscious reasons for his difficulties, and thus be able to relieve them. He had listened politely and with interest, went on to talk about himself, and then said that he had been at a fun fair the day before. He expressed his amusement about the showman, who had been proclaiming how marvellous his show was. Here the patient's unconscious train of thought showed me that while consciously he had appeared quite appreciative of my explanation, unconsciously he had criticised my description of the psycho-analytic method; he had unconsciously compared it with the boasting of the showman. When I told the patient this, he at once agreed to my interpretation, recognizing suddenly that this had been at the back of his mind. He enlarged on it by saying that actually the show had been wretched, and this again suggested that he had not only criticised my presentation of the treatment, but had also felt doubts about its prospects.

To understand the origin and the working of the unconscious mind and its relation to the conscious one, we have to go back to the developmental life of the baby. The phantasies and feelings of the infant do not fade away when he grows up and acquires new ways of behaviour and attitudes They are still present but mostly unconscious. They are active but they do not lead to the same pattern of behaviour and modes of reactions as in former times. Their influence is predominantly exerted in indirect ways and their presence can therefore usually only be detected by following the transformation of impulse, thought and imagining through a study of the various manifestation of the mind in the personal history of the individual and the emotional and intellectual life of the individual.

This realm of the unconscious mind is continuously increased by impulses, thoughts and imaginings which undergo repression because they are from earliest infancy onwards, repudiated by one part of the mind.

In the first few months of the baby's life, his bodily sensations are inextricably bound up with all his emotions. His first desires are connected with his mouth activities and pleasures, and thus his first and fundamental gratifications are bound up with his mother, who feeds and satisfies him. He loves her in a greedy way, and hates her if he feels unsatisfied. The mind of the infant is, as we know, predominantly ruled by his emotions, and love, greed and hatred alternate in him with lightning quickness. These mouth pleasures are an initial part of the child's sexuality. Our studies have shown that young children also experience genital feelings and desires, which relate first of all to the people nearest to them and most beloved, namely their parents. The girl, even at a very tender age, has desires towards her father which, though different in their manifestations from those of adults, are the ultimate source from which adult sexuality develops. The same applies to the boy and his feelings about his mother.

Thus a situation arises in which the little girl, who loves her mother and is dependent upon her in various ways; at the same time labours under strong feelings of hate and hostility towards her.

Another component derives from his excretory functions which are to him the source of both sensual pleasure and of intellectual interest. The little boy has similar conflicts and feelings in connection with his father.

Most of these very complex emotions and impulses – love, hate, greed, desire and jealousy – are incompatible with each other and the child is therefore helplessly exposed to pain, suffering and anxiety, from which he can find no way out. It is largely the painfulness of these conflicts which brings about the repression of those impulses, thoughts and feelings which are condemned and censored by one part of his personality, and are banished into the unconscious levels of the mind. Sexual desires are especially apt to be repressed, partly because they are also condemned by the adults, but still more because in the depths of the child's mind *they are bound up with feelings of love and hatred, remorse and guilt, and with the anxiety arising from these.* The very force of his desires which bid immediate satisfaction can thus cause him intense distress, driving him to rid himself forcefully of these desires by repressing them.

The powerful innate tendency to suppress whatever disturbs the equilibrium of the mind is enhanced by the demands which civilization necessarily makes on the child from his earliest days onwards. The child also feels that many of his desires are impracticable and unreasonable – and such verdicts by his critical faculty contribute to repression. Together with those desires and impulses which, the child feels, are dangerous and culpable, his conflicts between love and hate are to some extent shut off by repression in the unconscious part of his mind. The struggle however goes on in the depths, and is therefore, if repression be over-strong, liable to disturb the mental balance, just as (to take an example from the field of politics) subterranean activities are more likely to overthrow the regime than those which are allowed free expression.

The peculiarities of even the normal child, the ways in which his imagination works, the strangeness of the things he sometimes says, seeming to come from a different world, his emotional instability, his rapid change from happiness to unhappiness, his often unaccountable outbursts of naughtiness, and so on – these phenomena are so familiar that they are mostly taken as a matter of course. As a small illustration: a normal child of three years, after having played happily, is being put to bed and kissed good night by his mother, and says, looking under his bed clothes and shuddering, 'There are tigers there.' His mother tells him that this is nonsense, and probably with these words dismisses the strange and unpleasant incident from her mind. I shall offer an explanation of this child's fears later on.

The view, though true to some extent, that the child's intellectual immaturity, his inability to conceive the material world as it is and his lack of knowledge and experience, are responsible for his irrational behaviour takes account of one side of the picture only. It is only by considering his *unconscious* mind, and the conflicts and imaginings which are going on there, that we can understand many of the phenomena of his development.

The child, when dominated by his urges, has impulses to attack, injure and destroy the objects of his hatred, which are, however, at the same time the ones he loves most, namely his parents. As we know, quite violent and hostile tendencies in the child do sometimes find conscious expression; but the bulk of such impulses, the detailed aggressive imaginings which go with them, and the knowledge that they are directed against the people he loves most – all these elements of his mental life are repressed and become unconscious.

There is an additional fact which makes these repudiated feelings so terrifying for the child. It is characteristic of the young child's mind that he believes in the omnipotence of his thoughts and impulses, that is to say he feels that his aggressive tendencies and the imaginings going with them *do actually take effect.* He unconsciously believes, for instance, that when in greedy love or anger he wants to bite his mother, he does so in fact and thus injures or destroys her. This belief in his omnipotence makes such impulses absolutely real to him, and their being repressed only partly relieves his conscious mind. Unconsciously, these impulses remain active and give rise to powerful feelings of fear and guilt. Because of his destructive desires the child has strong fears of losing, either in the present or in the future, his loved parents, or brothers and sisters, and experiences strong apprehension and guilt on this score. Naturally the very presence, the affection and care of these loved people helps to disprove such fears, but they are liable to be aroused again in circumstances of stress.

If we consider from this point of view the relationship of the small child to his mother we find that his dependence on her, his clinging to her, is not derived from love and helplessness alone, but partly from fear. I imagine that you will find no great difficulty in agreeing with me so far, but I have now to put before you a much more difficult proposition, one which becomes understandable only through studying still more closely the child's unconscious phantasy life. His destructive tendencies have the effect of changing in his mind those people whom in phantasy he attacks, into attackers. To quote out of many instances one for which I am indebted to Dr Ernest Jones: A little boy of three, on seeing his mother's breasts, exclaimed 'Is this what you were biting me with?' He thus attributed to his mother's breasts his own impulses to bite them.

By this process of endowing others with his own impulses, the child who unconsciously feels as ravenous as a tiger may feel his parents to be tigers as well. In the unconscious mind there is a dread that the attacked person will retaliate upon the attacker in exactly the same way as the injury was done; the principle of 'an eye for an eye, and a tooth for a tooth'. In the child's phantasy, his father or mother turns into a tiger; and this in spite of his knowing, alongside these fears, that they are his kind parents whom he loves. Fears of this nature are likely to increase when the child is left by himself, particularly at bed-time. Then the imaginary, frightening figures, for instance the 'tiger-mother', gains in strength, since the real mother, who through her love and care counteracts fears of the kind, has gone. We see here another reason for the child's clinging to his mother. He feels that she protects him, not only against various objects of his fears, but that she counteracts and disproves in his mind the other aspect of herself, the imaginary mother whom he distrusts and fears. Though this terrifying mother is imaginary, in the depths of the child's unconscious mind she is very real; moreover, she cannot altogether be dissociated in his emotions from his other picture of her – the real mother whom he loves and trusts. Hence both trust and distrust of his loved ones exist in the child's mind, and for that matter persist to a certain variable extent in the adult as well.

In the instance of the child who imagined tigers in his bed we see that the content of the fear was to some extent conscious. The child knew he was afraid of tigers; but the fact that he was actually afraid of his own parents, who for the time being were represented by the tigers in his mind, was quite unconscious.

Infantile fears derive from their projecting their own aggression on to their parents and to other people – imagination thus colouring the facts. The nature of the facts however is of course of great importance in this process. The actual attitudes and personalities of the parents, the nature of their relation to the child and his experiences with them, play an essential part in the degree and the course the child's anxieties and apprehensions take. The ways in which in everyday life the adults deal with children are capable of disproving or diminishing such fears, or, on the other hand, of increasing them. [*Handwritten addition here:* To mention as an instance attitude of parents towards truth they confess.] Deprivations of various kinds are, it is true, inevitable in the child's life, since there are necessarily clashes between his powerful primitive urges, and therefore often impracticable desires, and the demands social life and education make on him. The attitude of the parents towards frustrating the 'good' or 'bad' reasons for (illegible) may add considerably to the pain of these deprivations or, on the other hand, they may lessen them, and thus also increase or diminish his hatreds and ensuing fears. At every juncture the influences from the external world and the apprehensions springing from his inner life are bound up with each other. In short, the irrational fears of children are the result of an interaction between his real experiences and his phantasy life and impulses.

It is surprising that even quite conscious fears are often concealed by children from the adults round them, even if they are friendly and understanding people. There is the obvious reason that children are afraid to appear cowardly and babyish. Again, when morning comes, the night-time fears have faded away, and the child tries not to remember them. But one deep and more powerful reason for the child's concealing his fears is the fact that in his unconscious mind he feels the frightening figures to be his parents themselves.

Furthermore, there is also an unconscious connection between his own aggressive impulses and his anxieties of being attacked in retaliation; for this reason he is afraid of betraying his own hostility if he shows his fears. These are some of the deeper motives which, unknown to the child, prevent him from revealing these apprehensive feelings. I know of many children of various ages who suffered cruelly from fears of all kinds and never told anyone about them. Such fears are largely responsible for many difficulties and idiosyncrasies children show; for instance, their dislike of going to bed, or their lack of appetite, 'food fads', difficulties over training in cleanliness and naughtiness of one kind or another.

One of the striking facts which the psycho-analysis of young children has brought to light is that such fears, which are a source of so much distress and suffering to the child, also act as a strong impetus to his interests, stimulate his wish for knowledge and have a vital effect on his intellectual, social and emotional development. The fear of having injured the people he loves, and his feelings of guilt on that score, gives rise very early to an intense need to make good, to make reparation for imagined injuries – a need which expresses itself in all the constructive aims and activities of the child.

This brings us to the wider issue – the fact that all of the interests and activities of children are bound up with their emotional life and rooted in their earliest relations and experiences, primarily in the relation to the mother. To begin with, the baby's satisfaction in being fed comes partly from the relief of his feelings of hunger, partly from the sensual pleasure he experiences when his mouth is stimulated by sucking his mother's breasts. The complex bodily and mental gratification which comes to the baby through the alleviation of his hunger and the close contact with his mother is the foundation of his love for her and for the feeling of security gained in his relation to her. Though his attachment to his mother is thus rooted in the mouth gratifications she affords him, his feelings of love soon extend to her as a whole person. Nevertheless, his mother's breast, and more specifically her nipple, remains ingrained in the mind as the fundamental objects of love.

At the same time as his love for his mother and for other people is developing, various things gradually come in the baby's mind to stand for the original loved thing – the nipple – because to him they are similar to it. For instance, any round thing may represent to him his mother's breast. This unconscious equation of objects with people or parts of people – the formation of symbols – is a fundamental process of the human mind. In this way, love and interest are partly transferred from people to things which have come to stand for them symbolically (Jones, 1918).

An object, the shape of which reminds the infant of the nipple or of the teat of the bottle, seems to have an irresistible attraction for him, and he will at once put it into his mouth and suck it. Step by step, with this bodily pleasure in sucking, love and interest, become partly transferred to those things which have taken on some qualities of the breast or bottle in his mind. Though first of all he likes sucking them, his love/attachment and interest persist even after he has given up the actual sucking.

I observed a baby, aged about 9 months, who repeatedly after his feed, and being quite contented, looked in a loving way at the empty bottle which stood near and carried on what could only be described as a conversation with it. He spoke to it, and then again and again stopped, as if waiting for a reply. It was the same kind of babbling talk which at this stage he often had with his mother – talk to which he actually expected her to respond. Not long after this, he would extend much interest to a humming top, being first attracted by its red knob, which he immediately sucked. This sucking relationship, however, soon led to an interest in the way it could be made to spin. He soon gave up his attempts to suck it, but his absorption in the top remained. When he was fifteen months old, it happened that another humming top, of which he was also very fond, fell on the floor while he was playing with it, and came to bits. The child was deeply distressed about this accident, even after the top had been put together again, and for a day or two did not even want to go near the toy cupboard where it was kept.

We see that partly by means of symbol formation, the individual achieves a relation to things which retain some of the features of the relationship to the people he loves. The child felt distressed at having broken the humming top and showed his concern in the way he did when he occasionally hurt his mother in a half-playful way, by attempting to bite her or by pulling her hair, and so on.

The process of symbol-formation is carried further into children's play activities in general, and elements of their emotional relation to people – love and interest, sexual phantasies and hostile impulses, the drive to restore, impulses and phantasies which are largely undergoing repression because they are fraught with conflicts – express themselves unconsciously in their play. Thus, through their play activities children are able to give vent to feelings and phantasies about people who play a vital part in their emotional life.

Most of these facts were discovered in the psycho-analyses of young children by means of a play technique which I devised. I shall now give a short account of a particular play of a child which occurred during a psycho-analytic session, and in which the conflicting feelings and tendencies in relation to his family found expression. (I may say that play of this kind is an everyday occurrence in the psycho-analytic playroom.)

Whilst with the grown-up the thoughts and feelings which he expresses in words are the chief material by which the psycho-analyst is guided in his work, in the analysis of children the various actions the child carries out with his toys, his whole behaviour, as well as what he says, are the principal means by which he manifests both his unconscious and his conscious thoughts and feelings. The kind of toys which the psycho-analyst puts at the child's disposal varies according to his stage of development.

A boy of about four years of age was playing with tiny houses, trees, people, etc on a table. Suddenly he tipped up the table, causing all the toys to fall on the floor, and remarked that an awful earthquake had occurred in the street. From what he told me it became clear that the calamity took place in the street in which his parents live, and also in the street where I live. He soon showed much concern about the condition of these people, picked them up, decided that some of them were uninjured and just needed a rest, and replaced the unharmed ones and some of the houses on the table. The number of the rescued people whom he then cared for corresponded to the number of people in his own family.

In this play the unconscious wish to destroy his nearest relatives and the counteracting wish to save and restore them – hatred as well as love – found expression. I may mention that on this day the child had felt frustrated at home for some apparently trivial reason, and this frustration contributed to his unconscious aggressive and vindictive desires and phantasies. We all know that play of this kind is quite ordinary, but to discover the unconscious conflicts and feelings underlying it is part of the work of the psycho-analyst of children.

Constructiveness in children's play springs from various sources. All of these, however, as for instance the child's pleasure in his developing skills, his satisfaction in creative activities, aesthetic pleasure, his wish to be appreciated by adults and to please them; all these are stimulated and constantly fed and influenced by the impulse to put things right, to undo harm done in phantasy and to make amends to loved people. With young children, a brick, for instance, can stand for a person, and putting a few bricks together may represent in the child's unconscious mind his uniting a number of people – parents, or brothers and sisters – whom for hostile reasons he has parted in his imagination. Or again, bricks or other toys may stand for parts of a person whom he has destroyed in anger and greed – eaten up or cut up – and who is now, through a gesture in the play, put together and made whole.

To speak of the more accomplished activities of children: when a child models a person or an animal, builds a house or draws a tree, he feels that he has actually created them, and can obtain bodily and mental pleasure in the creation. But the act of creation is always in some way a restoration and re-creation, for in his unconscious mind, these objects stand for the people he loves, whom he feels he has injured, and now wants to restore and bring back to life.

In his work with children the psycho-analyst obtains constant proofs that the child's pleasure in his play activities is greatly enhanced by the relief he obtains from giving vent to repressed impulses and imaginings in relation to people, while at the same time he knows that he does not actually injure and destroy the people themselves. And in so far as much of what he acts out in play is in his unconscious mind partly reparation and re-creation, his feelings of guilt and anxieties are again and again alleviated through his play activities.

As we see from this brief description, the child's unconscious mind shows great contrasts, violent and asocial impulses as well as highly social ones, which underlie his constructive and sublimated tendencies. This deep-rooted conflict between opposing forces in the depths of the mind governs human life in all its relationships, productions and manifestations. In the last analysis, it is the conflict between love and hatred towards one and the same object.

The psychological fact that loved people are also unconsciously hated, and that this is a fundamental source of conflict derived from infancy, is one of the important discoveries of Freud. This phenomenon has been termed ambivalence; more recently, the intensity and painfulness of this struggle in the infant, his feelings of guilt and powerful effects of these early conflicts on the development of the whole personality, have been adequately realized. These discoveries, arrived at in the psycho-analyses of young children carried out in the last fifteen years or so in this country, have led to a more complex picture of the unconscious and the conscious mind than was hitherto conceived. At the same time we have a better and a more profound understanding of the mode of working of that elaborate and dynamic structure which we call human nature.

The study of the young child's mind has shown me that the capacity for love, which is a natural impulse in the baby and grows in response to his mother's love and care, is soon greatly intensified and deepened by feelings of guilt and the fears of losing her through his hostile impulses. These emotions contribute to the drive in the child to protect the people he loves from his own aggression as well as from the harm done by others. To lose these loved people would mean to him the shattering of his whole outer and inner world. When anxiety increases, however, he feels as if he had actually lost them, and experiences great sorrow and deep feelings of guilt. Through these complex feelings a special element of anguish and deep mental pain enters into the struggle between love and hate, which has a bearing on our ability to understand and to sympathize with the suffering of others and enhances our capacity for compassion and helpfulness.

In normal development unconscious fears and conflicts are counteracted by the actual experiences of the child, by the love of the people around him, by the comfort he gains from finding day by day that he does not destroy and lose those he loves. Also, he can reconstruct and re-create them in his mind through his various activities and achievements, and thus gradually gain greater inner security and consequently greater stability.

I feel by now that you all want to tell me that this picture I have given you does not show normal children as we know them. Though you will agree with me that even normal children are easily distressed, are prone to fears and anxieties and even experience unhappiness, you may argue that these moods pass off quickly; that the child who has just been crying bitterly can feel jolly and happy a few minutes later. Therefore you may say that his sufferings cannot be so very painful and important. But I am suggesting to you that we are *a priori* inclined to minimize the signs which point to suffering in the child, and to overrate the indications of his happiness. For there are few things which adults in general, and particularly mothers, find more unbearable than knowing that a child suffers, without being able to remedy this completely. Now fortunately it is true that we can do a great deal towards relieving these sufferings. Our attitude towards our children from the first day of life can go very far to diminish and ease their conflicts and fears and to increase their happiness and feeling of security. Nevertheless, we are unable to eradicate the conflict between love and hatred in the child's mind at its source and we cannot spare it from all sadness and suffering.

I must remind you that in speaking about the anxieties of children I suggested that they often conceal these feelings to a very great extent from grown-ups, and I pointed out some of the deeper reasons for this secrecy. I should now like to add that the child unconsciously knows that the adults dislike his anxieties and unhappiness and are emotionally disturbed by them. He feels unconsciously that they try to dispel his anxieties and sufferings, not only for his sake but for their own as well; and the child has a very strong impulse to please and gratify those around him on whose love he is so very dependent. I think we cannot overrate the strength of this impulse and its effects upon his whole attitude, behaviour and development. His need to love and to be loved, to give satisfaction to the adults and to adapt himself to their wishes and standards is, however, greatly enhanced by feelings of guilt and the drive to reparation. Our own wish that our children should be happy, which leads us to minimize the signs of their unhappiness, thus coincides with their unconscious and conscious desire to gratify and to please us. But this implies that the child's own feelings of guilt and unhappiness often are being passed over and not allowed sufficient expression and discharge – in fact that to some extent his feelings are being sacrificed to the convenience and comfort of the adults around him.

The observation of babies shows that our smile will soon be reciprocated by theirs, and that they even seem to expect that their smiling at us will evoke our smile in return. This unconscious knowledge in the baby exists long before he can use words, even before he can understand our words. There are many ways in which the baby from the beginning is made to understand that we like him to be happy and do not want him to be unhappy; and it is a natural and essential part of our care and love for him that we do so. Nevertheless, if we are able to understand the inevitable sufferings of our children and to bear them with some equanimity and a minimum of anxiety we shall not increase, but are likely to diminish our children's difficulties. It is true that allowing the child greater freedom to manifest some of his difficulties may make him less manageable and adaptable in some ways. The child's adaptability, however, in so far as it depends upon his concealing conflicts from us, is often attained at great cost to himself. Some children who are too obedient, too good, as it were, and very easy to manage, are among those whose great mental difficulties and instability appear at a later stage of the development, especially in adolescence.

It is not easy to find the right compromise. The view that children should be allowed to manifest their feelings of hate and aggressiveness freely has been advocated by some modern educationalists, but this notion can be greatly overdone or wrongly applied. It is certainly a great relief to the child to be able to express hostile feelings towards us, without making us feel unduly injured or hurt or cross. The main point, however, is that we should not react with too strong feelings to what the child does and says. We can help our children most by our *attitude* in response to their expressions of feeling. If we can understand and bear the fact that children do experience hostility towards us at times and will express this through certain acts of hatred and destruction, and that they are often afraid of us, and therefore sometimes defiant and querulous – if we can realize these facts without too much worry and concern and without feeling hurt, then we are quite likely to find the right compromise. It is an old experience that things run more smoothly if the parent does not pay too much attention to the child's bad temper and 'naughtiness', and at times overlooks certain of his remarks and acts. On the other hand, there is a limit to this, and we should to a certain extent control the children's aggressive behaviour, and not let them run wild. If we did allow them complete freedom, this again would only arouse a feeling that we in our turn were afraid of their hatred and hostility, and this would make them feel still more guilty and unhappy.

Here we see one of the many reasons why it is so essential for children to have plenty of opportunity to play with other children. Among their contemporaries, they can manifest their aggressive feelings more freely, with less guilt and anxiety and also with less concern about the consequences. For instance, if

A hits B and B hits back, or if they break each other's toys occasionally, this may lead to a tussle, but one which usually soon passes and leaves them none the worse for the experience.

To return to my contention that children – and for that matter adults also – experience so much more unhappiness and conflict than is commonly recognized. The question now arises: Are conflicts and sufferings which are active in the unconscious mind felt as suffering by the conscious part? The answer would be that we are bound to feel our unconscious sufferings in one way or another. Though there is a strong barrier between the unconscious and the conscious mind, there is also a constant interaction between them. External and internal stimuli and experiences of every kind constantly affect our unconscious minds, our repressed conflicts and feelings. Earlier important situations are more or less strongly revived by present ones, and in turn influence, without our being in the least aware of this, our conscious feelings and impressions of the experience we are going through at the moment. The unconscious processes in our minds have a strong influence even on the ways in which we perceive and take in new experiences, and the significance they assume in our minds.

We may not be in the least aware what it is that worries us, makes us restless, disturbs our peace of mind, makes us sad for inadequate reasons, influences our actions (sometimes irrationally), inhibits us in carrying out useful and satisfactory activities, causes our tempers, disturbs our relationships with people, and yet we do suffer greatly under such states of mind and disabilities.

The influence of our unconscious conflicts and sufferings, however, upon our activities and conscious feelings, as I showed earlier, is by no means only painful and unfavourable, for in extremely elaborate ways, which influence all our activities and relationships, we transform unhappiness into happiness, and make constant use of our happy feelings and satisfactions in counteracting and overcoming our sufferings. The child, for instance, who cries because his mother has left the room, as I have often observed in my work with young children, may in his unconscious mind feel deeply distressed because he fears that as a punishment for his hate of her, or because she is destroyed by it, she may never come back again, and he will lose her altogether. It is true, children's growing capacity to understand and accept reality gradually counteracts such fears, but they do operate very strongly alongside rational understanding, and they are not only at the bottom of his unhappy moods, but also add to and intensify his joy and happiness when his mother returns. The satisfaction children gain from being loved by their mothers – and for that matter from receiving love in general – is thus increased, intensified and even altered in quality by their fears and feelings of guilt. We avoid feeling our unconscious unhappiness, which never altogether ceases, by constantly disproving, counteracting and diminishing it through our activities, interests and personal relationships; and these constant endeavours influence essentially the development and enrichment of our personalities.

In our drive to preserve and to re-create loved objects whom we have in our minds endangered, an impulse which expresses itself in all the manifestations of our lives, we counterbalance and diminish the early conflicts between love and hatred which persist, to a certain extent, throughout life. Sadness, sorrow and guilt are overcome and kept at bay through happy relationships to people, through the love we put into our work, through our devotion to ideals; and there is no activity, no interest, from the most simple to the most elaborate, which does not participate in this fundamental and pervading process of establishing harmony in ourselves as well as in the external world. Freud said, after he had discovered the unconscious sense of guilt [here Klein has written and then crossed out that 'we are not only more immoral but more moral than we know' and hand written above the line 'quotation 269 Epit.' She appears to be referring to the following passage from Freud (1923), which she may have found and quoted during the lecture itself:

> One may go further and venture the hypothesis that a great part of the sense of guilt must normally remain unconscious, because the origin of conscience is intimately connected with the Oedipus complex, which belongs to the unconscious. If anyone were inclined to put forward the paradoxical proposition that the normal man is not only far more immoral than be believes but also far more moral than he knows, psychoanalysis, on whose findings the first half of the assertion rests, would have no objection to raise against the second half.
>
> *(Freud, 1923, p. 52)*]

Similarly, it could be said that there is not only more hate and destructiveness in us than we know, but more love and creativeness than we realize. Feelings of love and helpfulness exist in the unconscious minds of all of us, though in some people they may be deeply buried, and find little expression in activities and relationships.

The unconscious mind is the soil from which all our constructive and creative impulses spring, out of which our deepest capacity for love develops, and with it kindness, goodness, compassion and fairness. I have tried to convey to you that our unconscious conflicts and sufferings which are the deepest cause of our unhappiness, are at the same time the very source from which the wealth of our inner life is increased, for it is linked up with our capacity to experience life, that is to feel; and only if we are able to feel unhappiness are we also able to feel happiness deeply and genuinely.

References

Freud, S. (1923). The ego and the id. In J. Strachey et al.(trans.), *The standard edition of the complete psychological works of Sigmund Freud vol. 19*. London: Hogarth Press.

Jones, E. (1918). The theory of symbolism, *British Journal of Psychology, 9*; reprinted in *Papers on psycho-analysis*. Hogarth Press. cf. The importance of symbol-formation and the development of the ego, Melanie Klein. *International Journal of Psycho-Analysis*.

4

SADNESS AND LOSS IN THE EMOTIONAL LIFE OF THE YOUNG CHILD

Melanie Klein (edited by Jane Milton)

Introduction

This previously unpublished pair of lectures is to be found in the Melanie Klein Archives at the Wellcome Library, in file PP/KLE/C.51 and can be viewed online. The lectures were given at the London Institute of Education in May 1939 as part of a series of three known as the Joseph Payne lectures, the overall topic of which was 'Psychoanalysis and Normal Development'. Chapter 3 of this book contains the first of the lectures. Like Klein's other lay lectures they are clearly and compellingly written, full of illustrative examples from the everyday life of infants. In file C.51 these lectures are called Part 1 and Part 2 and are separated by some summary notes that may have been Klein's first outline of the lectures. These notes will not be included in this chapter but may be consulted online.

The lectures

The role of feelings of sadness and loss in the young child's emotional life

Part 1

In my talks with you I am taking you back to the early stages of development which to some extent have already been dealt with by the former speakers. But I wish to discuss with you a particular aspect in the emotional life of the young child; and I think the general survey of development which you have been given will help you to understand this particular aspect.

Mrs Isaacs has given you an outline of the feelings associated with the infant's oral desires. She has described to you that the relation to the mother is first of all focussed on the mother's breast and that even in the earliest stages the gratification of being fed implies already the gratification of feelings of love. The mother's breast is the first love object. It is important to realise that while the alleviation of hunger gratifies the most dominant need in the baby, this gratification is from the beginning closely linked with the libidinal gratification derived from sucking which is the first manifestation of the infant's sexual life. The gratification derived from sucking is bound up with the importance the mother – first of all her breast – has as the first love object.

To the gratification of sucking are added the many elements which enter into the infant's relation with the mother. For, as Mrs Isaacs has described to you in more detail, the interest in the mother's face, the touch of her hands and the baby's pleasure in touching her breast, her face and her hands – all these are manifestations of a relation with the mother going far beyond the actual alleviation of hunger by her.

These feelings of love contribute to the picture of an object which can provide the highest gratification and satisfy all needs. The wish to possess for ever such an object plays a fundamental part in mental life. We find it expressed in the most elaborate ways in the adult mind, where it still persists as the fountain of all goodness and love. An optimistic or a pessimistic outlook in life is closely linked with the success or failure of the fundamental early relation to the mother.

Infants – even quite young ones, (though this becomes more apparent towards the middle of the first year) – vary a great deal in their attitude towards the people around them and, in their attitude towards gratification and frustration. A really happy baby, one who shows an increasing interest in the people and things around him and has much pleasure in taking food, is also capable of bearing frustrations. By this I mean that though he may cry vigorously at times of frustration, he is quickly comforted and his pleasure in food and his relation to people are not essentially disturbed. Though he enjoys, as early as from the second month onwards, the company of his mother and soon also of other people, he is in his waking periods also capable of being quite happy by himself. The fleeting expressions on the infant's face at such times indicate that a good deal is going on in his mind that the serenity – if one may speak of that in such a young being – is not vacancy but part of his successful adaptation to his external as well as to his internal world. Very important things go on in the young infant in such states when he appears to be happy by himself. As we know, such states of happiness by himself do not last long in very young infants, and again and again the baby will wish to see his mother, or to hear her voice or even her footsteps. I am not referring now to physical discomfort which necessitates alleviation by the mother, but to the infant's need to experience from time to time the presence of his mother, to see signs of her love, even to express his love; for these are the ways in which he, as it were, renews his relation with her. For only for relatively short periods can he keep this relation alive without her actual presence.

We see here an interaction between the child's relation to the mother as he sees and knows her and to his mental picture of her. To establish this picture of a good mother in his mind is one of the preconditions for the infant's happiness; this continues to play a part throughout life. This good relation to his mother established within the mind, becomes part of his inner world and has already in the young infant a bearing on the way he can suffer frustration, because frustration and deprivation are felt all the more strongly if to them is added anxiety and feelings of insecurity about the possession of a good and reliable object. Again, such attitudes can be observed in older children and in adults. For the degree of frustration people can sustain without getting bitter, resentful and hostile varies, as we know, very much with different individuals. It is very striking to see through what indescribable hardships some people can go and yet retain a fundamental trust and belief in goodness and faith in the future. Such an attitude goes back to the baby's happy relation to the mother's breast and becomes gradually more and more connected with her as a whole person.

I have repeatedly stressed now a real happiness in the baby and given you some criteria for such development. It is not difficult to distinguish between a baby who has difficulty over feeding who cries much, whose development in fact seems to go wrong, and a baby who thrives on his food and obviously enjoys life. But it is easy to mistake a baby who does not particularly dislike his food and cries little for a happy baby. And yet as development later on shows, some of these easy-going babies in fact are not really happy. Their lack of crying may be due to a kind of apathy, to something like resignation. It is difficult to account in so young a being for such a state of mind without allowing for a great complexity of emotions. But if we follow up the development of some of these babies in their relation to food and to people, we find that serious difficulties soon appear. They are often shy of people, particularly of strangers; their interest in the external world, in play and learning is inhibited, for instance they are often slow at learning to crawl and walk because there seems so little incentive. And they are in fact very often showing strong signs of neurosis as their development goes on.

There is another side, however, to this fundamental first relation. Even the happiest baby experiences aggressive feelings towards his mother. For love and aggression are the two predominant innate impulses, and they are both directed towards the first, and for some time unique, object – the mother. The resulting conflict is the cause for much mental struggle and for the feelings of sadness and fear of loss and feelings of guilt in the infant.

There are certain characteristics of the infant's emotional life which we have to keep in mind if we wish to understand the intensity of his conflicts. In his unconscious mind phantasies of a complete and immediate wish-fulfilment are very active. The infant is predominantly governed by his emotions and has not yet developed a relation to reality which would enable him to cope with his emotions. Early love is very greedy; cannibalistic desires and phantasies are, as Freud discovered, inherent in the infant's oral relation to his mother. They are reinforced at times of frustration and associated with feelings of grievance, resentment, and hatred. These desires to devour the mother's breast and the mother in hatred and resentment are the cause for anxiety and guilt in the infant.

There is another characteristic of the early mind which contributes to such feelings of guilt, namely the feeling of omnipotence of his thoughts and desires. When the infant has in his mind attacked his mother and devoured her, he feels that he has actually done so. But that implies to him that he has destroyed, or is in danger of destroying, any time his greed wells up, his most loved and indispensable object. It is true that an increasing degree of perception of reality again and again is evidence for the young child that his mother still exists and is unhurt. But such evidence is only relatively effective. For any time the child is longing to see his mother and cannot see her, or any time external or internal stimuli give rise to anxiety in him, he experiences feelings of loss, grief, sadness and guilt. These early feelings of sadness and guilt, as the analysis of young children and of adults has shown, are the foundation for feelings of depression in later life.

The strength of such feelings, the poignancy of the conflict, varies in children. The more securely the picture of the good mother is established in his inner world, the less acute will be the infant's feelings of grief, and the better will he be able to deal with them, but such depressive feelings are never missing.

What I am suggesting to you is that complex emotions are active even in young infants. One might say that there is something like a predisposition to experiencing feelings of loss, and that they attach themselves at once to the most fundamental first object, the mother's breast or the bottle given by her. That distress goes with such fear of losing the object.

But as you will have seen, I go further with my suggestions. In our view young infants experience sadness, that is to say depressive feelings, and guilt resulting from aggressive impulses directed against his loved object. Now such feelings of depression and guilt appear, we think, at a stage when the infant is able to take in the mother as a whole object, that is to say between four and six months. As you know, at this stage very definite changes in the intellectual and emotional development of the child become perceptible.

Another climax of such feelings arises in connection with the weaning, either from the breast or from the bottle, and it may become particularly strong at the time the last bottle is taken away. In this connection, the methods of weaning the child from breast to bottle, and from the last bottle, are very important.

Sadness and grief in infants have not yet been recognised at their full importance, while the unmistakeable emotions of anger and rage have been more generally observed. Yet grief is at times clearly expressed on the infant's face, and many an observant mother is aware of her child's distress (though she might not think of it in terms of grief). This is particularly evident when the infant begins to shed tears. The face becomes more expressive, the lines deepen, and something in his eyes indicates that his range of emotions has widened. In my view, the child's emotional development at this stage has progressed in the direction that the experience of guilt and depression is entering.

The infant's fear of loss and depressive feelings also link up with night terrors. For even with healthy and happy infants, who as a rule enjoy good sleep, it happens that under certain circumstances such as a change of surroundings – and sometimes without any ostensible cause – they may wake up from their sleep with actual terror. A striking instance of the emotions underlying such disturbances of sleep was reported to me by a mother. She said she found her baby daughter, who was as a rule happy and slept well, sobbing in her sleep at the age of ten months. She had observed this once or twice before. The evident feelings of sadness shown in this case contribute also to night terrors and other disturbances of sleep.

Feelings of sadness and fear of loss show themselves in many ways in infants if only we consider their attitudes sufficiently from that angle. For instance, fear of loss plays a great part in the severe though possibly short disturbance in the infant's relation to his mother, the complete withdrawal from her, which occurs in certain situations of anxiety, usually stimulated by the mother's absence. Provided we can fully appreciate the vacant look of the eyes, the movements of the body, the expression of the features, we shall see the loss of contact, the alteration in the infant's relation to his mother. We must also remember that after such an anxiety situation, though he child has already calmed down, the next feed is often disturbed.

The infant girl who sobbed in her sleep when she was ten months old, when she was five months old had been left crying longer than usual and was then found in what her mother described as a 'hysterical' state. She looked terrified, and the mother said she had no doubt that the child was frightened of her because she had not come when the child expected her. It took the child some time before she seemed to recognise the mother and re-established contact with her. What made this instance, which is quite an ordinary one, so interesting to me is that the facts which underlie such states were so clearly observable that the mother could not help recognising them. I have made similar observations on several infants at different stages from a few months onwards.

One of the outstanding features which one finds in analysing young children is the child's sense of insecurity because the parents seem to him so very changeable. As soon as his fears come up – and particularly when he is alone – the child is apt to feel that the 'good' parents have changed into the 'bad' ones, or else at times that they will never come back because they are destroyed by his own greed and hatred. This is one source of his early fears and conflicts.

Applying this analytic insight to the infant referred to above, we can say that her state was one of fear that the mother would never return because she was devoured or had turned into the 'bad' mother. This again helps us to understand what happens in a child's mind when the mother returns. Her very presence and signs of love re-establish the infant's belief in her as an unharmed and loving mother, though this evidence of her very presence may not be sufficient if the anxiety and his feeling of insecurity are very great. There is often some time needed until the effect of the evidence as it were can make itself felt. When the evidence of the mother being present and unharmed and loving is fully accepted unconsciously, that implies that his trust in the mother then is re-established and that his fear of persecution by a bad mother has decreased. For while the good mother is the greatest stand-by in the inner world of the child, and represents to him the means of allaying all his fears and troubles, the aspect of the mother in which she is felt to be bad and frustrating becomes the object of the greatest fears in the infant. These two aspects are very much split off from one another in the child's mind. The bad mother is not only in the child's mind dangerous because she is felt to be frustrating, but because she is felt to retaliate for all the attacks which in states of frustration – or when aggression predominates – are made in phantasy on her.

The good and loved mother is therefore all the more needed because she is to provide to the infant the evidence that she is good and not persecuting. This process of splitting the mother into a good and a bad one becomes more obvious in the way in which infants give their whole love to the mother and cling to her while they dislike and fear some other person, who then primarily stands for the bad mother. The fear of strangers, so often noticeable in infants, finds its explanation partly in these processes.

Many infants do not show this reaction to strangers, but this does not mean that this splitting process which I suggested to you is not active. When anxiety is not so acute, methods of dealing with it even in the infant are more successful. Also, such fears can be distributed more easily from objects on to other causes for anxiety. Let us say an infant who takes pleasure in food and shows no anxiety of strangers. On the contrary, is friendly and forthcoming to people as well as loving towards his parents. It seems that while the early feeding situation still exists, be it breast or bottle, so much reassurance against such anxieties is derived from it that they do not become very manifest. But with the complete weaning some of these anxieties may then be experienced in idiosyncrasies about food, or particularly be expressed in connection with habit training difficulties. Also such very happy infants sometimes in the first year, but very often in the second year, have certain disturbances of sleep. I suggested to you that night terrors of children are closely linked up with fear of loss and with grief. To give you one instance only of the content of such a night terror as shown in the instance of a girl of two. One night she woke up with a fright and cried bitterly, showing that she had wetted herself a very little. She was very much upset. After waking in the morning, she spoke of a lady, and then said with relief: 'lady gone'. There seems little doubt that there was a connection between the anxiety experienced during her sleep when she woke with a fright, and the lady she spoke about when she woke. The relief that the lady had not gone out of her mind was obvious and showed that she had been a cause of fear. In the light of what I have told you so far, this unpleasant lady represented the frightening aspect of the mother. The bed-wetting, her distress about it, and the frightening aspect of the mother were thus connected with each other in her mind. In her sleep, she felt the fear of having lost her good mother and was left with the bad mother, the lady she wanted to get rid of. Now this girl had shown very little of these splitting processes which I described to you, and yet no doubt they were active.

Now I am giving you an instance of a child in whom the splitting processes between good and bad mother and anxiety about the bad mother had manifested itself much more clearly even at an early stage. He had shown dislike or anxiety of strangers, and certainly a reserve towards them, a close scrutiny of them, even at the age of a few months (about the middle of the first year). When ten months old, he was held by his grandmother and was happily looking out of the window. In the same room were a few other people and one of them, an old lady, had come quite close to the grandmother holding the baby. As it happened, when the child turned round, the first thing he saw was not the face of his grandmother but the face of the old lady. He had a violent anxiety attack and only recovered from it when he was taken out of the room.

The same child, as I have been told, at eighteen months developed a strong phobia of an old lady in a guest house where he was staying with his parents. She was in fact not very nice, but friendly to the child and well meaning, rather too forthcoming and too much trying to please the child. But this could not explain the child's strong aversion to her. It amounted to his not being able to be in one room with her. Similar anxiety situations arose when he was two years six months old. Here the splitting of the mother into good and bad mother became very clear in relation to the grandmother.

To return to what I call the really happy baby. I would take it as one sign of inner security being in the process of being established that such interruptions in contact as I described do not last too long and do not occur too often, and that they would be overcome fairly easily, that they would not lead too readily to a disturbance in the feed following such an incident and in the relation to the people around him.

From this angle we get also a better understanding of the difficulties in taking food which are so frequent in infants and which in many cases cannot be accounted for by external circumstances. Here, however, I can only put forward a few general suggestions as to the reasons for the various feeding difficulties. Those children whose appetite improves when put on to the bottle prefer it because while the bottle symbolically stands for the mother's breast, it is further removed in their minds from the primary object – the breast – which they are afraid to destroy. If the anxiety is not too great (and much depends here on quantities of anxiety as well as on other factors) an infant might not refuse the breast and even thrive on it, and nevertheless his greed can be strongly inhibited. Some infants however do not succeed in the symbolic substitution of the bottle for the breast, and therefore even the bottle remains too vulnerable an object; this is one of the factors which contribute in my view to the inhibition in sucking. Some of such children can only allow themselves greed when solid food is offered.

One conclusion one might draw from what I am saying would be that since it is frustration which so obviously stirs aggression, one might prevent such conflicts arising by avoiding frustration. However, for one thing frustration is unavoidable, though one should of course not expose the child to unnecessary frustration. But if we could assume complete gratification, we would still find that the conflict between aggression and love is something so fundamental that its consequences cannot be avoided in the child. I am thinking for instance, of children whose breast feeding is not arranged according to a timetable and, as often happened in former times and still happens with many mothers nowadays, the baby is fed whenever it wants the breast. I have analysed such people who had such (one would say) complete gratification in babyhood, and I did not find that this had prevented, or even in some people diminished, this conflict. It is true that in the name of hygiene, with disregard of the psychological importance, much harm can be done. You know of course of all those books which in the upbringing of babies seem to consider only the physical point of view, and put the necessity of feeding according to timetable above anything else. I always think that a baby who has too great difficulties with five feeds in 24 hours should be given six feeds and that a baby which has too great difficulties with sleeping through the night should be given one feed in the night. But of course there are limits with regard to the mother's health and the physical needs of the baby. There is no doubt that a certain though flexible routine is necessary. But this routine should go along with a psychological understanding. When the baby cries and one has made sure that it has not got a pin sticking into it or that it has already been relieved of wind and it still is not happy, then one should not dismiss his crying as negligible. A great deal of comfort can be provided by the very fact that one picks up the baby, that one does show him love and friendliness, and very often after a little play of that kind the child will go happily to sleep. This shows that it is not only the food he wants; that the desire for the breast and for the feed is only part of the story. A baby also cries at times when he really does not desire food or could not even accept it. What moves him then is a feeling of longing for the mother which is mixed with anxiety, though this may not be apparent. His feelings of loss, the fear of not seeing the loved mother again, however primitively they are felt, are the reason why the baby needs love and attention and should be given it.

When all is said and done, we have to remain aware that very important processes and conflicts are going on in the baby's mind and that our understanding of these processes, even more than definite rules and regulations about the way the baby is taken care of, will help the young child to deal better with unavoidable conflict. It is not only the older child or the adult who senses a real understanding and sympathy with his conflicts, sorrows and sadness, but even in the infant in very early stages of development this understanding helps to establish this close contact which is one of the foundations for the baby's happiness as well as for his future stability.

Part 2

In my last talk, I tried to convey to you my experience that infants experience feelings of loss, of grief, and go through states of depressive feelings which are the foundation for depression in later life and can be the cause for even severe mental disturbance. I believe that is the origin of depression. Whenever later on strain or stress or external circumstances are bringing out depressive states, it is these particular situations in babyhood which lie at the bottom of it. That again does not mean that everything as it were is settled in babyhood. All through the important years of childhood – from birth to the fifth year – these depressive feelings can be reinforced and this would contribute to the strength and outcome of later depressive states. Even after the fifth year of life and all through life, experiences and circumstances would determine the strength and outcome of the illness. But I do think it is worthwhile keeping in mind that the roots of all that are in these conflicts and feelings of loss which I described to you in more detail in my last lecture.

You will agree with me that the conclusion to be drawn from that is that any means at our disposal to diminish these feelings of loss and insecurity at their root are of the highest importance prophylactically.

Speaking of the first years of childhood in which these fundamental relations to the parents which are so important in what Mrs Riviere described to you as the Oedipus Complex: these conflicts, to some extent inescapable, are very much accentuated and the outcome of the development in relations to people, first of all to the parents, is influenced by these depressive feelings. The little boy who feels hostile and jealous of his father and has death wishes against him will be better able to cope with this conflict between hatred and love for the father if he is less swayed by his fears of loss and by his depressive feelings. The same applies to the little girl in her relation to her mother.

Freud has found out that the ways in which young children deal with these conflicts has a bearing not only on their neurosis and personality but also on the sexual life of the individual.

To give you an instance: if a boy's feelings of loss and guilt in relation to his father are very great, he may retreat as it were from the heterosexual position, and his homosexual tendencies may be increased. As in every element of development, the attitude of the parents towards these conflicts is vital. Let us say a father who cannot bear any aggression or rivalry in his little son may turn the scale towards homosexuality. But considering all this from the angle of the internal life of the child, one would say that the strength of depressive feelings, insecurity and grief in the earliest stages are a contributory factor to his being able to bear these conflicts, and for that matter all conflicts, both in childhood and later on.

Now returning to the baby: I have discussed with you some difficulties in the baby from that particular angle. I shall now tackle this problem from another angle. What are the ways by which the baby deals with these feelings of depression and loss, and how does he overcome them as development proceeds? I stressed particularly in my last talk the connection between a greater feeling of security in his internal world and a greater capacity to bear frustration. The less security in his inner relations the infant can establish, the greater will be his tendency towards depression, and the less will he be able to cope with them successfully.

One might say that the ego of the infant from the beginning develops certain ways and methods of coping with such painful emotions.

I shall now consider some every day observations. It is common knowledge that infants expect praise and admiration for every new achievement. But it is less commonly recognised that he also wishes by means of these achievements to evoke love from his mother and to give her pleasure. How soon does he realise that his smile delights his mother, attracts her attention, keeps her near him, and at times serves this purpose better than his crying? There seems to be no doubt in analytic and non-analytic observers that when an infant cries, this is partly intended to bring his mother back to him; but that his smile and expressions of love could have a similar purpose has been less fully recognised.

I have seen a few infants, when they had woken with anxiety, using all their little tricks which they knew delighted the mother to keep her by their side. In one case an infant of ten months had woken with night terror, and the attempts on the part of her mother to put her to sleep were not successful. Every time the mother turned out the light, the little girl cried again with unmistakeable signs of anxiety. When the light was turned on once more, she clapped her hands, smiled, and did everything which she knew was pleasing to her mother. The anxiety behind this liveliness was quite apparent, as this playfulness and cheerfulness were different from the usual happy mood with which they were associated in daytime; the infant was obviously trying to avoid being exposed once more to anxiety. Actually, the mother decided to play with the child and to make her feel comfortable, and very soon the little girl went happily to sleep again.

In my view, an infant knows intuitively that his smile and other signs of affection and happiness produce happiness and pleasure in the mother and evoke similar responses from her. With older children and in adult life, quarrels are often followed by expressions of friendliness, which are felt in the unconscious – if not consciously – as the means of making amends and reparation. At the same time, they are also an essential method of gaining reassurance against anxiety and guilt, and thus partly serve defensive purposes. I believe that the same is true, mutate mutandis, of infants. One has only to watch the expression on an infant's face when his smile is not responded to and his attempts to please fail. The smile disappears, the light fades from his eyes, and something akin to sorrow and anxiety creeps into his expression.

We can also observe that the infant makes attempts to feed the mother in return for her feeding him. There are various things he expresses by putting his finger into her mouth. Sometimes he clearly wishes to explore the mouth, e.g. an infant of five months to whom I made noises corresponding to his own attempts to babble watched me with the greatest delight and interest and suddenly, while the sound came out of my mouth, he put his finger into my mouth – quite obviously an attempt to fetch the sounds out of it. At other times an infant indicates his wish for his mother to suck his finger or even playfully to bite it, which is partly an attempt to feed her. A little later on many an infant actually tries to feed his mother with his spoon. I am not concerned here with the extent to which the child imitates his mother, which no doubt he does; but my main point is that in this way he expresses his own feelings of love and gratitude towards her and his desire to feed her and give her pleasure as she gives him pleasure by feeding him. He also in my view makes reparation in phantasy and thus counteracts his feelings of guilt, which in a symptomatic way express themselves in feeding difficulties and phobias.

So far I have pointed out that an infant's expression of love, interest, pleasure, etc among other purposes serve the need for reassurance through his mother's love. Furthermore, that they express reparation, and thus are also the means of overcoming grief. Freud's observation of the eighteen months old boy with his cotton reel pointed in this direction. By means of this play the child was overcoming not only his feelings of loss, but, as I see it, also his grief.

There are various typical forms of play similar to the one of the cotton reel game. For instance, it is a general observation that children, sometimes even before the second half of the first year, enjoy throwing things out of the pram again and again, and expect them back. I observed a variation of this play in an infant of ten months who had recently begun to crawl. He was indefatigable in throwing a toy away from himself and then getting hold of it by crawling towards it. I was told that he had started this play about two months earlier when he made his first attempts to move himself forward. Another child, between six and seven months, once noticed while lying in his pram that when he lifted his legs, a toy which he had thrown aside rolled back to him, and he developed this into a game.

Already in the fifth or sixth month many infants respond with pleasure to 'peep-bo'; and I have seen infants playing this actively by pulling the blanket over the head and off again as early as 7 months. I observed an infant with whom the mother made a bedtime ritual of this game, thus leaving the child to go to sleep in a happy mood, which suggests that the repetition of such experiences is an important factor in helping the child to overcome his feelings of loss and grief. Another typical play which I found to be a great help and comfort to young children is to part from the child at bedtime saying 'bye-bye' and waving, leaving the room slowly, as it were disappearing gradually. I was able to observe repeatedly the effect of such experiences on the infant referred to above in daytime as well. Sometimes when the mother was about to leave the room, a fleeting expression of sadness came into the child's eyes, or she seemed near crying. But when the mother waved to her and said 'bye-bye', she appeared comforted and went on with her play activities. I saw her at the age between 10 and 11 months practising again and again the gesture of waving, and it was clear that the practice itself, even before she could actually achieve the gesture, had become a source of interest and comfort to her. 'Bye-bye' was also one of her first words.

The emotional experiences of losing the loved object and regaining it are an essential part of early mental life. The various methods the ego applies at different stages in dealing with feelings of loss are, therefore, criteria by which we could measure the development of the ego. Hallucination, which primarily serves wish fulfilment, is bound up with a sense of omnipotence and is either the basis of phantasy life or already part of it.

The bridge between the infant's sense of omnipotence and his adjustment to reality is the mother's breast which sometimes returns apparently at his wish, and thus confirms his belief in omnipotence. At other times, frustration forces him to submit this feeling, and his associated phantasies, to the testing of reality and thus weakens his sense of omnipotence. When an infant is able to feel that his mother will return, because his experiences of regaining the loved object have proved this to him, he has already make fundamental steps in the progressive testing of external reality, and thus in the growth of the ego; he is also beginning to overcome his depressive position. But while this adaptation to reality goes on, the infant has not by any means yet overcome his feeling of omnipotence and his belief in the magic gesture. In fact, to some extent, the actual experience of the loved person's return, while helping the infant to test reality, also substantiates his feelings of omnipotence. But the very fact that repeated experiences of frustration force the infant to subject this belief to the testing of external reality leads to its progressive devaluation.

In normal circumstances the infant's growing capacity to perceive the external world and to understand it increases his confidence in it, and his experience of the external reality becomes the most important means of overcoming his phantastic fears and his depressive feelings. For instance, the infant whose mother had introduced the 'peep-bo' game, and a little later the waving and saying 'bye-bye' at bedtime, showed a further important step in her methods of dealing with her feelings of loss and depression at 11 months. She thoroughly enjoyed crawling up and down a passage for hours on end and was quite contented by herself, but from time to time she crawled into the room where her mother was (the door had been left open) and had a look at her mother or attempted to converse with her, and returned to the passage.

When an infant is able first to sit up and then to stand in his cot, he can look at his mother and father whenever he likes, and this in some sense brings him nearer to them. This is still more the case when he is able to crawl and walk. The great psychological importance for the infant of standing, crawling and walking has been described by a few analytic writers. My point here is that these achievements are the means of regaining his lost objects as well as finding new objects in their stead, and thus help the infant to overcome the depressive position. To put it from another angle, the ego's striving to overcome the depressive position furthers intellectual interests and activities of all kinds.

To return to the infant who with his first attempts to move forward took to throwing a toy away from himself and tried to get it back without help. We can draw the inference that the meaning of this absorbing game, when he was able to crawl as well as at the earlier stage, was to regain his lost objects by his own efforts. It is interesting to watch the progress in the sense of reality as expressed in the stages of this play. At first, the infant threw the toy out of the pram and omnipotently expected it to come back. A little later he expected his mother to bring it back to him. This already implied great progress in his relation to reality. When he attempted to fetch the toy by moving towards it, he had achieved a greater power to test reality and actively influence, modify and control it. At the same time, since he was able to move towards his loved object (for which the toy stood) his hope to regain and secure it had increased. Thus he could gain greater reassurance as well as pleasure and a satisfaction of his interests. This is also an instance of the way in which the ego's struggle to overcome the depressive position gives added impetus to mental as well as physical development, for there is little doubt that the infant's desire to crawl was stimulated by his interest in this particular game. In the same way speech development, beginning with the imitation of sounds, is one of those great achievements which bring the child (physically and mentally) nearer to the people he loves and also enables him to find new objects. In all these achievements the infant's attempts to modify and control his objects – his internal and external world – play an important part. The co-ordination of functions and of movements is bound up with a defence mechanism which I take to be one of the fundamental processes in early development, namely the manic defence. This defence is closely linked with the depressive position and implies a control over the internal world. There is a constant interplay between the testing of external reality and the attempts to modify it, control it and come to terms with it on the one hand, and the relation to the inner world on the other. These two orientations, inwards and outwards, are gradually brought into harmony with each other; and the extent to which this is achieved is a measure of normal development.

Every step in ego development which enables the child to communicate with, perceive and understand the external world, helps him to gain greater security about his external objects. This again assists him in overcoming his fear of losing his good internal objects. If a satisfactory balance between these interacting processes is achieved, the child is well on the way to overcome his depressive feelings.

5

AUTOBIOGRAPHY AND REFLECTIONS

Melanie Klein (edited by Jane Milton)

Introduction

In this chapter two pieces of recently discovered material show Klein writing about herself and her work. The first item, a letter of 1955 from Klein to her friend and colleague Elliott Jaques, is a recent find which is not yet part of the Wellcome library archive. In this letter Klein expresses satisfaction about her work's reception at the recent Congress of the International Psychoanalytical Association in Geneva. She expresses hope mixed with caution about her scientific legacy.

The second is an autobiography from 1959 which has hitherto appeared in print only in an earlier and fragmented form. This fuller version, found in the archive of Klein's colleague Roger Money-Kyrle, had been considered but not included in Klein's *Writings* of 1975. Here, four years after the letter, Klein sounds altogether more confident about the survival of her work.

The letter to Elliot Jaques

This letter was found amongst some papers left with the Melanie Klein Trust administrator, Mary Block, and had probably been given by its recipient, Elliott Jaques, after Klein's death. It is not yet part of the Melanie Klein Archives at the Wellcome Library. Dated 7 August 1955, it is written on hotel headed notepaper, but the letter itself is handwritten by Klein.

Hotel Mont-Fleuri sur Territet-Montreux

RESTAURANT

Altitude 600 metres Telephone (021) 6 28 87 Funiculaire: Territet C.F.F.-Mt Fleuri

7th Aug. 1955

Dear Elliott,

Your letter and my p.c. crossed. So you know that I am well, enjoying my holidays and very pleased to have made such a good choice. I am very glad to know that the 'chateau Jacques' was no disappointment and that you are having a really good time and rest. The weather seems on our side, it is very pleasant here and so I hope it will remain kind to you too. I have as much company here as I want but apart from *very* stimulating conversations with a diplomate [sic], a Dr Joran, the minister for Israel at The Hague I have no particular wish for company. First I felt not to conform either with the definition 'to sit and think' or just to sit because I felt something in between – namely dreamy. – (Sorry to say that in contrast to Hazel's school report that when she is not dreamy 'she is vigorous in gym', – I am not particularly vigorous physically when not dreaming but rather focussing my mind on certain points; – perhaps vigorous mentally?) This brings me to one part of your letter about which I have been thinking a great deal. Yes, I have a solid feeling of enjoyment about the Congress, it was one of the most, or rather the most gratifying I have ever been to and I am still *very pleased* with the result. But even during the Congress and while I enjoyed the success for our group and became more hopeful about this work getting established I had some sceptical thoughts. You have seen me thoroughly enjoy also the personal tributes paid to me and this pleasure was quite genuine and yet–! When once during reading my paper I looked up and saw the faces of my friends lit up with pleasure and pride and felt that they not only like me personally but can be relied on to carry on this work – that meant much more to me than the oration which preceded my paper and followed it. I do not underrate the importance of more and more people getting interested in this work and this having shown *gradually* from 1949, – the Zürich Congress, – onwards but the future of this work and of Psychoanalysis as we understand it lies with the number of people who have penetrated enough deeply into it to *preserve* and to *hand it on* to others also in a deep and stable way. I have often told you and some of my other friends that I believe that psychoanalysts who really are steeped in the nature of the depths of the mind are bound to be forever a minority – but that would not matter if there are enough of them and if they can be relied on to carry on this work and to *continue* it. Much of the success which we saw, or at least a large part of it, is of a superficial nature, even the impression I made as a person had a share in it; – very useful indeed and as I said, I *did* enjoy it – but that in itself does not yet prove that the work is accepted or how deeply it has penetrated. It depends principally on how many people one can train and train *well*. – I am quite willing and I think able (for I feel stronger than I have felt for years!) to participate 'vigorously' in the fight ahead but this fight, which is *unending* is bound to be left to those who remain and come after me and whether it will be won or lost influences not only psychoanalysis but extends to many [word illegible] in human life. What a responsibility! – *Too great* I often felt for what I think in many ways is an ordinary and simple person but I don't feel alone any more in carrying it out. In Zürich, Amsterdam, less already in London – I had a strong feeling of loneliness in spite of success. But this time – and this is the most beautiful part of the gratification at this Congress – I don't feel alone any more and that is why looking at a few of my friends while reading my paper I had the feeling I described above. Only a handful – but very important. For many years, in spite of the support for which I am still *grateful*, – I felt at bottom to be in a minority of one. I only know it now fully that I *did* feel in a minority of one, – now no longer so. Lowenstein's remark in itself is unimportant but his, Hartmann's and Kris' attitude bars as I heard again and again the teaching of my work at the New York Society. This may and possibly will break down in time but it cannot be disregarded. – I received many sidelights on this as well as on the situation in our Society from Jones. They had lunch with me and stayed for hours and I was glad that the estrangement which I had felt for some time had given way to a much warmer personal relation for I like them and am grateful to him (he too has many reasons to be grateful to me though he does not realise this). But from a few remarks made I could gather a lot – I am still thought of internationally and in our Society as a dangerous person. No doubt certain emotions (cf Klein at Study of envy – etc.) play a great role and also the fact that he does not any more understand my work. By the way it is out of question that Freud's antagonism towards my contributions won't be mentioned in the 3rd volume of the Biography since Jones is going to make a good deal of various points on which Freud and he disagreed among others Freud's anger about the Symposium on Child Analysis (1927) and though Jones did not even remember that I already participated in it, – it is obvious that Freud's complaints how badly Anna has been treated by the Brit.Soc. will involve me and my work. I am not particularly anxious about this, – perhaps because it is going to show how partial Freud was towards his daughter. – tetogether [sic – should this be 'they together'?] don't believe that I am not fully aware of the success we had. In fact I am greatly looking forward to my work – first the full version of my Envy paper – the book about the child – but all the time I feel the paper on the Revision of Mental Structure calling within me to be done – perhaps in spite of everything for the next Congress! In the meantime I am lazy – but feel things growing internally. Best wishes, Yours Melanie Klein.

The autobiographical notes

These autobiographical notes were discovered by Robert Hinshelwood in the archives of Roger Money-Kyrle at the Wellcome Library and date from the end of 1959, the year before Klein died. Earlier fragmentary parts of the autobiography may be found in the Melanie Klein Archives in the Wellcome Library in file GBB/KLE/A.52. These were annotated and published by Janet Sayers and John Forrester (Sayers & Forrester, 2013). The authors were at the time unaware of the existence of this more complete version, which, following its discovery, was published on the Melanie Klein Trust website. The content of the 'Fragments' is similar to the present compiled version, though in the process of compilation Klein added some more details.

Hinshelwood's research showed that this fuller version was sent by Betty Joseph to Roger Money-Kyrle, who in 1962 was in charge of editing a complete edition of Melanie Klein's writing. This was eventually published in 1975 in four volumes as *The Writings of Melanie Klein*. A letter to Money-Kyrle from Betty Joseph in 1962 suggests that the 'Autobiography' might be included in *The Writings*. It appears in the 'wrong' archive because Joseph had clearly taken it from Klein's papers it to show to Money-Kyrle. In the event Money-Kyrle did not include the autobiography in Klein's *Writings* but retained the manuscript, along with Betty Joseph's letter, amongst his own papers. They thus came to be part of Money-Kyrle's own archives after his death in 1980 (Wellcome library PP/RMK/E.6/3:Box 11).

The autobiography covers 30 pages of foolscap typescript. It has been very slightly edited here for clarity.

Autobiography – Melanie Klein 1959

My father came from a very orthodox Jewish family and was what was called in Yiddish a 'vocher'. His father had been a business man, but, probably because the scientific capacity of my father was recognised, he was destined to be a Jewish scientist. He was married, according to the orthodox rites, to a girl whom he had never seen and only met on the occasion of the marriage. That marriage did not last long and was dissolved. I think at the time he was about 37. He had woken up to other interests and had revolted against his way of life. He had hidden under his Talmud books which gave him the possibility of matriculating. He went out one day without the knowledge of his parents and gained his matriculation at a gymnasium, as these schools were called. When he returned, his parents, particularly his mother, were horrified. He then declared that he was going to study medicine and I know from him that when he went in for his first examination, his mother was praying at home that he would fail. However, he passed and after some years he became a doctor. By that time he had completely broken with the whole orthodox attitude and had become independent of his family, though he never quite broke with them.

Cholera was raging at that time in the village of Poland and there were appeals for doctors to treat people. He answered the appeal, informed his family and, when he returned after several weeks or months, he found a letter from his mother imploring him not to go. In contrast to other doctors, who stood outside the cottage windows telling the villagers to take their pulses, he went inside, treated the people in the ordinary way and did not fall ill.

He met my mother, who came from Deutsch-Kreutz, on a visit to Vienna, where she was staying with people who had a boarding house. He at once fell deeply in love with my mother, who was twenty-five and an extremely beautiful girl. At that time he must have been about forty-four or forty-five. They married and for some time he practised as a physician in Deutsch-Kreutz, and then they decided to go to Vienna for my father to practise there. They moved to Vienna, but he could not make a living from his practice, and my mother therefore decided to have a shop, even though this was considered incorrect for the wife of a doctor. Here she sold plants, reptiles, etc. I know that she had a deep dislike of these creatures and that it was only through will-power that she could have anything to do with them. As I have said, she was very beautiful and some of her customers thoroughly enjoyed coming in and having conversations with her. One of my early memories is of going to the shop and I remember where it was in Vienna.

Then something happened. My father's father had been living, since his wife's death, with a daughter, who one day put him out onto the street. My mother at once agreed to take him in, and he lived with us until he died, apparently quite peacefully. When he died, he left them a few savings and a sweepstake ticket, which was quite a usual thing in the Austro-Hungarian Empire. As it happened, they won 10,000 florins and everything changed. My father bought the practice of a dentist and we moved into a flat, and I remember that I thought the change was very impressive.

Now I want to speak of my mother's family. I have already said that she was very beautiful. She had very black hair, a fair complexion, nice features and the most expressive and beautiful grey eyes. She was educated, witty and interesting. I have always been proud of the way in which she acquired her education. Her father was a rabbi in Deutsch-Kreutz. His father (my grandfather) was a very outstanding man: he was known all over the district for his knowledge and tolerance, being very liberally minded, quite different from the orthodoxy that characterised my father's family. He had all the German philosophers on his shelves, unlike the attitude of the bigoted rabbis.

There were three daughters, two of whom were beautiful, and they acquired their education by teaching themselves, by reading and I think probably also by discussions with their father. My mother even managed to learn the piano by herself. Of course she never played very well, but there was a burning need for knowledge in that whole setting. She also learned French. Many years later, when we lived in the country which is now a suburb of Vienna, she was taking the waters and I remember her walking up and down a large veranda with a little book in her hand which contained idiomatic French expressions.

As far as my mother's mother is concerned, I only knew her photograph which shows a lovely friendly old lady, and I know that I longed for her to be living, because I never had a grandmother, and I know that this was a nice, depraved, they are very much depraved. There is a connection with one of my earliest memories at this time, when he still left in the evening, and our maid, whose name I still remember, gave him his supper before he went. In the same way that he was faithful to my mother to such a degree that he would look at no other woman, so too was he conservative about food.

I remember very well the little rissoles which were what he had every night. The reason why the maid gave my father his supper was that my mother was not back from the shop. I cannot have been more than three when I have my first memory connected with my father having his dinner before leaving to go to the Orpheus. He was probably in a hurry. I remember that I climbed up on his knee and he pushed me away. That is a painful memory. Later, and this is a pleasant memory, when we went, from May to September, to Dorsbach on the Hensberg, which at that time was still countrified, though by now it is part of Vienna, he used to hold my hand walking up the hill on which we lived. My father was so set in his habits that he would never go to a restaurant by himself. He would always come home for what was then called a dinner and go back to his work afterwards, though it was quite a distance from his working place, and I fetched him coming home from school and we went up together. I also remember overhearing him, when I was just over thirteen, say to somebody that his youngest daughter would go to the gymnasium, and this definitely made me decide to go there, so I already had at that time some wish to study.

I was the youngest and he was already in his fifties when I was born. He was an old fifty. I have no memories of his ever playing with me. It was a painful thought to me that my father could openly state, and without consideration of my feelings, that he preferred my older sister, his first-born. On the other hand, I was very much loved in the family and very spoilt, in that I was given so much attention. My remarks were quoted and there is little doubt that I was thought to be good-looking and that the family were proud of me.

In some ways, until the relation with my brother and me developed into a deeper one, I did not feel I was completely understood, but at this time no one really thought that any special understanding of a child was necessary. But I think of my childhood as one of a good family life and I would give anything for one day of having it back again; the three of us, my brother, my sister and myself sitting round the table and doing our school work, and the many details of united family life.

I was the youngest of four children, the eldest, Emily, being six years older, my brother, Emmanuel, five years older, and the third, Sidonie, about four years older. I have no doubt, and this was told to me by my mother later on, that I was unexpected. I have no particular feeling that I resented this, because, as I have stated, there was a great deal of love towards me. My mother had no particular pedagogic principles, and no strict rules were kept. I do not remember ever having been punished, except on one occasion when I really provoked my father in a very cheeky way. He had suggested, when I did not want to eat something, that in his day children were made to eat it, and I replied that what was done some hundred years ago did not count today, which I knew would annoy him. He came over from his place and hit me on the shoulder. That is the only occasion on which I was smacked.

My mother had breastfed the three elder children, but I had a wet nurse, who fed me any time I asked for it. At this time Truby King had not yet done his devastating work. My mother's brother, Hermann, lived with us for some years whilst studying law. I was very fond of him and he, too, spoilt me very much. I heard him say many things, among them that, being so beautiful, a young Rothschild would have to come to marry me. He also had a lovely big dog, on which I rode.

I don't think I sufficiently understood my father, whose interest in me was not so great, because he had aged so much by this time. I admired certain things, such as his having done the whole of his medical studies by being a tutor, and having accumulated a large library and, what is more, learnt by himself ten languages, including Hebrew, in which he was a scientist. I know that he spoke Italian very well, because this was confirmed by an Italian who had a conversation with him, and that I could ask him for French and English expressions without bothering with a dictionary. His French was rather quaint and a little outdated, having fed on Moliere, Racine and the older poets. He also had had the opportunity of learning French from a veteran of the Napoleonic wars. I was told that it was rather classic French, but I admired his capacity to learn all this by himself. Actually he was a perfect scientist with very little capacity for practical life. Looking back, I understand him much better than I did at the time. He died when I was eighteen, and by that time had for years been somewhat senile.

I think that I had an attachment for my eldest sister in early childhood and that she was very fond and proud of me. I remember that, between ten and twelve, I felt unhappy before going to sleep and Emilie was kind enough to move her couch near to mine and I went to sleep holding her hand. Later on, when I developed intellectually, I found that we had little in common, and that remained throughout life.

Of my other sister, Sidonie, I have very pleasant and painful memories. I only remember her on her return from hospital, where she had been for scrofula. She was, I have no doubt, the best looking of all of us: I don't believe it was just idealization when, after her death, my mother maintained that. I remember her violet-blue eyes, her black curls and her angelic face. What I remember of her is her lying in bed, after her return from hospital, and her goodness towards me. At this time, and I must have been between four and five, the older ones had a knack of teasing me. They spoke amongst themselves of geographical things in a joking way, talking of Popocatepetl and other names, and I was entirely uncertain whether these were genuine or not. Sidonie, lying in bed, took pity on me, and she taught me the principles of counting and of reading, which I picked up very quickly. It is quite possible that I idealize her a little, but my feeling is that, had she lived, we would have been the greatest friends and I still have a feeling of gratitude to her for satisfying my mental needs, all the greater because I think she was very ill at the time. She died, aged about eight and a half, when I was about four and a half, and I have a feeling that I never entirely got over the feeling of grief for her death. I also suffered under the grief my mother showed, whereas my father was more controlled. I remember that I felt that my mother needed me all the more now that Sidonie had gone, and it is probable that some of the spoiling was due to my having to replace that child. It still fills me with grief that at that time we had no cure for TB, when now-a-days an entirely new treatment would have kept her alive, and I always feel that it was unnecessary that she did not live her life. My knowledge of myself told me that the very good relations with women and the capacity for friendship, which was always very pronounced in me, were based on my relation with this sister.

I have mentioned my relation to my brother, who seemed to me superior in every way to myself, not only because, at nine or ten years of age, he seemed quite grown up, but also because his gifts were so unusual that I feel that whatever I have achieved is nothing in comparison to what he would have done. From a very early age I heard the most beautiful piano-playing, because he was deeply musical, and I have seen him sitting at the piano and just composing what came into his mind. He was a self-willed and rebellious child and, I think, not sufficiently understood. He seemed at loggerheads with his teachers at the gymnasium, or contemptuous of them, and there were many controversial talks with my father. One of the always recurring topics was that my brother maintained that there was nothing in Schiller and that Goethe was everything that counted when my father grew very angry and quoted whole passages out of Schiller's work, which he admired. I remember him saying, in his anger, that Goethe was a charlatan, who tried to dabble in science.

My brother was deeply fond of my mother, but gave her a good deal of anxiety. The relation with my brother was, I think, a most important factor in my development. I date my deep friendship with him definitely from my ninth year onwards, when I had written a patriotic poem, and he took care about correcting it and seemed to appreciate it. From at least this time onwards, he was my confident, my friend and my teacher. He took the greatest interest in my development, and I know that, until his death, he always expected me to do something great, although there was nothing on which to base it. I remember that I wrote a little dramatic play when I was sixteen, and he even said that that was the beginning of something permanent, but it did not turn out that my capacity for writing, which was expressed in the beginnings of various novels and some poems (all of which I have destroyed) would ever have been to my satisfaction and probably not any good.

I deeply admired my brother, who had a genius as a writer and as a musician, and who often dictated to me what he was writing. I always thought that he had very much more creative capacity than I had, though he did not seem to think so. Later on, after his death, when I was twenty, I collected his writings together, with a great friend of his and mine, Irma Schonfeld, and managed to publish them. By then I was married and expecting my first child, and I travelled quite a distance to meet Georg Brandes, the literary historian, whom my brother had admired, to get a preface from him for this book, since he had refused by letter. Actually he had already left the house from which he had replied to me that he was too old and too tired to give any more prefaces or read any more books, but the friends with whom he had been staying, whose name I cannot remember, a woman writer and her sculptor daughter, seem to have been so impressed with me that their letter to Brandes produced the preface. Actually he used nearly all I had written about my brother in this preface. When, after a long struggle, I managed to get a publisher, and a good publisher, for him, it was a great grief to me that he went bankrupt soon after and the book was nearly lost. This book does not really give any idea of what my brother might have achieved, because we used every scrap in his notebooks, some of it quite immature, to put the book together, and it is a feeble picture of what might have come, although there are some beautiful things in it.

The illness of my brother and his early death is another of the griefs in my life, which always remain alive to me. I have said that he was a rather wilful child, though he could be extremely kind and was very fond of my mother and me. He had had scarlet fever when he was, I think, twelve years of age, and that was followed by rheumatic fever. I always heard from my mother with self-reproach, that, because all the family were going out to the Prater, he also would go, and this was supposed to have caused a relapse and occasioned the first fever. I do not know if this was so, but I have always felt that the family should not have gone and forced him to go with them. That rheumatic fever affected his heart and he had what was then known as double heart failure. It was always understood, and he knew it very well, that he could not live longer than some time in his twenties. This knowledge, of which he never spoke, must have had a great deal to do with his being rebellious and at times difficult. I have a beautiful letter from him, also one of the few things I have kept, in which he says that he hopes that what Fate will give me in years what it has deprived him of in days.

He studied medicine, but one of the reasons why he stopped his studies and got permission to do some travelling was that he felt that he wanted to use his gifts as a writer as much as possible. I know another factor which might have driven him away from home, but I will speak of that later on. He died in Genoa, on his way to take a ship to Spain. A postcard was found on his table, addressed to my fiancé, and he was notified of his death. He travelled to Genoa to fetch his luggage, which had already been deposited by my brother for shipping, and no receipt was found to show which it was. The luggage had been described to my fiancé, who was looking through an enormous hall full of baggage for it, when he saw a periodical protruding from a case. It was a number of *Fackel*, by Krauss, of whom my brother thought well. He then claimed this lot of luggage and was given it, and it contained manuscripts which I want to put together into a book. He was twenty-five when he died. Here again I have the feeling that had one known more about medicine, one might have been able to do something and keep him alive longer, but I have been told that even now rheumatic heart diseases are not always curable. I don't know whether this is true or not, but it left me with the same feeling that I had about my little sister, that many things could have been done to prevent his illness and early death. Writing now at the age of seventy-seven, and he was five years older than myself, I cannot imagine him as a man of eighty-two. In my memory he remains a young, strong-minded man, as I knew him, strong in his opinions, not minding if they were unpopular, with a deep understanding of art and a passion for it in many ways, and the best friend I ever had. My oldest son, Hans, who died at the age of twenty-seven when mountaineering, had, particularly in his early years; quite a resemblance to my brother, as I think has also Eric. I think also that my grandson, Michael, has something of his appearance, but I may be wrong, because all these figure had so much in common in my feelings.

The relation to my father was complex, partly because he took, so I felt, relatively little interest in me and so often professed that my older sister was his favourite. In addition, not only was my father old for his age, but I think that in his sixties he must have had a stroke and he became rapidly senile. He certainly was so when I was twelve or thirteen years of age.

My relation to my mother has been one of the great standbys in my life. I loved her deeply, admired her beauty, her intellect, her deep wish for knowledge, no doubt with some of the envy which exists in every daughter. Up to the present day, I still think a great deal about her, wondering what she would have said or thought, and particularly regretting that she was not able to see some of my achievements. I wonder often what she would have thought about these. Although she was extremely ambitious for me when I was a young child, when she grew older and things became more difficult – my father had largely become senile and my brother's illness had got worse, and she had really to keep the family going – I often heard her say that she didn't care for any greatness, she would wish him to be healthy, even if he had been a wine merchant or something like that. I am convinced she felt similarly about me, and that her great wish was for me to be happy, and yet I have a feeling that she would have been proud had she been able to realise what I have actually done.

Again, it is difficult for me to picture that by now she would have been 110 years old, because I still see her as she was before she died. She died in my house, having lost, through circumstances, everything to my sister, whose husband had taken over the practice my father had before. She died when the 1914–18 war had begun and was very much concerned because my brother-in-law had by then been taken prisoner by the Russians, or rather, when the Premsyl fortress was being beleaguered by the Russians. My husband and others told her that this fortress was practically impregnable to take, but I wonder whether she believed them. She had at this time grown very thin and she was X-rayed and examined at the clinic in Budapest, where we then lived. She complained that the room where she was examined was icy cold, though it was late autumn, and she felt that the bronchitis which followed on that examination was due to the room being so cold. At that time one of the assistants at the clinic where she was examined told me that the X-ray did not show anything about cancer and he suggested that she should, in a few months, be examined again. I have since come to the conclusion that she must have had cancer, which caused her loss of weight.

I remember still how we walked up the hill in Bade, where we had a very nice flat. She was a little in front with my husband, and I was behind. I could hardly keep back my tears and was full of grief. Of course I felt, as one would, that I might have looked after her better, though living in the house with her grandchildren was obviously the best thing for her. Eric was four months old when she died and she enjoyed the baby, but ever since my brother had died, and that was much more distinct than after the death of her husband, she had to a large extent lost interest in life. This did not show in an unpleasant way: she still remained interested in everything concerning me and other people, she still took an interest in my clothes and in my books, but, looking back, I know that she withdrew more and more her interest in life as far as she herself was concerned. I never imagined anyone could die the way she did, completely in possession of her faculties, calm without any anxiety, and obviously not at all afraid or reluctant to die. I nursed her for some of the time, but we had a nurse for the last week. She was ill for about three weeks. The only thing in which I saw something of her anxieties having come up was that she told me that the nurse was strict. When she saw me so deeply grieved about the approach of her death, she said 'If it means so much to you, make a gruel and I will eat it,' because by that time she took hardly any food. Being an excellent cook, she told me how to make a chicken broth and forced herself to take it. It was quite obvious that she attempted to go on living for my sake. Even then she had not lost interest in me and my activities, my children, my home. I had a wet nurse for Eric, due to circumstances which I might mention later, who behaved very badly and terrorised the whole house. When I told her about this, she suggested that I should put up with everything and have the child fed only about nine or ten months, and I followed her advice. I remember that, with a certain feeling of guilt that I might have done more for her, and we know that such feelings exist. I knelt down by her bed and asked her forgiveness. She replied that I should have at least as much to forgive her as she to forgive me. Then she said 'Don't grieve, don't mourn, but remember me with love.' I have since seen my sister die, full of anxieties and feelings of persecution, and heard of other people die, where anxiety was very prominent; I did not imagine that one could die in such a serene way, completely without anxiety and regret, no accusation against anyone, and friendliness towards my sister, though there she did actually have cause for complaint. But I never heard her complain about my sister in the preceding years and everything she had left from the pocket money my husband gave her she sent to my sister, who needed it. She has in many ways remained my example and I remember the tolerance she had towards people and how she did not like it when my brother and I, being intellectual and therefore arrogant, criticised people. She would not agree with us. She had never had any particular feeling that she was in fact an outstanding woman; she was modest and when the question arose about something concerning the maid, she used to say 'Well, I would not like to do that, why should she?' Of course, at that time, maids did not have the same treatment as they have now, but, in the best sense of the word, I think my mother was a socialist. As far as her means went, she really tried to make a relation with the maids, and we had one for many years, who was on equal terms. Sometimes she was taken advantage of, but she did not seem to mind that.

I am not sure of the relation between my parents. It was a very united family life. My father even travelled from the Martinstrasse where we lived and he walked to Dorsbach for his lunch. It would never have occurred to him to go out alone or even to go to a restaurant. My mother was extremely dutiful, both as a wife and as a mother and everything was done for the education of the children. I do not remember any occasion when my parents went out by themselves. However, whereas my father was deeply in love with my mother, until his death, and extremely jealous, which was quite noticeable, I am not sure whether my mother was in love with him; in fact I do not believe she was. She looked after him, she was good with him, but occasionally I saw signs of dissatisfaction in her. In my phantasy, or was it perception, she had been in love with that student in her little home town, to whom I have referred earlier, who died of TB. Of course, in those days marriages were not simply ended as is the case today. She had respect for my father and appreciated his qualities, and it seemed a good thing to accept his proposal. Sometimes I thought that perhaps she was glad, but I have never been able to get to the bottom of this, whether she was simply not passionate or not passionate as far as my father was concerned, but I do believe that occasionally I saw a slight aversion against sexual passion in her, which might have been the expression of her own feeling and upbringing etc.

I have already referred to the change in circumstances, which was extremely important to my feelings. I have no memory of the place where we lived before our fortunes improved, but it seems it was not good. I was very proud when we moved into a very nice flat with a balcony, which I remember very well, when I was about five years old. There is something of which I am not sure. I don't know whether my sister died before we moved, but I believe she died in the flat. I remember that I was extremely happy about the jewellery, silver and canteen which my mother received and about the flat being so nice, and I also had new clothes. My happiness was very much increased when my parents decided to buy the house where the dentistry practice which my father had bought was carried out. I remember that an old friend of my mother, Mrs Hennier, also mortgaged some money on this house, and it seemed to me an onerous thing that my parents should actually own a house. The pride and happiness that I felt about these changes made it clear to me that I had been worried about the financial difficulties; I would almost say poverty, which preceded the moves.

I had begun to go to school from the flat in the Alserstrasse and was very happy there. I never was shy; I liked the company of children, which I had not had until then, as at this time one did not go to kindergarten. I gave no trouble at school and also liked acquiring knowledge, and soon became a very ambitious pupil, paying great attention to the marks I received and to the one thing which at this time expressed the teacher's satisfaction, the words 'worde belobt'. No detailed reports were given, only marks, and, in the case of a very good pupil, these particular words. I remember the first day at school, when the teacher, dealing with a number of timid and anxious children, asked them their name in the following way. When she asked 'Who is called Marie?' the little girls called Marie had to put up their hands and say 'My name is Marie.' I waited anxiously for my turn to come, though a number of children were under the benches, being so anxious, and had to be dragged out, to tell their names. My name, being a little unusual, did not come, and being unable to wait any longer, when the teacher said 'Who is called Marie?,' I put up my hand; when she said 'Now say nicely "My name is Marie",' I said 'My name is Melanie.' She looked at me little reproachfully and said 'Your turn hasn't come yet' and I felt rather ashamed, though actually there was no other Melanie and my turn would not have come.

It was at this time that I had French governesses. The first one was Mlle. Chapuis. My parents engaged her through some agency from a convent, and I know that she was very religious. She was very kind and I have no memory of any unpleasantness about her. But she did not stay long because she got very homesick. She recommended a young girl also from this convent, Mlle. Constance Sylvester. She still had plaits, was nineteen years old and at first was very timid and anxious, but blossomed out very quickly. She was very good with me and took an interest in my thoughts, whereas the other members of the family spoilt and admired me, but were not particularly interested in what went on in my mind. Mlle. Chapuis had taken me repeatedly to church with her and I knelt when she did. I felt extremely guilty about that, because I felt convinced that my parents, being Jewish, would not have agreed to my kneeling in a Catholic church and participating in the services. However, I did not want to give Mlle. Chapuis away, since she was otherwise very kind to me and I liked her and also I had a feeling of attraction to those Catholic services. There must have been, in fact I know there was, some revolt against my Jewish origins and an attraction to something else. Constance did not do that. She soon seemed to lose some of her fervour and became extremely gay. I was her favourite because not only did she understand me, but I thought I understood her better than the others. I know that my brother teased her a lot. My sister Emilie was a bad pupil, and, since she had no trouble with me, my relation with her was quite a close one. I had another secret which I did not tell my mother and which made me feel very guilty, and that was, when she went out with me, according to the Viennese fashion, young men would talk with her and on a few occasions she allowed them to walk with her on the street. I was quite sure my mother would disapprove but my loyalty to Constance would not let me report it. She gave it up herself as a certain point, probably feeling that it was wrong.

This attraction to the Catholic Church, which was stimulated by Mlle. Chapuis, led later on, when I was nine or ten, to some things which tortured me and which I could only confess to Constance. That was the feeling that I would one day become Catholic and how I would hurt my parents. I remember I told her 'I don't want to do it, but I shall have to,' and she replied very understandingly, 'Well, if you have to do it, you can't help it.' This Catholic attraction showed itself at school, where I felt deprived when I saw the Catholic children running to the priest and kissing his hand. I remember that on one occasion I plucked up my courage and also kissed his hand. He patted me on the head in a very friendly manner, but that occasion I did not mention.

I had decided at about fourteen that I would study medicine, but I may have been stimulated by hearing my father say to a patient that I was going to the gymnasium. At that time this was not true, because I was then going to a lyceum (lycee), where I learnt French, English and all the things that a girl of good family was expected to know. At that very moment, I decided that I was going to change over to the gymnasium, and, since it was the middle of the year, my brother taught me Latin and Greek, to keep up with the subjects taught at the Gymnasium. I still remember, with amusement, that, though he was very keen to help me, he was a most impatient teacher. My prep from one day to the next was to learn the four conjugations in Latin, and, when I muddled them, he cried out in anger 'You want to study! You must become a shop assistant.' Still, with preparation, I was able to pass the exam, which consisted mainly of Latin and Greek, and life took on an entirely different aspect for me.

I must have been longing to study, or to do something, without having been aware of it. Now I knew that I was going to study medicine and had even thought of psychiatry. I was extremely happy in that school, where the girls' intelligence was above the average, and where the teachers were much more interesting and interested than at the previous school, and I was looking forward with great happiness to further studies at the University, though at this period the financial situation at home was very stringent, as my father had become more and more senile, and the house was kept going by the indefatigable capacities of my mother. I bore all sorts of deprivations, in comparison with those of my schoolmates, fairly easily. It was on rare occasions that I got a new dress and theatres and concerts were also rare occurrences, but I had a lively and happy connection with my schoolmates and was soon introduced to friends of my brother. It was altogether a very intellectual circle in which I lived and I blossomed out. This was also a time when I read passionately whatever I could get hold of, deep into the night. My mother did not know this, as my room was apart from hers. I know that I did my prep largely in the tram, which was at the time still horse-drawn. I got behind in geometry, which was a subject I did not like, and a friend of my brother undertook to help me. He fell deeply in love with me and at the time I also had opportunities of meeting a few other young men, and, when I was seventeen, I met my future fiancé. At that time there were actually four young men in love with me, all of which I know would have wished to marry me. I was very much impressed by my fiancé, who seemed to me to be intellectually outstanding, and again I am afraid that I was influenced by my brother's opinion, who made friends with him. He was a second cousin and had visited us for that reason, but he fell in love with me and very quickly decided the issue by proposing to marry me.

While being intellectually very forward at this time, well-read and stimulated by a very intellectual circle, and therefore believing myself mature, I was in many ways only a child. At this stage, intellect was what impressed me most. I think I was both flattered and impressed by my future fiancé's proposal, though it was clear we should have some time to wait. He already had his degree as an engineer, but still had his way to make. I accepted his proposal and it did not take very long for me to fall in love with him. From that time I was so loyal that I refrained from any entertainment where I might have met other young men and never expressed a feeling that I already had in my mind, that we were not really suited to one another. Both loyalty to my fiancé, with whom I was up to a point in love, and circumstances prevented me from mentioning this to my mother or my brother. I often wonder whether my brother, with whom I had such a deep and close connection, did not realise that I was doing the wrong thing, and whether he did not unconsciously know that I was going to make myself unhappy. He soon left his medical studies and, with very little money, travelled and could not bear to remain in Vienna any more. Certainly I had not spoken of my doubts either to him or to my mother, so, though they may have thought my fiancé a difficult person, they also knew that I was in love with him, and thought that I did not mind him being difficult. I must allow for the fact that, since my sister's marriage and brother-in-law's taking over the dental practice, the whole financial situation had become worse and it would not have been easy for me to return to my studies, which I was longing to do. Whether or not this was the main factor of my doing something which I knew was wrong – my marriage – I cannot say, but it must have been an important reason.

When I became engaged, my fiancé had finished his studies as a chemical engineer, but had still to have more practice and to make a position for himself, so the marriage was planned for two or three years later. I used this time for attending courses at the Vienna University in art and history, but even then I felt that I was not doing what I actually wanted to do, which was to study medicine. My engagement lasted four years and I was married the day after my twenty-first birthday. My husband had a position in a paper factory, partly owned by his father, in Rusemberck, which at that time was part of Hungary, but with a predominantly Slovak population. After the war it became part of Czecho-Slovakia.

My first child, Melitta, was born ten months later, on the 19th January 1904, and I was very happy with her. She was very attached to me as well as to her nannie, who was a good Slovakian peasant woman. At that time I learnt

Slovakian, and spoke it fluently. Melitta was a beautiful and fairly easy baby and soon showed herself to be very intelligent.

I threw myself as much as I could into motherhood and interest in my child, and my mother, who had more or less lost her home through different circumstances, came to live with us, which was a very great comfort. I know all the time that I was not happy, but saw no way out.

Considering how little I had travelled as a girl, I had two important travels: one when Melitta was one year old, with my husband to Trieste, Abbasia and Venice, and the second more impressive journey in May 1906 to Rome, Naples and Florence, which opened up a new world. I was entirely indefatigable about seeing paintings and sculptures, and these journeys, of which my husband also was very fond, gave me a good deal of happiness. My honeymoon, too, had been an experience along the same lines, because we travelled to Zurich and, on the way, went to Constanza. It was all very new and impressive to me, as I hardly travelled before.

Three years after Melitta's birth, my son Hans was born, on 2nd March 1907. He developed well and I also fed him. He showed in the early stages of his life a precociousness and intellectual ability which was quite outstanding. At eighteen months, he could speak Slovakian (I had spent the first three years in a Slovakian town, where my husband was engineer in a paper factory) and German, which I cultivated in the beginning, in such a way that he could turn from speaking German to me to speaking Slovakian to the nurse without any difficulty.

When Melitta was three years old, six weeks after Hans was born, my husband got a better position as director of several factories in Silesia, and we lived in Krappitz, a small provincial town without any charm, and I felt very unhappy, as I could not find anyone with whom I could even converse. I was very much strengthened by my mother's living with us. This was a great help to me, as the incompatibility between the characters and views of myself and my husband was becoming increasingly obvious. I am glad to say that he liked her and never had an objection to her living with me, since she was a very retiring and quiet person. There was no trouble between him and her.

Then, partly because I felt unhappy there, he accepted a position which centred on Budapest, where he was also the director of several factories, and I found life entirely different. There were relatives of my husband there, to whom I became attached, and altogether life in Budapest, with theatres, parties and pleasant company, was in complete contrast to the three years I had spent in the little Silesian town, which seemed inhabited by narrow-minded people, with whom I had nothing in common.

My third child, Eric, was born a month before the First World War started and, when he was five years old we left Budapest. This war, from the Hungarian point of view, was carried out without any interest. People knew very well that the Austrian Hungarian monarchy was doomed, something I heard long before the war started. There was plenty of food for people who could pay for it, and the idea that was so important in the Second World War in England, that one should not buy things when others could not afford them, did not exist. Civilians were in no danger, the war was happening somewhere else. When the short-lived but very stringent Communist regime started in 1919 at the end of the war, we left Budapest and I went to live for a year in Slovakia with my parents-in-law, with whom I had always been on very good terms, especially my mother-in-law, and my husband found a position in Sweden. Having been by birth an Austrian subject, I had now become a Czecho-Slovakian subject. My husband, having settled in Sweden, soon managed to become a Swedish subject since he was not keen on being Czecho-Slovakian. In this way I became a Swedish subject, which, at a later date, was very useful to me. This was the preliminary of our actually parting from one another, and lasted until 1922, when we were divorced. I took with me my youngest son, who was then only eight, and nominally I also had the right to have my other two children, but that was not practical at the time, as I was still financially dependent on my husband.

While living in Budapest I had become deeply interested in psychoanalysis. I remember that the first book of Freud's that I read was the small book on dreams (not *The Interpretation of Dreams*) and, when I read it, I knew that that was it – that was what I was aiming at, at least during those years when I was so very keen to find what would satisfy me intellectually and emotionally. I entered into analysis with Ferenczi, who was the most outstanding Hungarian analyst. Technique at this time was extremely different from what it is at present and the analysis of negative transference did not enter. I had a very strong positive transference and I feel that one should not underrate the effect of that, though, as we know, it can never do the whole job.

During this analysis with Ferenczi, he drew my attention to my great gift of understanding children and my interest in them, and he very much encouraged my idea of devoting myself to analysis, particularly child analysis. I had, of course, three children of my own, at that time, and, as I said, I had not found that the information that education and understanding could provide the whole understanding of the personality and therefore have the influence one might wish to have. I had always the feeling that behind that was something with which I could not come to grips. There is much that I have to thank Ferenczi for. One thing that he conveyed to me, and strengthened in me, was the conviction in the existence of the unconscious and its importance for mental life. I also enjoyed being in touch with somebody who was a man of unusual gifts. He had a streak of genius. Also he strengthened in me the desire to turn to child analysis and he carried it out in fact by telling to Abraham at the Congress in 1920 in The Hague.

I heard – a memory which is very important to me – Freud at a congress in 1917 between the Austrian and Hungarian societies, and I remember vividly how impressed I was and how the wish to devote myself to psychoanalysis was strengthened by this impression. By 1919 I had already done some psychoanalysis with one child and I read a paper to the Hungarian Psycho-Analytical Society, which aroused great interest (it was the first one in my book *Contributions to*

Psycho-Analysis). It was following this paper that I became a full member of the Hungarian Society. I never had any supervision.

I remember with gratitude Anton von Freund, who was most encouraging and quite convinced that here was a blossoming talent that should be used. I am sorry that he died young – of cancer – I always felt that he would have been friends and he remains one of the good figures in my life. On that occasion he put certain questions to me, which I could not answer at the time, but which in retrospect seem quite relevant to a deep understanding of children, which was then not so pronounced in me.

After I had lived with my parents-in-law, who were most hospitable, for a year, I decided to go to Berlin. By that time, the estrangement between myself and my husband had very much increased. My reason for going to Berlin was that I had met in the autumn of 1920 at the congress at the Hague, already as a member of the Hungarian Society, Abraham, who strongly encouraged me to settle in Berlin and to devote myself to child analysis, and provided me his support, a promise which, like others he made, he fully kept.

So I arrived at the beginning of 1921 in Berlin. My daughter, who had passed her matric[ulation] in the Slovakian town where I had lived with my parents-in-law, joined me and my three children were with me. She went to Berlin University to study medicine, and I began slowly to gain ground in Berlin as a psycho-analyst. A description of how I soon got access to the deeper layers of the mind in children is given in my paper 'Play technique and its history and significance', in *New Directions*. I have often been asked how it was that I tackled the children in the way I did, which was entirely unorthodox and, in many cases, in contrast to the rules laid down for the analysis of adults. I still cannot answer what made me feel that it was anxiety that I should touch and why I proceed in this way, but experience confirmed that I was right and, to some extent, the beginning of my play technique goes back to my first case.

My interest in children's minds goes back a very long way. I remember that, even as a child of eight or nine, I was interested in watching younger children, but all that was still dormant until it became alive in my psycho-analytic work. Or, rather, it had become very much alive in my relations to my own children. Maybe the fact that many ideas about education did not have the effect that I aimed at contributed to my conviction that there was something which lay deeper – the unconscious which has to be tackled if one wants to bring about changes in the difficulties of children. From 1922, when the divorce became effective, my practice in Berlin grew, and I had opportunities of analysing children, also some of my colleagues; and some of the fundamental approach which I used has remained true until today. No doubt much has been added, but this is all shown in my papers and books.

Dr Hug-Hellmuth[1] was doing child analysis at this time in Berlin (later she became the wife of Muller-Braunschweig) but in a very restricted way. She avoided completely interpretations, though she used some play material and drawings, and I could never get an impression of what she was actually doing, nor was she analysing children under six or seven years. I am quite sure that we had very little in common and she was most reluctant to have anything to do with me. I do not think it too conceited to say that I introduced into Berlin the beginnings of child analysis. I was successful in my work and I treated, though his analysis was broken off, a child sent by the school authorities. All this contributed to my practice widening. I believe that, if I had persisted in staying in Berlin and had had the further support of Abraham, child analysis on my own lines would have been stabilised.

So I worked on my own in Berlin and I only remember one important occasion on which I asked Abraham's advice. This was when the anxiety in a child grew in a way which frightened me. Abraham more or less advised me to go on, some quite important changes in the child happened, and it turned out that I had been at a climax and that a few days later the anxiety went down again. This experience has been definite in developing my methods of approach. I knew now that it was anxiety that one had to analyse, and that, if one could find the unconscious reasons for it, with all the implications, one could diminish it. I met Ernest Jones at a congress in Salzburg in 1925, where I gave my first paper on the technique of child analysis, an approach which was entirely new, completely controversial and strongly doubted by many analysts. Ernest Jones was very much impressed by it and I remember that, when I asked whether he would publish a paper of mine in the *International Journal of Psychoanalysis*, he said he would publish a book if I wrote one. This was very encouraging and so was Abraham's impression of the value of my work with children. He was very cautious, the real scientist, who would weigh carefully the pros and cons, uninfluenced by emotion, but who seemed to feel that something here was growing which might be of great importance. It was unforgettable that, when I participated in 1925 in a congress, he said at the end of the paper I read (Erna's history), which later made one chapter in *The Psychoanalysis of Children* [see Klein (1975[1932])] that the future of psycho-analysis rested with child analysis. He had never before expressed his opinion so strongly to me and, since I was really in those first years unaware of the importance of the contribution to psycho-analysis that I was making, his saying so came to me as a surprise. I felt that I was working in the only way one would work with children, though I was of course gratified by results and by some papers which I had already written. I did not evaluate my contributions in the way in which they have since by many people been judged and in which I now myself judge them, considering how much light they have thrown, not only on the child's mind, but on the whole development of the adult, and that they have become the approach by which really ill people can be cured or improved, and that many children who might never have been cured have been made better in this way.

In 1925 Ernest Jones, stimulated by the opinion of Mrs James Strachey,[2] who at that time was in analysis with Abraham in Berlin, and Mrs Riviere, who from the beginning took a great interest in my paper, invited me to give lectures on child analysis in England. By that time I had been able to have analysis with

Abraham, feeling very strongly that what Ferenczi could not do might be done. This was a very important factor in my development. At this time I was still unhappy, feeling my divorce, and both in need of some help and driven by the urge to know more. When I approached Abraham with the request for an analysis, he told me that it had become a principle with him not to analyse anyone remaining in Berlin. He was referring to some very unhappy situations which had resulted from broken-off analyses with colleagues who had become hostile to him. I don't know where I found the courage, but my answer was 'Can you tell me of anyone in Berlin to whom I could look up in such a way that I can go to them for analysis?' He never replied to that question, but he accepted me for analysis. I had to wait a few months and the analysis started at the beginning of 1924 and came to an end when Abraham fell very ill in the summer of 1925 and died at Christmas of that year; a great pain to me and a very painful situation to come through.

To return to Ernest Jones' invitation to give lectures on child analysis, I had neglected to write the paper on my work with children in the form of lectures. I had six weeks to write six lectures, which were at the time translated into English by Mrs Strachey and one or two other people who helped. In 1925 I had the wonderful experience of speaking to an interested and appreciative audience in London – all members were present at Dr Stevens' house[3] because at that time there was not yet an institute where I could give these lectures. Ernest Jones asked me whether I would answer in the discussion. Although I had learnt a lot of English privately and at school, my English was still not good and I remember well that I was half guessing what I was asked, but it seemed that I could satisfy my audience in that way. The three weeks that I spent in London, giving two lectures a week, were one of the happiest times of my life. I found such friendliness, hospitality and interest, and I also had an opportunity of seeing something of England and I developed a great liking for the English. It is true that later on things did not always go on so easily, but those three weeks were very important in my decision to live in England.

In 1926 Ernest Jones invited me to come for a year to England to analyse the children of some colleagues. It was first a question of six children, including Ernest Jones' two. I remember that my Berlin colleagues said that I was absolutely mad to undertake this, as it was sure to lead to catastrophe with my colleagues, but I did not feel this was so. In fact apart from one case where I had some difficulty with the mother, things went quite well. I had already in Berlin started to analyse adults as well, and that I continued in London. After a few months Ernest Jones asked me, and here I think the influence of Mrs Riviere and Mrs Strachey also came in, if I would settle in London. I was quite free to decide about my future and I accepted his suggestion, in particular as, since Abraham's death in 1925 the Berlin society had begun to deteriorate and support for my work had become very questionable. Three months after I had come to England, I was able to take my son, Eric, whom I had left behind with the family of a schoolmaster in Frankfurt, to England. He was then twelve and a half and when he was thirteen and a half, after being tutored privately and at the Hall, he passed his examination into St Paul's, where he finished his schooling. My son, Hans, had chosen to be an engineer and paper-maker, and had become more or less independent from his father. My daughter Melitta had finished her medical studies, but decided to become an analyst, had married and settled with her husband in England in 1932.

When at the beginning of the thirties, there was a possibility for me in the United States I did not even consider it. England had become my adopted motherland. Since the situation in Austria, both from the analytical point of view and from other angles, was not attractive any more (in 1926 appeared Anna Freud's book, which started the everlasting controversy against me, and the Viennese society was extremely hostile to me and my work), there was nothing to attract me to live in Austria. My mother, who had lived with me, died in 1914, at the beginning of the war, and my only bond with Vienna was my sister, who lived there, but this tie was not strong enough to take me back. So more and more I have really accepted England as my country and went through the Second World War with all the feelings of English people at that time. This was very much increased by Hitler having destroyed so many of my friends in various lands, and Germany having become a country I abhorred. In spite of some many difficulties developing in a psycho-analytical society in England from about 1935 onwards, I have never regretted coming to England, working here and founding a school of thought and approach to child and adult analysis, which I do not think will ever be killed by controversial trends. Within the limits of human capacity, I feel that I have done something which perhaps in the future may prove to have been a great contribution to the understanding of the human mind. All that is bound up with my attitude towards England, and I remember with gratitude Ernest Jones standing by me until 1935, when he began, even before the war, increasingly to retire from conflict.

My memory is, as I have so often said, that I was in some ways spoilt and conceited, and I did not feel that I was completely understood. I certainly very much wanted praise and liked to be in the picture. In a sense I was the opposite of being shy and I was rather what one would call in German 'verlaut'. Another feature, which was linked with the desire for praise and admiration, was that I was very ambitious. From the moment that I entered school it was very important to me to get the best possible marks, and that attitude, I remember, I had until I went to the gymnasium. There I had begun to be very interested in the subjects themselves; I had very interesting teachers, very intelligent schoolmates, and I think my ambition had already abated there. When I started psycho-analytical work, I was, I think, still very ambitious; it is contradictory that, at the same time, I had no idea I was really putting forward entirely new contributions to theory and I really felt that that was something that was self-understood. I was not conceited at that time, because I felt that no other conclusions could be drawn in analysing children and in following what Freud had laid down. Nevertheless, for years to come, I still felt very ambitious, and the struggle which I had against my critics – this became very strong after Abraham's death and in particular when Anna Freud's book, which denigrated my work, appeared – referred not only to my work, but also to myself. That is to say, at the beginning of my psycho-analytical work, the old ambition was still there. The further I progressed the less it grew. My own psycho-analysis, which played such a large role in my development, must have contributed to that, because more and more I lost my personal ambition, which probably applies more to the thirties, and concentrated on the interest of producing what I know to be an extremely important contribution to psycho-analysis. This change over from personal ambition to protecting my work must have gone with great changes to myself.

There is no doubt that I had become, from the beginning of my analytical work, dedicated to psycho-analysis, and the feeling that that was the main object to be protected diminished the old interest in personal ambition. The older I got, the less my personal ambition became, and it is true that personal experience contributed to my becoming resigned, and even resigned about the protection of my work, which I took really to be the protection of the development of psycho-analysis. For years I was still working and went to all the Congresses from 1922 onwards, except the one in 1936 in Marienbad, and always did my duty by psycho-analysis, but I became more and more doubtful whether my work would survive and whether the depth to which I was able to take psycho-analysis was something which many people could bear, and whether there were many people who would carry out analysis to such a depth. I became very sceptical as time went on about the survival of my work, but in recent years, with a group of outstanding colleagues, who have the capacity to protect this work and who can and will continue it after my death, I am again hopeful. In all these years up to now, I have actually never shirked my duty to psycho-analysis, even in recent years – I am speaking in November 1959, very near my 78th birthday – I have hardly ever cancelled a session and have attended nearly all meetings, even when I knew that the paper was not worth while, because I felt that in the discussion I might be useful and because I felt that my presence and my voice might have some influence on the younger people, even those who do not belong to this group.

That change from strong personal ambition to the devotion to something which is above my own prestige is characteristic of a great deal of change that went on in the course of my psycho-analytic life and work. When I abruptly finished my analysis with Abraham, there was much which had not been analysed and I have continually proceeded along the lines of knowing more about my deepest anxieties and defences. I have now a mixture of resignation and some hope that my work will perhaps after all survive and is a great help to mankind. There are of course my grandchildren who contribute to this feeling that the work will go on, and when I speak of having been completely dedicated to my work this not exclude my also being completely dedicated to my grandchildren. Even now, when they have become much less close to me, I know that I have been a very important figure in the first few years of their lives and that this must have been of great benefit to them. All three loved me deeply until six or seven years old, and Hazel even up to nine or ten, and I believe that they have kept some affection for me, though unfortunately they are far less in contact with me; except Michael, who has in recent years become much closer to me again and who I know has at least unconsciously, and perhaps partly consciously, the feeling that I am of great value and also that he can speak freely to me.

Notes

1 This is a curious passage, since Hermine Hug-Hellmuth worked in Vienna, the first woman in the Viennese Society; and she was never married to Carl Muller-Braunschweig, remaining unmarried (see Maclean & Rappen, 1991). So far as Hinshelwood can ascertain these are the only inaccuracies in the autobiographical notes. They are rather glaring mistakes, and there may be a reason for it. Hug-Hellmuth was the centre of a couple of serious crises in the psychoanalytic world around 1920. Firstly she forged a supposed diary of a young girl, which confirmed psychoanalytic theories about sexual development, and secondly she was murdered in 1924 by her adopted son whom she had brought up according to psychoanalytic principles. These incidents can be discovered in Maclean and Rappen's book. It is not surprising that such incidents would impact with some disturbing effect on psychoanalysts in general, and on someone such as Melanie Klein especially interested in the impact of psychoanalytic ideas on children. There were in fact several other people in the Berlin Society who were working psychoanalytically with children at the time. One was Ada Schott who did marry Carl Muller-Braunschweig, probably in 1925.

2 See *Bloomsbury/Freud* (Meisel & Kendrick, 1986), which contains the letters between James and Alix when she, Alix, was in Berlin during her analysis with Abraham in 1924–25, and which gives a view of the Berlin Society including Melanie Klein.

3 This refers to Adrian Stephen, though Klein spelled it incorrectly. He was the younger brother of Virginia Woolf (nee Stephen).

References

Klein, M. (1975[1932]). An obsessional neurosis in a six-year-old girl. In *The psycho-analysis of children. Volume 2 of The writings of Melanie Klein*. London: Hogarth.

Maclean, G. and Rappen, U. (1991). *Hermine Hug-Hellmuth: Her life and work*. London: Routledge.

Meisel, P. and Kendrick, W. (1986). *Bloomsbury/Freud: The letters of James and Alix Strachey, 1924–25*. London: Chatto and Windus.

Sayers, J. and Forrester, J. (2013). The autobiography of Melanie Klein. *Psychoanalysis and History, 15*, 127–163.

PART 2

Studies from the Melanie Klein Archives

6

ON MELANIE KLEIN'S CONTEMPORANEOUS REFERENCES TO HITLER AND THE SECOND WORLD WAR IN HER THERAPEUTIC SESSIONS[1]

Claudia Frank

Introduction

It is often assumed that Melanie Klein leaves external reality more or less unconsidered in her works. With reference to some unpublished Klein archive documents from the 1930s and 1940s and held in the Wellcome Library, I show this assessment to be a prejudice. During the Second World War years, Klein did not focus exclusively on the inner world but examined the interplay between the external and internal worlds. In her treatments, particularly in the transference and countertransference, Klein regularly considered the political situation and the 'Hitler in us', as well as indicating how, in politically critical and extreme situations, internal fears and destructive identifications are connected with outside events. By giving detailed quotations from unpublished documents from Klein's estate concerning the Austrian *Anschluss*, the Munich Crisis, and documents from 1940, I largely allow the texts to speak for themselves.

In her paper 'The Oedipus complex in the light of early anxieties', published in English in 1945, Klein mentions her 10-year-old patient Richard's identifications with the 'bombing and dangerous Hitler-father' (Klein, 1945, p. 14). Here Klein is primarily concerned with the representation of aspects of the Oedipus complex that had mainly been revealed by her child analyses. With reference to two case reports, the analysis of Richard and the treatment of the 2¾-year-old Rita (cf. Frank, 1999), she describes the situation with boys and girls. I am citing this publication here from a perspective that Klein herself did not explicitly formulate either in this or in other publications, namely the way in which the contemporaneous historical circumstances, especially the international situation conditioned by Hitler and National Socialism, emerge in analyses and how she dealt with them. I would therefore like to quote in more detail a passage from this paper that makes some of this clear. We know today that Richard's three-month analysis was conducted in 1941 (May to August) in Pitlochry (Scotland), where Klein was living at that time. The analysis was interrupted for a few days because she went to London, with Richard's knowledge.

> Richard's attempts to restrain his hatred and aggressiveness and to deny his grievances were not successful. The repressed anger about frustrations in the past and present came out clearly in the transference situation – for instance, in his response to the frustration imposed on him by the interruption of the analysis. We know that by going to London I had become in his mind an injured object. I was not, however, injured only through being exposed to the danger of bombs, but also because by frustrating him I had aroused his hatred; in consequence he felt unconsciously that he had attacked me. In repetition of earlier situations of frustration, he had become – in his phantasied attacks on me – identified with the bombing and dangerous Hitler-father, and he feared retaliation. I therefore turned into a hostile and revengeful figure.
>
> *(Klein, 1945, p. 14)*

It is worth noting here that the Klein archive relating to Richard also includes some correspondence between Klein and Richard's mother from 1941 to 1942, which demonstrates Klein's interest in Richard's further development. These letters are moving to read and I think they convey among other things how 'digestibly' Klein perceived even destructive phantasies. She writes, for example, on one occasion that the mother should not take her son's remark that he wants to be a dictator so seriously, that it is nothing unusual for children in a period in which fears of dictators were proliferating in such a way to try to play the dictator themselves. She continues:

> I can only say one thing: as long as you maintain your belief in him, in his gifts and good qualities, which are present alongside the obvious flaws, this will be a great support to him and as I know has been until now the greatest support.
>
> *(letter of 24 October 1941)*

This accommodating way of being able to look directly at destructiveness, which many describe in her, may be better conveyed by this letter than by her notes from memory, in which she mostly describes her own interpretations in a highly condensed form. This correspondence, from archive file B.41, is not available digitally at present, as for confidentiality reasons access is restricted until 2043.

Twenty years after this short analysis of Richard, Klein published her detailed notes made from memory (along with some observations) in *Narrative of a Child Analysis* (Klein, 1961). This book vividly portrays how Richard is immediately concerned with Hitler in the opening sequence of the first session, the role

Hitler constantly plays in this analysis and how Klein variously names her patient's identifications with a bombing and dangerous Hitler and also interprets them when she herself is identified with Hitler. (When I emphasize this aspect of the analysis here, it may give the impression – and reinforce the preconception – that Klein was only concerned with this aspect of destructiveness. The book itself, as well as Meltzer's (1978) paper, 'Richard week-by-week', which elaborates various aspects of the psychoanalytic process, nevertheless conveys an essentially more multi-faceted picture, which is why it is referenced.)

It was several decades before any reference could be made to a 'Hitler in us' in psychoanalyses in the Federal Republic of Germany. For instance, Anita Eckstaedt tells us in the introduction to her book *Nationalsozialismus in der 'zweiten Generation'*, published in 1989, that she was deeply horrified in 1980 when Judith S. Kestenberg, with whom she was discussing one of her cases, used the interpretation 'That is the Hitler in your patient' (Eckstaedt, 1989, p. 13f.). It was only decades after Hitler's systematic destruction of the European Jews and all the National Socialist crimes, that destructive identifications of this kind were gradually being perceived, interpreted and worked through in the analytic situation. This was meanwhile being documented in various ways. For the most important literature on this subject, the reader is referred to Ludger Hermanns' impressive overview (2001) of the German Psychoanalytical Association over a 50-year period. Here he traces the individual stages and states that – after the invitation to hold the IPA Congress in Berlin in 1977 was declined in Jerusalem and after the Bamberg Conference of Central European Psychoanalytic Associations in 1980 – the German Psychoanalytical Association (DPV) conferences were successfully turned into a 'place for the successive self-confrontation with the "Nazi-introject" in our psychoanalytic identity', in which meetings with Hillel Klein and Herbert Rosenfeld made a vital contribution (Hermanns, 2001, p. 45).

Nevertheless, Chasseguet-Smirgel diagnosed the situation as early as 1987 in her 'Reflections on the Hamburg Congress' on the basis of her experiences before, during and after this first IPA Congress to take place after the Second World War on German soil, in 1985. Here she observed that most of the German analysts lacked the basic theoretical, clinical and technical knowledge of identification processes. Instead of 'guilt', the word 'shame' kept persistently emerging. 'This is to say that it is not a matter of assuming responsibility – by identification with the parents, and possibly with the analytical parents – for what happened in Germany' (Chasseguet-Smirgel, 1987, p. 437). Further on, she wrote:

> *What is one to do with a Nazi father?* Apparently, the only solution is to reject him. If you speak of the need to integrate your identifications with that father, you are immediately treated as a Nazi yourself. But in the absence of identification, where there is only counter-identification, there can be no genuine choice between acceptance and rejection, and sublimation becomes totally impossible. In order to become a human being in

> the full sense of the term, we have to be able to discover, confront and own the Hitler in us, otherwise the repressed will return and the disavowed will come back in various guises.
>
> *(Chasseguet-Smirgel, 1987, p. 437)*

While not everyone would concur with her assessment here, there was certainly a lack of the necessary space for the perception, the interpretation and the working through of corresponding destructive facets of object-relations in the German Federal Republic (among other places). Martin Wangh states in his paper on the working through of the Nazi past in the German psychoanalytic community that the 'intergenerational scotomisation' was gradually being penetrated. 'At the same time even today the embarrassment and defensive behaviour of younger German psychoanalysts towards colleagues of other nationalities still evinces the symptomatic consequence of that scotomisation' (Wangh, 1996, p. 111f.).

This contrasts sharply with Melanie Klein's plainly self-evident engagement even by the 1940s with the 'Hitler in us' in the transference and countertransference, which will now be examined more closely.

Klein's notes in their historical context

When Melanie Klein (1945) published clinical material explicitly referring to the 'Hitler in us', this was certainly not self-explanatory. Of course there were also works at this time by other people (outside Germany) whose case report extracts include a reference or two to Hitler. The PEP Archive makes it possible nowadays to obtain a fairly quick rough overview of the major English-speaking journals. This search does produce some, if not many, papers in which Hitler appears in the patient's material and is addressed in some way.[2]

I have not found anything though that is comparable to Melanie Klein's (1961) *Narrative of a Child Analysis*, which gives a detailed account of how this aspect was taken up in the transference and countertransference and interpreted. Even Limentani – who in his 1989 paper 'The psychoanalytic movement during the years of the war (1939–1945) according to the archives of the IPA' expresses his disappointment at finding out so little about what it was like to be an analyst in wartime in Great Britain – only mentions Klein's portrayal of a child analysis as a notable exception (Limentani, 1989). This published record of contemporaneous references to Hitler is certainly noteworthy but would hardly justify my title, since Klein published no further case reports from which anything apposite could be quoted. If we also consider the prejudice that external reality is neglected by Klein (and by Kleinians in general), it may be surprising to discover the extent of her concern with the contemporaneous background that is attested for the pre-war and wartime period in the Melanie Klein Archives. I am omitting here the sometimes detailed treatment notes that exist not only on Richard but on many other patients, both adults and children/adolescents. There are for example almost 300 typewritten pages of the analysis of 'Dick', which had been resumed in Autumn 1941, that provide a gripping account among other things of the preoccupation with Hitler and how this was understood by Klein (see Chapter 13 of this volume).

I am restricting myself here to the material that Klein herself explicitly compiled under the category of how the world situation characterized by Hitler was expressed in patients' reactions and how these were to be understood. Prior to this she had from her earliest beginnings in the 1920s not only been recording individual patients' material in the form of notes made from memory, but at the same time always collecting and annotating material that especially interested her with specific key words. For the area that is of interest there are essentially three distinct collections in the Archives, some of which can be further subdivided – these mainly consist of typewritten, dictated pages. There is sometimes a note made by the secretary that there is something she has not understood, and accordingly there are repeated gaps; the A4 pages had been only partly improved and amplified by Klein in handwriting. These collections are as follows:

> Firstly, approximately 30 pages which refer to patients' reactions to the so-called annexation of Austria (*Anschluss*). In the Archive these documents are labelled as concerning 'Crisis I: Reactions of patients to events in Austria' (PP/KLE/B.84).
>
> Secondly, at least 100 pages relating to the period before and after the Munich Agreement in September 1938, summarized in the Archive as 'Crisis II: Before and after the crisis' (PP/KLE/B. 85).
>
> And thirdly, and last, a letter from Joan Riviere of 3 June 1940, in which she puts the suggestion and request to Klein that she should present her reflections on the current political situation, as well as the nine-page manuscript that Klein, partly using key words, prepared for this meeting and that is headed 'Was bedeutet der Tod für das Individuum?' [What does death represent to the individual?] (PP/KLE/C. 96).[3]

Whereas the third item I have listed explains the immediate cause and purpose that led Klein to write down her reflections, it is unclear why she might have assembled the documents concerning the first two items. As she anonymized the reference to the individual patients in these notes, for example by identifying the patients alphabetically with A, B, C in the first 'bundle', it seems probable that she had in mind a 'more official' use. With the documents in which she initially only collected material under specific key words for herself, she generally proceeds not by anonymizing but by writing the name of each patient who is the source of the material. No external impetus for collecting the documents concerning the patients' reactions to the Austrian *Anschluss* has yet been possible to determine. However, among the documents concerning reactions to the 'Munich Crisis', the following letter from Klein's Secretary Hilda Lawrence can be found. On 25 November 1938, Lawrence writes to Dr Glover: 'Mrs. Klein asked me to send you the enclosed notes on reactions of patients to the crisis, which are a further explanation of the notes already sent to you' (file B.85, image 90).

It can be gleaned from this letter that not only the documents stapled to it, which are marked 'Please return to Mrs K with compls. Gl' (B. 85 image 56) but also the documents concerning the Munich Crisis, which had very obviously been assembled previously, were sent to Glover. (Of course we cannot exclude the possibility that she also sent the documents concerning Austria to Glover; but there is no conclusive indication that this was the case.)

Why were these documents sent to Glover? There is some information about this in Glover's (1941) publication entitled 'Notes on the psychological effects of war conditions on the civilian population I'. We learn that the Institute of Psycho-Analysis began to investigate the psychology of the civilian population immediately after the Munich Crisis (Glover, 1941, p. 133). The practising and associate members of the British Psycho-Analytical Society had been sent questionnaires about reactions to the Munich Crisis, as observed during analytic, therapeutic and consultative practice. Furthermore, these were also to include observations that every analyst made in everyday life. The results were then represented in a tabular form and discussed at the Society's meetings, following which a further list of questions was sent out. In the reports from the local Societies that were all printed in the *International Journal of Psychoanalysis*, these meetings are also recorded.[4]

With regard to the Munich Crisis, Glover summarizes that the majority of the patients 'reacted' to the crisis. Most of them were unsettled by it to various degrees and in various ways. Some reacted with an improvement, albeit temporary, in their previous symptoms. A minority was unaffected, being apparently indifferent, or almost ostentatiously ignoring the whole situation. This summary is then further subdivided; sometimes individual analysts with their results and assessments are also identified by name. In a footnote (Glover, 1941, p. 135) all 20 analysts who reported on reactions to the crisis are listed in alphabetical order, however Klein is not among them. Is this attributable to tensions between Glover and Klein? Did she perhaps not complete the questionnaires? Given the wealth of material that she evidently made available to him, it is in any case a surprising discovery.

Unpublished documents by Melanie Klein

Documents relating to the Austrian Anschluss

In the first half of this bundle of approximately 30 pages, B.84 (containing, in addition to the manuscript pages, separate notes on paper with amplifications to specific passages), there is a tidied-up typewritten text including some handwritten corrections. The second half is more uniform, apparently with a few missing pages, and the collection of material concerning the patients is rather more like a 'work in progress'. Unlike the earlier pages, these include an indication of the date: 'In the week of the 19th–25th the following material appears'. Under the date 19.3.38 Klein then begins with a patient's dream. I will focus next on the presentation of the first half of the manuscript.

Klein introduces her collection of her patient's reactions to the Austrian *Anschluss* in early 1938 by remarking that the phenomenon of entire nations subjugating themselves to dictators is fundamentally more interesting than the psychology of the dictators.

> We get to understand this better if we study the reactions of people who are not directly implied, but stirred in their feelings by happenings like the overrunning of Austria. I shall now give some material, following these events, from several patients, and later on draw my conclusions.
>
> *(File B.84 image 1)*

Klein then presents six patients in varying degrees of detail. To give an impression, I will select extracts from three patients.

She first presents the session of a Patient (A), who opened the session by telling her about the feelings he had had over the weekend. He reports his sympathy with Austria, the Jews, then with psychoanalysis, which he supposed was being suppressed, and with Freud in particular whom he greatly admired. A few critical comments follow about his own [i.e. the British] government. Finally, he related his sympathy specifically with Klein, knowing her to be Austrian.

> In the course of further assocns. in speaking about his own psychology he said in passing by 'The main thing would be that my feelings would come out' – without paying much attention to this remark which was not quite understandable from the context. The next day he started straightaway with criticism of psycho-analytic writings, an external stimulus being that he had recently read some analytic books. It appeared that this criticism veiled the one of Freud, and that feelings of hatred which came out quite clearly in another connection made clear that triumph and satisfaction with the situation of analysts in Vienna had been covered up the day before by more superficial feelings of regret and sympathy. Hatred and the wish to see me humiliated, deprived of the possibility of working, jealousy of what the patient felt as my superior knowledge to his own had come to the fore [. . .] It now became clear that Austria and myself were standing for the mother who had been raped, injured and humiliated, and that sadistic fantasies of this kind had been strongly aroused in the patient through this event. The remark of the day before, the meaning of which had not been clear at the time, could now be understood in the following sense. The main thing would be that K. should receive real, good feelings of sympathy while the patient unconsciously felt that these were to a large extent not true. At the end of the 2nd hour [. . .] the patient had not only

> realised his sadistic wishes against K. and Austria, but also noticed that he really enjoyed these feelings – a thing which he had not been so capable of understanding on former occasions. In leaving me he said quite unexpectedly to himself and me 'I feel as if I had had an undeserved holiday'.
>
> *(B.84, images 1–4)*

On the third day, Patient A displayed a completely different reaction, namely guilt. Klein summarizes as follows: he could not even in phantasy take up the fight against an aggressive father figure because he felt that he himself wanted to injure the mother and was therefore no better than the aggressor in any respect. Because of this dynamic it was impossible to oppose the Hitler-father.

Whereas Patient A refers directly to the political events, Patient B, whom I would next like to present, utters not a single word about the current situation, as Klein observes, but is despondent and hopeless with regard to his own analysis:

> Criticises me extremely sharply, that I am incapable of helping him, am quite useless and even accuses me of knowing that. He declares strongly in an unusually decided manner that he must give up his analysis and he can't go on any longer. The only interpretation I suggest after these remarks which had taken up the greatest part of the hour, is that we have no real explanation for his change in attitude from one day to another, and that this newly created situation about Austria seems to have had an influence on his feelings about analysis. He denies this absolutely, and gives me various reasons why he should be entirely indifferent. I suggested that my uselessness, my incapacity to help, which had been so strongly emphasised on this day, were connected with his feeling that Austria and I had been injured and that therefore no help could be expected any more from me. B. denies this, but leaves me obviously less tense. Something however was noteworthy which spoke to the contrary of this whole attitude. B. had on this very day a morning hour, which only happens once a week. For weeks on end he had missed about half of this hour – sometimes even more. On this day he had been only 15 minutes late and started the hour by saying that he is rather late and that he left his breakfast for this reason. I did not interpret this in the hour, but in one of the following ones I interpreted this as the wish to see as much as possible of me.
>
> *(file B.84 images 5–7)*

Later on, Klein summarizes as follows: 'The accusations against me, the increase of hatred because of frustration were used as a means to deny the value of the object, which for his feelings could not be saved' (B. 84, image 9).

In this example, Klein spontaneously conveys the patient's attitude to her and the analysis that suddenly change with the political events, and how the patient seems to have experienced them in relation to his analyst. Consciously, the patient certainly disputes a connection, but the tension abated through this evidently being understood. I will not pursue this case further here either and would now like to present some extracts from the material of a Patient (C):

> Patient was very depressed – expressed strongly her horror and her disapproval of what has happened and though she is English feels closer to the matter since she has friends in Austria. She is also concerned about me. The following day she reports a dream which had extremely worried her.
>
> Dream: She was in Germany and was talking to Goering. She wanted to shoot him, but could not make use of the pistol, because she has no knowledge of using one (true), whereby it was unclear whether she had a pistol or not. Goering remained quiet and became actually quite friendly, explaining to her how one uses a pistol. The patient couldn't help feeling a certain attraction for Goering and was aware that she was on the way to starting to flirt with him. But then other people came in and Goering had her arrested; so it seemed he had really only pretended. She was to be shot, but before that happened Goering took up a little sand from the floor. It was only a little and she couldn't really make much out of that.
>
> *(B.84, images 11–12)*

Klein interpreted the degree of ambivalence here and how it might also mean that a bit of sand was not actually harmful.

> C. now recognises that actually in the dream it seemed that Goering's taking up the sand was the preliminary to her being shot, and that the sand was really put there by herself [...] this little sand which one could not do much with meant a subtle attack on Goering [...] The emphasis which the patient had laid on the fact that she could not manipulate a gun [...] obviously expressed [...] her harmlessness. The little detail however that she was shooting with faeces was well hidden away. The interpretation could be linked up with the general attitude of the patient – a deep feeling of being insincere even though there is apparently not much ground for it. The dangerous father who at the same time was an object of attraction and whom she wanted to please and take away from her mother, she at the same time wanted, for reasons of jealousy and of fear, to poison and to kill by means of subtle anal attacks – one basis for her feelings of insincerity, thus never knowing whether her feelings were true. [...] These subtle attacks and phantasies were also the basis for her fears of persecution by people. Actually she had been very much disturbed by this Austrian business, identified herself with Austria and also myself, and hated Hitler very strongly. But the fact that he also represented the F. whom she wanted to [...] take away from M. had again disturbed in this connection the truth of her feelings of sympathy. Before leaving me the pat.

confesses something extremely shaming to herself, and says that she felt there was a certain pleasure in her over the sensation (in the sense of a thrill through sensational news) which this event stirred in her.

(B.84 images 12–14)

I think this sequence from the analysis of a woman who, as Klein writes, hated Hitler but discovers her susceptibility to an exciting flirtation with these machinations shows in an exemplary way how the internal situation could be understood in the analysis against the background of the external situation in international politics.

While Klein had mentioned at the beginning of her collection that she is also anticipating that the analysis of her patient's reactions will yield some information about the phenomenon of entire populations subjugating themselves to dictators, she does not explain this in the extant documents specifically in relation to the *Anschluss*. Her ideas take shape implicitly through the description of the various patients – of which I have only presented a selection. But in both the next two bundles (from 1938 up to the Munich Crisis of 1940) we learn something specifically about what is now to be discussed.

Documents relating to the 'Munich Crisis'

Most of the material archived under the heading 'Crisis II' consists in collections of a combination of detailed summarized session sequences and summarized passages from analyses mainly of adult patients (file B.85). In the most detailed ones, Klein sets out five patients' reactions to the 'Munich Crisis', constantly adding amplifications and with individual patients, sometimes choosing sub-headings such as 'Patient S. before the crisis' or 'Patient S. after the crisis'. She has also presented some relevant material, albeit less extensively, from the analyses of a female patient and a 'small girl'. However, here I would like to focus on the 16 pages (as well as some pages with amplifications) that she – as mentioned above – sent as a supplement to Glover in November 1938. They contain the summary of her experiences and reflections from her analyses in this period:

> With most of my patients the situation before the crisis activated deep anxiety-situations, their fears about the actual external dangers thus becoming much more acute. This was shown by the fact that at the time of the greatest strain the analysis of internal anxiety-situations, with these patients, relieved some of the tension [and] fears aroused by the international state of affairs. They then became more capable of judging and dealing with the external situation, and of making decisions, etc. I should like to differentiate here between the days when war seemed very probable, the first stage, and the last two or three days preceding Munich, when the war seemed practically definite, the second stage, then again, the

> time which followed the Munich agreement, the third stage. In those days when war seemed inevitable, with most of my patients there was a striking alteration in their feelings and attitude. The early anxiety-situations which had been aroused were still active. Yet the patients became less anxious and seemed to accept the position with a certain amount of resignation and determination, and the wish to help and co-operate had become stronger. Obviously this was due to the feeling of indignation over Hitler's attitude at Godesberg, which seemed to leave no doubt that Britain had to defend itself and freedom in general against him.
>
> *(B.85 images 56–57)*

The deeper processes underlying this change in attitude, as Klein explains, come into four categories. Firstly:

> The external dangers, since war was apparently inevitable, had become more real and less phantastic, less vague and indefinite, than in the previous days. Thus a process by which anxieties connecting with the unknown and dangerous internal situations may be alleviated when a definite external-danger situation becomes operative. As is well known, this can be carried to extremes, and the mechanism of seeking external dangers in order to relieve internal ones, is characteristic of a manic attitude. In the cases of which I am speaking, however, this mechanism was not very strong, and, moreover, certain elements present brought about a whole constellation of feeling which was not of a manic character.
>
> *(B.85 image 58)*

Secondly, Klein explains:

> a special element in it was the identification with a good father – Chamberlain – which came about after Godesberg, for a very short time only, when he was felt to stand up to Hitler and to protect the attacked people. This identification with a good and just father went along with the freeing of hatred and aggression against Hitler – standing for the bad and destructive father and the bad id-sadism and hatred thus becoming ego-syntonic, while love for the 'good' objects and the wish to protect them came out to the full. This showed very clearly in the transference situation also, when concern and interest in my well-being appeared more strongly.
>
> *(B.85 images 58–59)*

Klein then adds that the identification with a good and strong father, moreover, allowed the 'reparation element' to gain in strength and scope, since the impulse to reparation (in the present situation concerned with the attacked and weak peoples) at the same time was felt to undo damage done in the earliest situations. Finally some relief of anxiety and guilt derived from these early anxiety-situations and depressed feelings were obtained, and all this contributed to the alteration of feelings before-mentioned (see B.85 image 59).

On the following pages, Klein summarizes in general terms the early development of children, which she uses as a basis for understanding, among other things, how good and bad mother- and father-figures initially determine the unconscious phantasy situations. When the ambivalence then diminishes, the strict separation between good and bad objects then eases:

> Yet the ways in which the early hatred against a 'bad' father figure (or 'bad' mother figure), who are felt to be harmful and dangerous to other loved objects, is dealt with by the ego remains of fundamental importance for the attitude to right and wrong and moral courage in later development. If this hatred, which ultimately is the hatred against one's own 'bad' and violent tendencies against the bad Id, has become bound up with the love for the good objects which are to be protected against the bad aggressors (ultimately against oneself) the foundation is laid for an attitude in which hatred will be turned against what is felt to be unfair, bad, wrong, violent, not only to oneself but to people or things one loves and who need protection. Of course the 'good' causes in the service of which this attitude can be used, vary as we know in different epochs, with different peoples, and even with the different sections of the same people.
>
> *(B.85, images 63–64)*

Finally, she states:

> This description seems rather schematic and also to lead us away from our topic, but I am aiming at a special point, important for our subject, namely the constellation of feelings, the mental attitude, which makes for identification with the dictator or against it. The reinforced idealization and admiration of the sadistic father as an escape from fears and conflicts is an element, tending to increase homosexuality, and bound up with deep denial of psychic reality, which is important in character disturbances. The capacity to stand up against the bad father-figures or rather, what he has come to stand for, namely, badness, wrong-doing and violence in the outside world, which goes with love for the good one who protects mother, has a bearing on uprightness of character, and also tends to further heterosexuality.
>
> The fact which my material proves clearly, however, is that the necessity to bow to the dictator-father, to plot and side with him, at the expense of the attacked and loved mother and the other children, is due to the internalization of these figures. The anxieties are so much intensified, therefore, because the fight with an internal father is so overwhelmingly dangerous – much more than any fight with the external father-figure could be. Thus, giving in to the external father-figures is to a large extent the result of these

internal fears. But if the anxiety of an internal father is much stronger than that of an external one, so, also are the guilt and the conflicts resulting from the desertion of the internal good mother and her children.

In the patients I am referring to, the tension, guilt and fears of this internal situation, and the despair which arose out of it, in the first stage, became to a certain extent relieved in the psychological situation setting in after Godesberg in the second stage. Their being able to identify themselves with the good father against the bad one, and their wish to protect the mother, definitely relieved guilt and some anxiety. The hatred against Hitler, when allowed to come out with all details of sadism as an ego-syntonic reaction, also allowed the love part – repressed and warded off together with the hate – for the good father and mother to extend to the oppressed objects, felt to be the 'good' loved ones.

(B.85 images 67–71)

Whereas at the beginning of her account relating to the Austrian *Anschluss* Klein had asked how the subjugation to dictators such as Hitler may be motivated, through this document we get to know her reflections. In summary it can be stated: the fears and conflicts that are connected with an internal bad father figure can be felt to be intolerable. A possibility of apparently resolving the conflicts consists in the idealization of this internal 'strong' father figure, which is accompanied by a denial of destruction, sadism and the corresponding fears. An attempt is sometimes made to stabilize this defence by subjugation to an external strong dictatorial father figure such as Hitler.

When we now come to the third item, the documents from 1940, we find some further reflections of this kind.

Documents from 1940

These include a letter of 3 June 1940 by Joan Riviere that seems to have been the impetus for Klein's manuscript 'What does death represent to the individual?'

My dear Melanie,

When the first official mention of invasion began, the possibility of our work all coming to an end seemed so near, I felt we should all have to keep it in our hearts, perhaps, as the only way to save it for the future. Also of course I was constantly thinking of the psychological causes of such terrible loss and destruction as may happen to mankind. So I had the idea of your telling me (and then a group of us) everything you think about these causes, so that all of us who can understand these things at all should share and know as much as possible, to help preserve it.

My idea is that you should tell us first what you think about the *causes of the German psychological situation*, and *secondly*, of that of the *rest of Europe* and

> mainly the Allies, since the last war. To me the apathy and *denial of the danger* in the Allies especially England is not clear. (I never shared it.) How is it connected with what I call the 'Munich' *complex, the son's incapacity to fight for mother and country, and his homosexual leanings*?
>
> These are the sort of questions I wanted you to speak of. I thought we would have no discussion – the only questions should be to get your meaning clear – I asked people to send in questions beforehand, which I can probably arrange in some order to bring up at a moment when you are dealing with that kind of point. If there is time I would send you the points before. Do you go to 9 Manchester Square on Saturday before this meeting? Or where will you be?
>
> *(C.96 image 1–2)*

The letter ends with the remark: 'I am so looking forward to Saturday – psa is a great anodyne in all this anxiety!' (C.96 image 2).

Klein's manuscript, which may have served as preparation for this meeting, begins as follows:

> The increasing danger of a terrifying death brings out in individuals both the deeper reasons of their fear of death as well as their methods of combating this fear. Instances A. Patient of very religious upbringing in whom the fear of Hell had played a great part in childhood, a fear which had intellectually been entirely overcome is revived in the present situation. The internal hell which could not be overcome by love as demanded by religion because devil and helpful God were so very much the same in his unc. mind. In this case and others it became clear that terror of own destructiveness, murderousness and nervousness, fear of having arranged for Hitler to destroy the world, and especially the incapacity to dissociate the evil father and parents from the good ones, to dissociate love from hate, and therefore to turn hatred against the evil thing – love and protection towards the loved and good people – that all this has a paralysing effect in the relation to external dangers. One conclusion: a) An important step in development is the capacity to allow oneself to split the imagos into good and bad ones which goes with the capacity to trust one's constructive tendencies and love feelings. Only thus is it possible to hate with full strength what is felt to be evil in the external world – to attack and destroy at the same time protecting oneself with one's good internal object as well as external loved objects, country, etc. against the bad things. To be able to achieve this is also dependent on b) The relative strength of internalized relations versus external ones – or rather the balance between internal situations and relations on the one hand and externals on the other.
>
> If the feeling that external war is really going on inside – that an internal Hitler is fought inside by a Hitler-like subject – predominates, then despair results. It is impossible to fight this war, because in the internal situation

> catastrophe is bound to be the end of it. This depends also on the ways and means in which the subject is carrying out the internal war. If he feels to out-Hitler Hitler, then it will all end in complete destruction inside. If there is a better balance between internal happenings and external happenings the war inside is not predominating, then one can turn with strength and determination against the external enemy. There are many other factors at work which all work towards greater trust in one's own capacity to love and construct as well as in the good object and determine this balance between internal and external.
>
> *(C.96 images 3–5)*

Klein goes on to explain that the current situation is proving to be a very strong stimulus for re-experiencing anxieties connected with early phantasies and how impressed she is by the effect that analysis can have under such circumstances:

> One very typical thing was the guilt about the attraction towards this [sic] to the destructive and dangerous penis which Hitler's murderous weapons represent. In men it appeared that quite hidden passive homosexual phantasies, plotting and scheming with the destructive father, came to the fore. a) They had instigated Hitler to this destructive intercourse and enjoyed it sadistically. b) Terror of being destroyed and identification with the threatened mother reinforced the tendencies to scheme and plot with the dangerous father. To this is added the anxiety of the internal destruction by this dangerous father who becomes more and more internal the more the external reality proves his dangerousness. The guilt about the sadistic alliance with the dangerous father is one important reason for denial: but I see the most various methods used against it.
>
> *(C.96 images 5–6)*

Later on, she writes:

> Fear of death decreased when trust in me, in analysis, and more generally, in the survival of goodness in spite of all dangers to values, increased. The feeling that goodness cannot ultimately be exterminated, which may be a denial of danger in external relations, was based on a better balance between facing danger and yet relying more on internal goodness and trust in some good object. The question of balance so often stressed appears as the ultimate decisive factor. Optimum between external and internal, love and hate, and the methods used against anxiety. Certain amount of temporary denial obviously unavoidable and necessary. We look at nature, we read a book, we play with a child, we enjoy food, etc. and we have to remind ourselves that our life and country is at stake. In between the good experience has helped us to deny the danger. If the denial predominates in the attitude, it may lead to complacency, flight to

> the good inner objects, etc. If the help provided by the fact that such good things we just enjoy exist, the belief in the good objects and in goodness ultimately, is not too much denial of the bad things, it may help us to take steps to preserve goodness externally, and may internally help us to remain calm in the face of danger.
>
> *(C.96 images 8–9)*

In terms of the treatment technique, Klein finally records the 'confirmation about the main principles of our work; even now reassurance does not seem to be of great value (certain exceptions and rather limited). But an undisturbed keeping or holding fast to analyse aggression, guilt, which disturbs the belief in constructive and reparative tendencies seems most helpful' (C.96 image 10). She reminds us of the need to remain aware of the constant interplay between the present external situation and the internal past situation and therefore also past experiences.

Concluding remarks

The question nevertheless remains as to how far Klein's reflections, which have been transmitted to us through the documents presented in extracts and that she, at least in part, may have shared and discussed with colleagues, have left verifiable tracks of any kind. At the moment I can only make some very speculative connections in this regard, which I would not therefore wish to explain in detail. One idea is that they may have had some influence on Jones's (1941) paper about the psychology of Quislingism. Jones sees this phenomenon as being based on the incapacity to understand an enemy, which is accompanied by the denial or sanction of his aggressiveness. Some of his reflections resemble those of Klein, but these may of course have been present generally in this group. There is I think a further possible line of speculation concerning Money-Kyrle, who published his paper 'Some aspects of political ethics from the psycho-analytical point of view' in 1944 (Money-Kyrle, 1944). In a preliminary overview, he distinguishes various types: there is the aggressive self-righteousness of the paranoiac, who delusionally imagines that he is being persecuted; as an opposing extreme he identifies the denial of a danger that is only too real. Referring back to Klein's published observations; he sees them as rooted in a feeling of internal persecution. Whereas mechanisms of projection seem to be one of the key determinants of the Nazi ideology, Money-Kyrle (1944) writes that mechanisms of disavowal were one of the key determinants of the disarmament policy up to 1934. He calls this the ideology of the scotomists (p. 167). He distinguishes some further types that he also describes in more detail in a subsequent paper.[5]

Regardless of how far Klein's ideas more or less directly influenced colleagues' later publications, I was struck by the way in which she kept on the track of destructive identifications, did not evade them, and how this enabled her to allow some space for trusting and loving object relationships. The difficulty of doing that – in any international political situation – is of course not limited to pertinent Hitler identifications. Freud wrote as early as 1933 [1932] in his lectures that were not held, the *New Introductory Lectures on Psycho-Analysis*:

> Our hypothesis is that there are two essentially different classes of instincts: the sexual instincts, understood in the widest sense . . . and the aggressive instincts, whose aim is destruction. When it is put to you like this, you will scarcely regard it as a novelty. It looks like an attempt at a theoretical transfiguration of the commonplace opposition between loving and hating . . . But it is a remarkable thing that this hypothesis is nevertheless felt by many people as an innovation and, indeed, as a most undesirable one which should be got rid of as quickly as possible. I presume that a strong affective factor is coming into effect in this rejection. Why have we ourselves needed such a long time before we decided to recognize an aggressive instinct? Why did we hesitate to make use, on behalf of our theory, of facts which were obvious and familiar to everyone?
>
> *(Freud, 1933,* S.E. *22, p. 103)*

To this day there remains 'a strong affective factor' that still influences the discussion about this concept, the rejection of the death drive.

In her late monograph *Envy and Gratitude*, Klein (1957) identifies a factor that in my view makes the strong affective rejection in connection with the death drive somewhat more comprehensible; we know that it took Klein herself about ten years to refer back to Freud's concept of the death drive in order to conceptualize her experiences adequately.

> For the urge even in the earliest stages to get constant evidence of the mother's love is fundamentally rooted in anxiety. The struggle between life and death instincts and the ensuing threat of annihilation of the self and of the object by destructive impulses are fundamental factors in the infant's initial relation to his mother. For his desires imply that the breast, and soon the mother, should do away with these destructive impulses and the pain of persecutory anxiety.
>
> *(Klein, 1957, pp. 179–180)*

The wish to be free of destructive identifications then fosters the need for an inexhaustible, ever-present breast, an omnipotent object.

In the meantime, many analysts have contributed to making it possible to work through, reflect on and discuss destructiveness in the countertransference; a precondition in my view. Only a few voices will be quoted here, which seek to conceptualize the difficulties of dealing with such large-scale identifications. Grubrich-Simitis (1981) states:

> [when] atrocities of an unimaginable order of magnitude, worse than the worst imaginable oralcannibalistic or anal-sadistic fantasies, under conditions in which all highly organized defense structures and mature superego demands had been destroyed, these events must have signified the downfall of the secondary process and the 'seizure of power' by the primary process.
>
> *(Grubrich-Simitis (1981, p. 438)*

With reference to Bion's concept of caesura, Loch (1993) explained that it seems probable that for large groups overwhelming catastrophes such as the Holocaust, for example, are a caesura that leads to mutations in the psychic structure (Loch, 1993, p. 63, fn. 20). As one representative example among many, I would only wish to cite Appy (1992), who in his paper 'Was bedeutet "Auschwitz" heute?' allows us to participate very deeply in the process of working through in the countertransference. Is it too optimistic, if we concur with Klein's supposition that patients' courage grows, the depression diminishes and their capacity to make decisions and so on increases when hatred and guilt, which are connected with early phantasies, have been further analysed (C.96 image 5)?

Notes

1 An earlier version of this chapter was published in Frank (2003) 'Zu Melanie Kleins zeitgenössischer Bezugnahme auf Hitler und den Zweiten Weltkrieg in ihren Behandlungen'. *Psyche – Z Psychoanal.*, 57: 708–728. This translation is by Sophie Leighton.

2 For example, Bak (1946) cites in his paper, 'Masochism in paranoia', a patient's dream in which Hitler, Mussolini and Hirohito are to be executed. The patient offers to stand in for Hirohito, who cannot be found. The execution is a form of decapitation, with the scalp being separated from the skull, and they stick a knife into the back of his head. Bak comments that the patient was able through masochistic identification to become the father, the powerful and beloved enemy. The price that he had to pay was castration (Bak, 1946, p. 296). Bornstein also reports passages in a child analysis in which the patient was preoccupied with Hitler (e. g. Bornstein, 1945, p. 154), but does not interpret this in the transference. Geleerd (1943) explains a girl patient's play phantasy in which the analyst was Hitler and the patient a policeman. As far as I can see, however, she does not interpret this scene in the transference.

3 To the best of my knowledge, reference has only so far been made to this manuscript in publications, namely in the book *Reading Melanie Klein*, edited by Phillips and Stonebridge, 1998. Zaretsky (1998) and Stonebridge (1998) each refer in a passage to this manuscript but not in terms of the aspect that I am choosing here. [Editor's note: this document is also to be found on the Melanie Klein website blog number 14, date November 2018.]

4 17 November 1938: Symposium on 'Psycho-analytical aspects of the war crisis' with contributions from Mrs. E.F. Sharpe, Dr. M. Brierley, Dr. S. Payne and Dr. M. Schmideberg. 25 May 1939: 'Discussion of war mental emergency measures'. Mr. E. Kris: Summary of relevant literature; Dr. E. Glover: Outline of existing approved schemes; M. W. Schmideberg: Treatment of panic in casualty areas and clearing stations; Drs. Carroll, Scott and Gillespie: Treatment of acute states in hospital – differential treatment of pathological types – importance of early diagnosis; Dr. J. Rickman: On varieties

of treatment. 7. June 1939: 'Continued discussion on treatment of sub-acute and chronic war neurosis'. Dr. E. Bibring: Summary of relevant literature; Dr. E. Glover: Further report on organisation; Dr. W. A. Brend: Administrative problems; Dr. Mira (by invitation): War experience in Spain: Dr. S. Payne: Treatment of 'shock' by hypnosis with or without light anaesthesia and drugs; Dr. D. Carroll: Report on subcommittee and treatment of acute states with special reference to drug treatment. 4 October 1939 in Memoriam Sigmund Freud. 'Discussion of war-time emergency measures'. 12 June 1940: Symposium on 'Psychological factors in war-time morale with special reference to the "quisling" type of situations that induced his reactions, opened by Dr. E. Jones'. 18 October 1940: Discussion concerning the psychological effects of the air raids. Introductory lecture: Mr. W. Schmideberg. 15 January 1941: Dr. E. Stengel: On experiences during internment. 5 March 1941: Discussion concerning the impact of war and social hardship on morale. Introductory lecture: Dr. W. Hoffer.

5 It is also interesting in this connection that in 1946 Money-Kyrle was a member of the control commission 'German Personnel Research Branch'. Using psychiatric interviews, this commission tried to find people who could be entrusted with responsible posts. Money-Kyrle summarized his impression at that time in 1951 in a postscript on 'Some aspects of state and character in Germany'. He described a widespread feeling of collective guilt of a truly depressive kind, albeit sometimes manifesting itself through an accentuation of denial. He felt that these people's tragedy consisted in having to deal with the feeling that they had devoted their aggression – tenaciously and heroically – to the defence of something that they themselves in their innermost hearts felt to be connected mainly with something dark and sinister. 'It was therefore often of great therapeutic importance to them as individuals – and probably also for the future of their society – to be allowed to participate in the protection of what they could feel, both consciously and unconsciously, to be a better object. The idea of Western culture threatened from without had already begun to play the rôle of an object of this kind, and in the idea of its defence they had begun to seek an outlet for an unconscious reparative impulse. But there was also a tendency to turn against these new ideas in moods of fresh despair. In other words, very many Germans in 1946 were in a depressive phase which could be succeeded either by an impulse to constructive reparation or, if this failed, by a renewed paranoidal attack on the objects they had injured' (Money-Kyrle, 1978, p. 244). In the paper itself, Money-Kyrle distinguishes two groups of characters that he encountered in his interviews: the so-called 'authoritarians' and the 'humanists'. With regard to the problematic that concerns us here, he impressively summarized his findings to the effect that with the humanists the sense of guilt related to not having put up enough resistance, whereas in those who trusted in authority the guilt feelings related to the inner rebellion against an increasingly reckless kind of politics.

References

Appy, G. (1992). Was bedeutet 'Auschwitz' heute? (What does 'Auschwitz' mean today?) In R. Moses and F.-W. Eickhoff, eds, *Die Bedeutung des Holocaust für nicht direkt Betroffene.* (The meaning of the Holocaust for those not directly affected.) *Jahrbuch der Psychoanalyse*, Beiheft 14. Stuttgart: frommann-holzboog.

Bak, R. (1946). Masochism in paranoia. *Psychoanal. Quart.*, *15*, 285–301.

Bornstein, B. (1945). Clinical notes on child analysis. *Psychoanal. Study Child*, *1*, 151–166.

Chasseguet-Smirgel, J. (1987). 'Time's white hair we ruffle'. Reflections on the Hamburg Congress. *Int. Rev. Psycho-Anal.*, *14*, 433–444.

Eckstaedt, A. (1989). *Nationalsozialismus in der 'zweiten Generation'. Psychoanalyse von Hörigkeitsverhältnissen.* (National Socialism in the 'Second Generation'. The psychoanalysis of master–slave relationships.) Frankfurt/M: Suhrkamp.

Frank, C. (1999). *Melanie Klein in Berlin: Her first psychoanalyses of children*. E. Spillius, (ed.). Trans. S. Leighton (Ch. 1, S. Young). London: Routledge.

Frank, C. (2003). Zu Melanie Kleins zeitgenössischer Bezugnahme auf Hitler und den Zweiten Weltkrieg in ihren Behandlungen. *Psyche – Z Psychoanal.*, *57*, 708–728.

Freud, S. (1933). New introductory lectures on psycho-analysis. In J. Strachey et al. (trans.), *The standard edition of the complete psychological works of Sigmund Freud vol. 22*. London: Hogarth Press.

Geleerd, E. (1943). The analysis of a case of compulsive masturbation in a child. *Psychoanal. Quart.*, *12*, 520–540.

Glover, E. (1941). Notes on the psychological effects of war conditions on the civilian population (1). *Int. J. Psycho-Anal.*, *22*, 132–145.

Grubrich-Simitis, I. (1981). Extreme traumatization as cumulative trauma. *Psychoanal. Study Child*, *36*, 415–460.

Hermanns, L.M. (2001). Fünfzig Jahre Deutsche Psychoanalytische Vereinigung. Zur Geschichte der Psychoanalyse in Deutschland 1950 bis 2000 (Fifty years of the German Psychoanalytical Association. On the history of psychoanalysis in Germany from 1950 to 2000). In W. Bohleber and S. Drews (eds), *Die Gegenwart der Psychoanalyse – die Psychoanalyse der Gegenwart* (Present-day psychoanalysis – the psychoanalysis of the present day). Stuttgart: Klett-Cotta, pp. 35–57.

Jones, E. (1941). The psychology of quislingism. *Int. J. Psychoanal.*, *22*, 1–6.

Klein, M. (1945). The Oedipus complex in the light of early anxieties. *Int. J. Psychoanal.*, *26*, 11–33.

Klein, M. (1961). *Narrative of a child analysis*. London: Hogarth Press.

Klein, M. (1957). *Envy and gratitude and other works 1946–1963*. M. Khan (ed.), London: Hogarth Press.

Limentani, A. (1989). The psychoanalytic movement during the years of the war (1939–1945) according to the archives of the IPA. *Int. Rev. Psychoanal.*, *16*, 3–13.

Loch, W. (1993). *Deutungs-Kunst* (The art of interpretation). Tübingen (Ed. diskord).

Meltzer, D. (1978). Richard week-by-week. In D. Meltzer: *The Kleinian development*. Perthshire: Clunie Press.

Money-Kyrle, R.E. (1944). Some aspects of political ethics from the psycho-analytical point of view. *Int. J. Psychoanal.*, *25*, 166–171.

Money-Kyrle, R.E. (1951). Some aspects of state and character in Germany. In *The collected papers of Money-Kyrle*. Perthshire: Clunie Press, 1978, pp. 229–244.

Phillips, J. and Stonebridge, I. (eds) (1998). *Reading Melanie Klein*. London/New York: Routledge.

Stonebridge, L. (1998). Anxiety in Klein: The missing witch's letter. In J. Phillips and I. Stonebridge (eds), *Reading Melanie Klein*. London/New York: Routledge, pp. 190–202.

Wangh, M. (1996). Die Durcharbeitung der Nazivergangenheit in der deutschen psychoanalytic community. Versuch einer Einschätzung aus naher Ferne. (Working through the Nazi past in the German psychoanalytic community. Attempt at an assessment from a close distance.) *Psyche – Z Psychoanal.*, *50*, 97–122.

Zaretsky, E. (1998). Melanie Klein and the emergence of modern personal life. In J. Phillips and I. Stonebridge (eds), *Reading Melanie Klein*. London/New York: Routledge, pp. 32–50.

7

'ON REASSURANCE'

An unpublished paper by Melanie Klein (1933)[1]

Claudia Frank

Introduction

In this chapter I present Melanie Klein's paper 'On Reassurance', which may be found in her Archives in the Wellcome Library, file PP/KLE/C.67. I show that it was a contribution to Edward Glover's investigation on psychoanalytic technique in the 1930s. I discuss the paper against the background of the technical discussions conducted in London at that time (including contributions from Melitta Schmideberg and James Strachey) and of Klein's relevant publications. Although Klein consistently considered the 'correct' interpretation to be most effective means of reassurance, she occasionally also accepted a non-interpreting approach. In this respect the paper presented here goes further than any other of her published writings.

As a result of her experiences in child analysis, anxiety quickly became a core clinical and theoretical issue for Klein. Her observations concerning depressive and paranoid anxieties are of continuing relevance today, with the treatment technique continuing to be controversial. In *A Dictionary of Kleinian Thought*, Hinshelwood (1989) sums this up as follows under the heading 'Anxiety and technique':

> Klein's interest in the content of anxiety led to her technique of deeply penetrating interpretations. In contrast, the classical technique evolved by the ego-psychologists was concerned with analysing the ego's defence mechanisms (and adaptation mechanisms) and led to criticism of Klein that her deep interpretations were themselves the cause of anxiety because they must be experienced by patients as intrusive and therefore persecutory, with the result that Kleinians are confronted with a great deal of persecutory anxiety.
>
> *(Hinshelwood, 1989, pp. 119–120)*

The development of analytic treatment technique has been little researched. I have decided to construct another small building block here, which belongs in the domain just outlined of 'anxiety and technique' but places a question-mark over the widespread idea that all the contributions to this discussion have been controversial in the sense of ostracizing or defamatory. My historical context is the first study of psychoanalytic technique that Glover published in 1940 under the title 'An Investigation of the Technique of Psycho-Analysis' (Glover, 1940). In 1955 the article was reprinted in Glover's book, *The Technique of Psycho-Analysis* (Glover, 1955), and I am referring to this edition in my quotations. The questionnaires themselves, however, are only contained in the 1940 edition, so the dates of its despatch are taken from this earlier version. In a review of Glover's original report, Fenichel (1942, p. 230) emphasizes that literature on psychoanalytic technique is very incomplete and that teaching it, then as now, is based on oral tradition, which makes contemporary research more difficult. Studies on this subject are therefore, more than with other themes, reliant on unpublished literature and analytic case notes.

I present here one of these unpublished contributions. The Melanie Klein Archive file PP/KLE/C.67 consists of four undated typewritten pages that have been partly corrected and amplified in handwriting. The original document can be consulted online through the Wellcome Library. It is untitled; on page 1 there is only a (typewritten) 'B'. Diagonally to the left at the top is also – not in Klein's writing – the handwritten addition 'Klein Supplementary'. The Archive catalogue describes this file as 'Contributions to discussion on reassurance' and dates it as 1941. This temporal classification does not seem very plausible to me because as far as can be ascertained there was no (official) discussion about reassurance in 1941. But such a discussion probably did take place in connection with Glover's above-mentioned investigation that began in July 1932, when questionnaires were first sent out to members of the British Psycho-Analytical Society, and ended in 1938 when the final responses were collated. In my view it was Glover's investigation that almost certainly formed the impetus for Klein to record her thoughts at that time on reassurance.

Klein's discussion paper 'On reassurance'

Here, crossed-out phrases that are mostly illegible are not reproduced and corrections have been incorporated into the text without commentary. The text, written in English, is as follows:

> I take it that reassurance is an essential part of analysis. Of course I speak of correct reassurance as well as in speaking of interpretation I mean correct interpretation. They are correct if they follow out of the analytic situation and are grounded on certain analytic rules. A few of them I have suggested in my book p. 139/40. [Klein is referring here to her 1932 book *The Psycho-Analysis of Children* (Klein, 1932)]. Shortly, the interpretative

work is directed at that part of the material associated with the greatest latent anxiety. Furthermore each interpretation following a little way the threats of the Superego, the impulses of the Id and the attempts of the Ego to reconcile the two i.e. defence mechanisms.

You see as yet I have not made any distinction between reassurance and interpretation. They seem to me to have something in common. To sum up what the interpretation does: While the interpretation uncovers the latent anxiety and goes on to connect it with the particular fantasies underlying it, so it stirs first anxiety, and after having done so, resolves it. Another suggestion which I made is that by uncovering the anxiety of the fantastic Superego, the Ego becomes able to compare the fantastic picture of the analyst which was at the time in his mind with the real person. The eye [it seems likely that the homophone 'I' was intended here] is able to make a reality test (Realitätsprüfung). Now through this test the anxiety gets diminished, or, for the time being entirely resolved, but the outcome of this is the fact that the analyst has changed from an enemy to a helper, from the bad mother into the good one. In my paper 'Personification in the Play of Children' (Jones number p. 203) [This means Volume 10 of the *International Journal of Psychoanalysis* edited by Jones, in which the paper appeared (Klein, 1929).] I come to the conclusion that as the analyst assumes the hostile roles which the patient attributes to him and subjects them to analysis, there is a constant progress in the development of the anxiety inspiring Imagos towards the kindlier identifications with their close approximation to reality.

Now the correct reassurance makes only one part of the different steps which I have described in connection with the interpretation. By some means – words or actions –the analyst gives the proof that he is a good object. If the reassurance is actually to be effective, this proof must follow out of the analytic situation, and must include a bigger or smaller number of proofs in connection with anxiety situations which are standing in the foreground. Of course the larger the scope of those proofs is, i.e. the more anxiety situations are disproved, the more effective or lasting reassurance will be. One result which the interpretation produces, i.e. to strengthen the belief in the good object is effected by the correct reassurance as well, but the reassurance does not effect a diminishment of the anxiety of the bad figures, which is the most important part of the analytic work. The reassurance, therefore, seems to me an important means to allay anxiety through the temporary increased belief in the analyst as a good object. It thus enables the analyst to uncover anxiety and diminish it lastingly. I have found that every interpretation which works its way is felt by the patient as a reassurance as well, as it proves, through the relief of anxiety, that the analyst is a 'helper'.

A lot could be said about the wrong reassurance, but that is not the point. The point is that reassurance cannot be applied much with quite a number of people and that its value varies very much in different stages of the analysis. I think that this is due to the fact that every proof that the analyst is a good figure is taken as a libidinal gratification (you remember, perhaps, that in my view the helping figures are derived from the good mother who gives libidinal gratification). Thus every proof of this kind satisfies but raises at the same time more libidinal wishes, so that patients who cannot tolerate their libidinal wishes for the analyst and are afraid of them cannot get an allaying of anxiety through reassurance. (Of course there are still a lot of other reasons why people cannot accept reassurance, anxiety of getting disappointed, mistrust etc.)

Those people will only react to the interpretation which resolves anxiety of the bad figures. They also cannot tolerate for a long time the fact that through the interpretation the analyst becomes too much of a good figure and therefore anxiety is stirred up again very soon. Of course the more anxiety is diminished the more they can bear the fantasies connected with the good objects and can appreciate kindness as such. But that, of course, is only one type of patient. It seems to me, to speak more generally, that with patients in whom the belief in good figures or in a good figure is very strongly used as a cover against the anxiety of bad ones, reassurance will be more likely to be effective. Those people who use the flight to the good object very much as a defence can be quite as ill (can be full of mistrust etc.) as those who have developed other ways of defence. Now even with those people with whom reassurance is effective, reassurance ought only to be used as a means to help the main purpose-the complete cure. No doubt that some people can be greatly influenced by effective reassurance but of course that is not the aim of analysis. That is clear. But the point in question is how much reassurance, how much interpretation is one to use during the course of the treatment? I think this very largely depends on the case, but, I think, still more on the analyst. The very fruitful discussion following your questionnaire has shown what a wide scope one must allow for differences in technique even if one might one day (let us hope!) come to the result of agreeing with fundamental principles.

The way of interpreting, as well as the whole technique, is so much an outcome both of the personality and the analytical ways of the analyst that I do not think one will be able to come to a definite rule as to how much reassurance to use. One might surmise that an analyst might be able to interpret things earlier and in such a way (laying out all those connections before the patient) that he feels less necessity to use so much reassurance. Another analyst might find his way better by putting more reassurance in between his interpretations. Still, I have got quite convinced in thinking this point over in connection with my cases that reassurance is an essential part of analysis and not only an emergency measure.

(PP/KLE/C.67 images 1–4)

In this text, Klein tries in general terms to understand and define the necessity and the limitations of reassurance as closely as possible. It is for her self-evident that in the state of knowledge at the time no fixed rule can be formulated about reassurance. She strives hard to account for the practice with various patients and by various analysts. But in all this she holds on to the crucial point, which is that actual reassurance only happens when the phantastically charged bad figures can be brought as such to an analytic investigation and are gradually subject to changes through this – so ultimately reassurance of anxiety is effected through interpretation. But she also considers that it may be necessary or essential on the way there to be available sometimes as a good object, as a 'helper', to relieve the anxiety temporarily so that the ego is not overcome by anxiety and can continue to function. Klein conceptualizes this point (or one aspect of it) theoretically not long afterwards as a manic position that is part of every person's development and enables the ego that is still weak to grapple progressively with depressive despair without becoming completely overwhelmed and paralysed. I think it is also perceptible in the quoted text that she is trying to capture in words the difficult balance between the necessity of reassurance in the service of development and its tendency quickly to become counterproductive (like the manic defence).

To which discussion context does this paper belong?

Glover's investigation of psychoanalytic technique in the 1930s

Glover had already published some detailed 'Lectures on Technique in Psycho-Analysis' in 1927, perhaps wanting to rectify what he considered to be Freud's omission in never having written a systematic description of the technique of his own analyses (Glover, 1927, 1955, p. 262). In the preface to his 1930s study, Glover explains that his first intention after being appointed as the 'Director of Research' at the Institute of Psycho-Analysis in London was to establish the therapeutic practice in the regions (Glover, 1955, p. vi). To this purpose, he drafted a questionnaire that was based around questions that had repeatedly been put to him over the years by candidates but also by experienced analysts. In his evaluation, he divides the material into ten main areas. Four of these concern interpretation (1. the general methods of interpretation, 2. the interpretation of anxiety, 3. various problems in interpretations, 4. free associations, forced phantasies and 'active' advice) and three concern the transference; the others address termination, psychotic cases and the relationship between theory and practice.

This questionnaire (Glover, 1940, pp. 143–147) was sent out on 8 July 1932 to 29 analysts, of whom 24 responded. The results of the initiative were then circulated to the British Psycho-Analytical Society for discussion. On 30 September 1933 a 'Supplementary Questionnaire' was sent out (Glover, 1940 p. 147; cf. Glover, 1955, p. 268), containing questions that had not been thought about in the first version. Afterwards some further discussions took place, and the results, together with some lectures that had been given at that time at the Society, were incorporated into the concluding report. This procedure is open to methodological objections – and the study has also been criticized accordingly, first by Fenichel (1942) in a review and more recently by Fine and Fine (1990). But *one* goal was nonetheless in my view achieved by Glover, namely that the investigation generated a stronger scientific concern with technical questions and discussion of these and so remedied a lack that he had complained about in his introduction (Glover, 1955, p. 261).

One point on which great uncertainty and obscurity evidently prevailed – as it turned out from this investigation – was the problem of the 'deep' interpretation and reassurance (cf. Fine & Fine, 1990), 'the reassurance problem was clearly unresolved' p. 1019). I would like to add here that in my original German article (Frank, 2005) I followed Strachey (1934) 'The nature of the therapeutic action of psychoanalysis', by translating 'reassurance' as 'Angstberuhigung' and the translator of his article, Valerie Merck, who points out in a footnote to the German translation (Strachey, 1935) of this groundbreaking paper:

> There does not seem to be any German word that means exactly the same as the English word 'reassurance'. In everyday speech it is similar to 'Beruhigung'. But it has come into use in psychoanalysis to describe attempts to alleviate anxiety directly through the patient's ego as opposed to the method of interpretation.
>
> *(Strachey, 1935, p. 505, translated quotation)*

The latter point – namely reassurance as opposed to interpretation – is Strachey's definition. Certainly though the use of 'reassurance' as a term was not always so completely uniform. A random sample from the English translations of Freud's works reveals that 'reassurance' was chosen for various German words, e.g. in 1922 in 'Dreams and telepathy', for 'beruhigende Versicherung', in 1932 in 'The acquisition of power over fire' for 'Trost', in 1936 in *Inhibitions, Symptoms and Anxiety* for 'versichert sein wollen gegen'. As far as I can tell, the concept does not appear in Freud as a technical term and seems to be occasionally mentioned otherwise but – at least in publications – hardly to have been discussed in more detail. If we then look for instance through Glover's (1927) *Lectures on Technique in Psycho-Analysis* we find 'reassurance' twice in a treatment-technical sense, for instance, in his observations concerning the opening stage of analysis. Here he states that it is not very helpful just to say to the patient at times that he is showing resistance, and then continues: 'The explanations we give at the commencement of analysis should where possible embody some interpretation along with reassurance, and it is here that the usual method of expressing early unconscious defence can be ventilated' (Glover, 1927, p. 332). He does not further explain at this point the nature of the encouragement but returns to our theme in a later section in connection with resistance. This concerns the fact that when a patient is silent we should first try to encourage him to talk (Glover, 1927, p. 513). At other places in the lectures, where Glover has used 'reassurance', the word has no treatment-technical meaning. It is similar with

Ella Freeman Sharpe's (1931) paper 'The technique of psycho-analysis' (my thanks to Ulrike May for the reference to these lectures). Here too there are colloquial uses as well as a technical discussion of when 'reassurement' is appropriate, when the patient very anxiously asks, 'I shall be all right, shan't I?' (Sharpe, 1931, p. 36).

In the first questionnaire of Glover's investigation 'reassurance' only appeared as a secondary point in the question about methods of dealing with anxiety. It had then, Glover reports, emerged in the context of the discussion about 'deep' interpretations that some further important issues were connected with it. The first concerned the relation between interpretations and the patient's anxieties, hence the question about the appropriate means of dealing with these anxieties (Glover, 1955, p. 282). The advocates of 'deep' interpretations regarded precisely these interpretations as the best means of dealing with anxiety; others argued for phased interpretations; and some had the feeling that in stages of prevailing anxiety a certain degree of psychic reassurance was necessary. Altogether the discussion generated much confusion and was the stimulus for addressing the problem again through the 'Supplementary Questionnaire'.

This second questionnaire enquired under the heading 'B. Additional to the Principles of Interpretation' about the respective definition of 'reassurance' (Glover, 1940, p. 147). The wording was as follows:

1 (Since the use of terms such as 'deep interpretation' and 'reassurance' may introduce some artificial distinctions.) *What do you understand by the term 'reassurance'?*
2 If you accept the term as distinct from interpretation, do you regard it as an essential part of analysis, or it only an emergency measure?

It emerged how differently the concept was defined individually, with most understanding it to refer to a reduction of anxiety not by interpretation but by means such as suggestion or reference to reality. Most respondents considered reassurance as an emergency measure; two regarded it as 'rare'. Most concurred in the view that a degree of reassurance was unavoidable in certain stages of the analysis.

Obviously Klein's observations reproduced above are to be categorized in this context. These may have been her response to the question in the second questionnaire about the use of reassurance. That is suggested, as well as by the content, by the fact that 'B.' is on p. 1 as well as the title 'Klein Supplementary'. Also on page 3 there is an explicit reference to the questionnaire and discussion: 'The very fruitful discussion following your questionnaire has shown what a wide scope one must allow for differences in technique.' We know from the printed meeting minutes of the British Psycho-Analytical Society that Glover presented the summary of the questionnaire responses on reassurance in analytic technique on 7 February 1934 (Int. Zschr. Psychoanal., 1934, p. 281). In my view it is therefore most probable that Klein wrote down her reflections on this subject, which are transmitted on the four pages presented here, between October 1933 – the second questionnaire having been sent out on 30 September – and January 1934, and gave them to Glover.

It would be interesting to read through the other analysts' answers as well and compare them with Klein's observations. Unfortunately, however, there are no written answers in the British Psycho-Analytical Society Archive from this questionnaire study (my thanks are due to Polly Rossdale for this information). In the Archive documents there are also no detailed discussion minutes available. The meeting minutes contain only summarizing comments. For example, they state on 5 April 1933:

> Glover then gave a Report on the Questionnaire on Technique sent out the previous year. A discussion followed, opened by the President and continued by Mrs Klein, Dr Schmideberg [. . .]. It was decided to continue systematic discussion at subsequent meetings and that a resume of the Report should be distributed before such discussion.

And on 3 May: 'A discussion of the Report on Technique was resumed, opened by Dr Glover,' and so on.

In his assessment of the questionnaire initiative, Glover concludes that the question of dealing with anxiety is in no way resolved and that there is only so far an emergent understanding of the complex nature of anxiety (Glover, 1955, p. 288). Klein's view at that time seems also to have entered into this statement. We can however describe the development of this discussion that led to this (provisional) result in more detail, since Glover also gives a detailed account of the lectures in 1932–1934 that were devoted to the subject of 'reassurance' at the British Society. As far as can be seen there were two evenings after the first, but still before the second questionnaire was sent out, in which this question was discussed. First Melitta Schmideberg, Klein's daughter, presented a short paper on 18 January 1933, in which she intervened in favour of reassurance at the beginning of the analysis of young children who show anxiety. Klein and Searl then emphasized in the discussion that reassurance is unnecessary when correct interpretations are given at the right time and that it often impairs the later analysis (Glover, 1955, p. 285).

On 13 June 1933 Strachey presented his now famous paper 'The nature of the therapeutic action of psychoanalysis' (Strachey, 1934). As already quoted above, he unambiguously defines reassurance as an exertion of influence in order to alleviate anxiety directly by means other than the method of interpretation. He states that reassurance can be described as 'behaviour on the part of the analyst calculated to make the patient regard him as a "good" phantasy object rather than as a real one' (Strachey, 1934, p. 148). He gives some reasons that lead him to doubt the advisability of this behaviour. He then sums up:

> his anxiety may be reduced; but this result will not have been achieved by a method that involves a permanent qualitative change in his super-ego.

> Thus, whatever tactical importance reassurance may possess, it cannot, I think, claim to be regarded as an ultimate operative factor in psycho-analytic therapy.
>
> *(Strachey, 1934, p. 148)*

It is slightly surprising that Klein does not mention Strachey's work in her observations, which, as becomes clear from her 1936 technique lectures (published in Steiner, 2017), she esteemed, and quotes in detail there. Of course Strachey's lecture was, however, not then yet available in printed form.

On the same evening of 7 February 1934, on which Glover put forward the summary of the responses on reassurance from the second questionnaire initiative, Melitta Schmideberg presented a more detailed paper on reassurance as a tool of analytic technique (the printed version was published in 1935). In it she discusses a great many issues to which I cannot do justice here. The advantage of her text is that it also contains examples that illustrate the framing of the problem. One of her key statements, which she does not however stringently maintain, is that theoretically as it were reassurance can always be avoided if the anxiety is dissolved by an interpretation. But in practice it repeatedly occurs that an analyst is unable to give the necessary interpretation. Schmideberg (1935, p. 316) emphasizes that she always analyses the anxiety as well as using reassurance, and hereby differentiates herself not least from Ferenczi's active therapy, which in her view did less to reduce anxiety than to increase acting out. Schmideberg felt that reassurance can only have the time-limited aim of momentarily easing the situation, and cannot be used to influence the patient's character or symptoms (p. 317). What she means by this can be clarified with the following example that concerns a case of her husband's (p. 308): a patient with severe hysteria came for treatment not by her own impetus but for the sake of her boyfriend's wishes. She began the analysis with a strong resistance and had great difficulties in speaking. Every other day she did not speak at all. In one session she was silent again and complained of severe headaches. The analyst gave her some pills for her headaches and advised her to remain quiet. Her immediate reaction was to begin to speak without any difficulty and thereafter the analysis proceeded more easily.

After Schmideberg's presentation, a discussion took place that Glover describes as reserved yet friendly (Glover, 1955, p. 288). Of the various standpoints that he presents, I will give only that of Klein. First Herford had recalled Abraham, who had explained the need to keep the analytic situation free and relaxed; and then, Glover states: 'Klein agreed that the correct form of reassurance was just as important as the correct form of interpretation and emphasized the importance of the analyst's own attitude towards the patient. Excessive anxiety was detrimental to the treatment' (p. 288). This essentially corresponds, as we have seen, to Klein's written response to the second questionnaire.

So whereas on the first evening (January 1933) there is evidence that Klein and her daughter held opposing views on reassurance (against and in favour, respectively), their principles and goals seem in the course of the discussion to have brought them closer together. At the beginning of 1934, both considered reassurance by interpretation to be desirable while also taking account of clinical difficulties in which this path is not always open, where it can then also be temporarily helpful to make recourse to reassurance. In terms of their clinical practice though, they will have adopted differing approaches, as the quoted example at least suggests.

Here also the limitations of this kind of questionnaire study become especially clear. As Fenichel (1942) has demonstrated, many questions (so also the answers) are far too general to be of any value – apart from the fact that some questions could not be answered by consultation but only by research. As concerns our particular issue, Fenichel writes: 'The answers to the questions concerning anxiety, especially about interpretation of anxiety versus reassurance against it, tell us nothing that was not clear beforehand: analytic interpretation of anxieties would be the method of choice, but reassurances often are unavoidable' (Fenichel, 1942, p. 232).

Interestingly in the British Psycho-Analytical Society Archives there is another document by Klein entitled 'Notes for General Meeting' (CIB/F01/51) – again typewritten and partly hand-corrected – in which she returns to Glover's investigation and specifically to the matter of reassurance. These 'notes' are also unfortunately undated, but it is clear from the content that they were written during the War. The catalyst for them seems to have been Glover's (1940) first publication of his findings, which also led to more general criticism of his administration. Here I would only like to quote the passage on reassurance, since it substantiates the possibility that the manuscript 'On reassurance' originates from the context I have supposed. Klein criticizes the fact that her attitude to reassurance is only represented with two sentences in the summary of the discussion of 7 February 1934 (see the above quotation). She suggests that the reader may in her case – as of course also with the other discussants – conclude that these sentences represented her assessment of the problem at that point in time, whereas her response to the questionnaire provided a more comprehensive commentary, in which she also emphasized the disadvantages and dangers of reassurance. If she had been asked, she would have suggested also the following point in her answer for publication in 1934, and here she quotes verbatim a sentence from the paper printed above:

> One result which the interpretation produces, i.e. to strengthen the belief in the good object, is effected by the correct reassurance as well, but the reassurance does not effect a diminishment of the anxiety of the bad figures, which is the most important part of the analytic work.

Klein therefore raises the question as to why the written answers have only been incorporated in anonymized form into the evaluation, whereas this was not the case with the summaries of the discussion points.

Klein's contribution in the light of her relevant publications

What is the relationship between Klein's contribution to the discussion in archive file C.67 and her published observations on the subject? She refers in her contribution to two publications – her 1929 paper on personification and her book *The Psycho-Analysis of Children* (Klein, 1932). In 'Personification in the play of children', Klein describes the point that concerns us here in almost identical terms. She states that 'the analyst assumes the hostile roles required by the play-situation and thus subjects them to analysis' (Klein, 1929, p. 203). The gradual dismantling of the excessive severity of the superego is thereby achieved in the play analysis and the development of the anxiety-inducing imagos progresses 'towards the kindlier identifications with their closer approximations to reality' (p. 203).

In 1932 Klein sets out the situation rather more comprehensively. She works from the premise that one of the child's greatest psychic achievements, which takes up a large part of his psychic energy, is mastering anxiety. The child therefore unconsciously values the objects above all according to whether they alleviate or arouse his anxiety. Accordingly he applies to them his positive or negative transference. In treatment technique this means that:

> [the analyst] should ensure the continuance of analytic work and establish the analytic situation by relating it to himself, at the same time referring it back, by means of interpretation, to its original objects and situations, and in this way resolve a certain quantity of anxiety. His interpretation should intervene at some point of urgency in the unconscious material and so open a way to the child's unconscious mind [. . .] Thus by making a *timely* interpretation – that is, by interpreting the material as soon as it permits of it – the analyst can cut short the child's anxiety, or rather *scale it down*, in those cases too where the analysis has started with a positive transference. [. . .] It follows from what has been said that not only a timely interpretation but a *deep-going* one is essential. If we have an eye to the full urgency of the material presented, we find ourselves obliged to trace not only the representational *content* but also the anxiety and *sense of guilt* associated with it right down to that *layer* of the mind which is being activated. But if we model ourselves on the principles of adult analysis and proceed first of all to get into contact with the superficial strata of the mind – those which are nearest to the ego and to reality – we shall fail in our object of establishing the analytical situation and reducing anxiety in the child.
>
> *(Klein, 1932, pp. 51–52; my italics)*

Both publications are primarily concerned with the reduction of anxiety by interpretation – that was Klein's discovery, her innovation. But it can be inferred that she also has reassurance very much in mind to some degree, for example from her statement that a precondition of work for many cases in the age of puberty consists in this, as some of these often difficult analyses fail 'unless we sufficiently take into account the adolescent's need for action and for expression of phantasy and are careful to regulate the amount of anxiety liberated and, in general, adopt an exceedingly elastic technique' (Klein, 1932, p. 139). (Both the above papers were certainly also known to Schmideberg and Strachey. In some of her reflections – compare for example the regulation of anxiety – Schmideberg probably referred to Klein's book. Strachey refers explicitly in his paper to Klein, including to *The Psycho-Analysis of Children.*)

At first then nothing essentially new is formulated in the unpublished contribution discussed here. All the same, the text reveals a consideration of various aspects that does not appear as such in the publications. It can be observed in the contribution that Klein is trying again to account to herself for exactly what is at stake in reassurance, that she is grappling with the problem and does not 'just know' (as a common prejudice against her would have it). It is worth noting in this context that Klein's remarks about 'correct'/ 'right' and 'wrong' interpretation or reassurance may be taken to mean that she was thinking about right and wrong. In my view the context makes clear though that Klein uses these words as short-hand for the necessity in 'correct' interpretations or reassurances for the analytic situation to have been understood in its essential dynamic connections. Cf. here also Fenichel's (1953) introduction to his essay 'Concerning the theory of psychoanalytic technique':

> In discussing the 'theory of technique' it is unfortunately still necessary to discuss the justification of this concept. There exist some views about the 'irrational' nature of psychoanalytic technique which oppose any attempt at constructing a theory of its technical principles [. . .] such conceptions must in the final analysis lead to that method itself being regarded as irrational, losing every characteristic of science and becoming pure art.
>
> *(Fenichel, 1953, p. 332)*

Klein's insights also emerged from a concerted endeavour in the analytic situation. We know for instance that in the earliest child analyses she had also at first spontaneously tried to use 'reassurance' – for example by telling the 2¾-year-old Rita a story or offering her handbag to her to search through when the small patient wanted to leave the room again (see Frank, 2009, p. 115ff., p. 125, p. 134). But increasingly she discovered that when she understood and interpreted the children's anxiety, this was the more effective means of reaching them and alleviating their anxieties over the long term.

Let us take another look at the period after the document was written. At the time of the discussion so far considered in the British Psycho-Analytical Society, Klein had not yet clearly differentiated the two fundamentally different – paranoid schizoid and depressive – anxiety-situations. This did not happen until a few years afterwards and it facilitated a subtler consideration of each of these situations, which however did not remove the fundamental dilemma. In Glover the issue of reassurance recurs in connection with psychotic patients. He reports a discussion of 2 May 1934, where there were obviously very diverse assessments of the advantages and disadvantages of reassurance with such patients (Glover, 1955, p. 336). Glover attributed this among other things to the uninspired form of the questions, but it was probably also due to the still inadequate theoretical conceptualizations that in these cases led to some further difficulties. What can be inferred from Klein's later publications about her views 'On reassurance' after the 1930s?

Klein's (1961) *Narrative of a Child Analysis* is both clinically and theoretically the most detailed source here. It is to the best of my knowledge the only later paper that also constantly discusses the issue of reassurance explicitly in relation to case material. Klein as is known conducted the four-month analysis of the ten-year-old Richard in 1941 in Scotland and recorded the sessions in detailed notes made from memory. The time limitation was clear from the outset and Klein was therefore also constantly under great pressure. This certainly contributed to her sometimes spontaneously making recourse to reassurance, without in every instance realising this herself (cf. the explanation of such an example in Frank, 2002). I am selecting two episodes in which she herself mentions this point.

In the 38th session there is some talk among other things about Klein's planned journey to London, which Richard knows about. He is worried about it and afraid that she will be caught in a bombing raid. Klein answers that 'the part of London where she was going to stay was not particularly unsafe'. And she adds in brackets: 'Obviously this reassurance had no effect' (Klein, 1961, p. 181). In the second annotation to the 65th session, she then records in a general way:

> I have repeatedly remarked that, in spite of not deviating in essentials from my technique, I sometimes answered questions, which had the effect of reassuring Richard. In this particular session I had not only answered a question but had given a very direct reassurance which I on the whole deprecate. What caused me to do this was that the child not only unconsciously feared the end of his analysis but consciously realized his urgent need for it. My knowledge that he might not, for years to come, have any opportunity for analysis, and the particular circumstance that his father had fallen seriously ill, no doubt had an influence on my counter-transference. The question will probably arise how far this affected the course of the analysis. I find it difficult to decide [...] But as a matter of principle I wish to repeat that even in this case it would have been more useful to have avoided this occasional reassuring attitude.
>
> *(Klein, 1961, p. 326)*

She further explains how reassurance led to the idealization of her person and monstrousness was split off and projected outwards. (This example is later also quoted by Feldman, 1993, in an article on reassurance.) There are situations then in which Klein consciously (or spontaneously) makes recourse to reassurance. However, in the examples that she presents she reflects on this critically: she describes the difficult countertransference situation in which she found herself, how she wanted to do something good for Richard, tried to do this by answering questions, encouragement and so on and how it did not actually have the desired effect.

In her monograph *Envy and Gratitude*, Klein discusses the same point in further detail. She talks about some analysts' attempts 'to strengthen feelings of love by taking the rôle of the good object which the patient had not been able to establish securely in the past' (Klein, 1957, p. 225). She emphasizes how greatly such a procedure differs from the technique 'which, by helping the patient to achieve a better integration of his self, aims at a mitigation of hatred by love' (p. 225). According to her observations, techniques based on reassurance are rarely successful in the long term. There is in every person a deep need for reassurance rooted in the early relationship with the mother. For the analysis that means:

> This longing for reassurance is a vital factor in the analytic situation and we must not underrate its importance in our patients, adults and children alike. We find that though their conscious, and often unconscious, purpose is to be analyzed, the patient's strong desire to receive evidence of love and appreciation from the analyst, and thus to be reassured, is never completely given up. . . .The analyst who is aware of this will analyse the infantile roots of such wishes; otherwise, in identification with his patient, the early need for reassurance may strongly influence his countertransference and therefore his technique. This identification may also easily tempt the analyst to take the mother's place and give in to the urge immediately to alleviate the child's (his patient's) anxieties.
>
> *(pp. 225–226)*

So there is an understandable wish for reassurance or confirmation, which we may share in the countertransference (and that we are also urged to share) – it seeks the avoidance of anxiety or pain. But actual strengthening results from the experience that the object does not have to avoid these anxieties, pains, disappointments and so on, that these can be tolerable and a way of dealing with them can be found.

Closing remarks

The impetus for Klein, probably in Autumn or Winter 1933, to write rather more than three pages 'On reassurance', was the investigation of psychoanalytic technique that Edward Glover initiated and conducted in the 1930s at the London Institute of Psycho-Analysis. The document reproduced above is a further testimony to Klein's committed participation in the activities of the London Institute, of which I presented two years ago another example from the late 1930s. At that time she made available to Glover extensive anonymized analytic material in the context of a study of reactions to the Munich Crisis (Frank, 2003).

At the end of his report, Glover made a summary of the findings and formed three categories: 1. areas about which there was almost complete agreement; 2. points on which two thirds of those surveyed could agree about general tendencies; and 3. questions about which there were marked differences of opinion. He ascribes the findings of the enquiry about reassurance to the second category and records that the general tendency was to understand *reassurance* as the reduction of anxiety by non-interpretive means; it is considered as an unavoidable recourse in certain stages of analysis, and it is seen as an additional measure, not an alternative to interpretation (Glover, 1955, p. 346). Klein's contribution can also certainly be subsumed into this category. Klein's balanced discussion of this set of problems may, however, have surprised some people and does not appear as such explicitly in her publications.

Finally I would like to note that to my knowledge there is little more detailed literature on reassurance following this period. However from the Kleinian side, Feldman (1993) has published an important clinical study.

Note

1 An earlier version of the chapter was first given as a lecture at the 17th Symposium on the History of Psychoanalysis held on 13–15 February 2004 in Tübingen. It was then published as Frank (2005): 'Angstberuhigung' – Zu Melanie Kleins unveröffentlichtem Beitrag 'On reassurance'. In *Luzifer-Amor. Zeitschrift zur Geschichte der Psychoanalyse*, 36, 23–41. This translation is by Sophie Leighton.

References

Feldman, M. (1993). The dynamics of reassurance. *Int. J. Psychoanal.*, *74*, 275–285.

Fenichel, O. (1942). Review of an investigation of the technique of psycho-analysis. E. Glover (ed.), with assistance of M. Brierley (1940). *Psychoanal. Quart.*, *11*, 230–234.

Fenichel, O. (1953). Concerning the theory of psychoanalytic technique. In H. Fenichel and D. Rapaport (eds), *The collected papers of Otto Fenichel, first series*. New York: Norton.

Fine, S. and Fine, E. (1990). Four psychoanalytic perspectives. A study of differences in interpretative interventions. *J. Amer. Psychoanal. Assn.*, *38*, 1017–1041.

Frank, C. (2002). Verstehen und Missverstehen. Zur Entwicklung vom 'Wisstrieb' und seinen Hemmungen bei Melanie Klein zu 'Konzeptionen/Misskonzeptionen' bei R. Money-Kyrle. (Understanding and misunderstanding. On the development of the knowledge drive and its inhibitions in Klein to 'conceptions/misconceptions' in Money-Kyrle.) Semester-Journal, special issue of the Karl-Abraham-Institut/Freie Universitat Berlin, *Studiengang Psychologie, Fragen an die Sphinx*, U. Engel, L. Gast and A.-K. Oesterle-Stephan (eds), pp. 21–37.

Frank, C. (2003). Zu Melanie Kleins zeitgenossischer Bezugnahme auf Hitler und den Zweiten Welkrieg in ihren Behandlungen. (On Melanie Klein's contemporaneous references to Hitler and the Second World War in her therapeutic sessions.) *Psyche*, *57*, 708–728. Also in this book Chapter 6.

Frank, C. (2005). 'Angstberuhigung' – Zu Melanie Kleins unveröffentlichtem Beitrag 'On reassurance'. *Luzifer-Amor. Zeitschrift zur Geschichte der Psychoanalyse, 36*, 23–41.

Frank, C. (2009). *Melanie Klein in Berlin. Her first psychoanalyses of children.* E. Spillius, (ed.). Trans. S. Leighton, and S. Young. London: Routledge.

Glover, E. (1927). Lectures on technique in psycho-analysis. *Int. J. Psychoanal., 8*, 311–338 and 486–520.

Glover, E. (1940). *An investigation of the technique of psycho-analysis. Research Suppl. 4 to Int. J. Psychoanal.* London: Balliere, Tindall and Cox.

Glover, E. (1955). *The technique of psycho-analysis.* New York: Int. Univ. Press.

Hinshelwood, R. (1989). *A dictionary of Kleinian thought.* London: Free Association Books.

Int. Zschr. Psychoanal. (1934). Minutes of the British Psycho-Analytical Society, 7 February 1934. *Internationale Zeitschrift für Psychoanalyse, 20*, 281.

Klein, M. (1929). Personification in the play of children. *Int. J. Psychoanal., 10*, 193–204.

Klein, M. (1932). *The psycho-analysis of children.* London: Hogarth Press.

Klein, M. (1935). A contribution to the psychogenesis of manic-depressive states. *Int. J. Psychoanal., 16*, 145–174.

Klein, M. (1961). *Narrative of a child analysis. The conduct of the psycho-analysis of children as seen in the treatment of a ten-year-old boy.* London: Hogarth Press.

Klein, M. (1957). *Envy and gratitude.* In M. Khan (ed.), *Envy and gratitude and other works, 1946–1963.* London: Hogarth Press.

Schmideberg, M. (1935). Reassurance as a means of analytic technique. *Int. J. Psychoanal., 16*, 307–324.

Sharpe, E.F. (1931). The technique of psycho-analysis. *Int. J. Psychoanal., 12*, 24–60.

Steiner, J. (2017). *Lectures on technique by Melanie Klein: Edited with a critical review by John Steiner.* London: Routledge.

Strachey, J. (1934). The nature of the therapeutic action of psychoanalysis. *Int. J. Psychoanal., 15*, 127–159.

Strachey, J. (1935). Die Grundlagen der therapeutischen Wirkung der Psychoanalyse. *Internationale Zeitschrift für Psychoanalyse, 21*(4): 486–516.

8

'IS IT AN ANIMAL INSIDE?'

Melanie Klein's unpublished 'Don Juan' paper (1939)[1]

Claudia Frank

Introduction

Melanie Klein had been asked to contribute an article to the issue of the *International Journal of Psychoanalysis* celebrating Ernest Jones' sixtieth birthday. In this chapter I describe how she hurriedly wrote a text about Don Juan which, however, was rejected by the editor. The material is to be found in the Melanie Klein Archives at the Wellcome Library in file PP/KLE/C.91, also available online. I discuss the manuscript in the context of Klein's published work as well as of the relevant contemporary literature. In Klein's view, Don Juan's genitality is determined by oral impulses and fears. He attempts to ward off a depressive breakdown through a manic acting out. The chapter ends with some reflections about why Klein, contrary to her intention, failed to revise her manuscript for later publication.

First conceptual draft and the context of the project

In archive file C.91 it seems that Klein first set down the idea that was to be realized in her unpublished Don Juan paper in a handwritten page in German with some English words, to be found in image 79 of the file. The paper itself exists in fragments in the first part of the file. Finally in its fullest form, in typescript with handwritten deletions, amendments and additions and marked 'Don Juan better copy', it forms the latter part of the file, from image 96 onwards. As both the handwritten fragment below and the full paper are undated, I cannot ultimately prove my hypothesis that this mostly German fragment in image 79 is the embryonic form of the later project. However, the nature of the annotations suggest that this is the case. The text reads as follows:

> Ich u. Es Obey
>
> *Freud s. 404 Todesangst des Melancholikers – DonJuan der stirbt, – weil [er] das Aufgefressen – werden seines guten Objektes nicht erträgt – kann gutes Objekt nicht festhalten – Untreue zur Frau weil –* [er] *das bose Obiekl kontinuierlich fiittem muss – (who has got the other women when he satisfies himself with one woman?) – urspr. Gier die auf böses fressendes Objekt projiziert ist sowohl rivalry u. Gier live*

In English this reads:

> Ego & Id Obey
>
> Freud p. 404, the melancholic's fear of death – Don Juan who dies – because [he] cannot tolerate his good object being devoured – cannot hold on to a good object – infidelity to woman because – [he] must continually feed the bad object – (who has got the other women when he satisfies himself with one woman?) – orig. greed that is projected on to bad devouring object as well as rivalry & greed live

To readers unfamiliar with the material, this page may be only partly comprehensible. Purely linguistically, the first striking feature is the few English words embedded in the predominantly German text – whereas the full-length 'Don Juan' manuscript is entirely written in English. Is Klein possibly reverting – in relation to a first creative idea – in a two-fold way to her roots: to Freud, to whose collected works she has obviously referred in the original and to her mother tongue? Let us consider the individual words.

The word in the heading on the right 'Obey' stands for the play *Don Juan* by the French author André Obey, which Klein has chosen as the basis for her reflections on Don Juan. More immediately accessible are the words in the middle of the heading, 'Ego and Id'. We might at first consider them to be an association to her theme, which would of course make sense, especially to the Id as the site of the drives. But the second line makes it clear that this refers to Freud's text *The Ego and the Id*, in which Klein has evidently read about the fear of death in melancholia. As a reminder: Freud wrote here:

> The fear of death in melancholia only admits of one explanation: that the ego gives itself up because it feels itself hated and persecuted by the super-ego, instead of loved. To the ego, therefore, living means the same as being loved – being loved by the super-ego, which here again appears as the representative of the id.
>
> *(Freud, 1923, p. 58)*

The point that was relevant to Klein in this context is therefore not connected with what we generally understand as relating to the drives but refers to a highly specific superego problematic that is nevertheless entirely charged with the drives.

Then follows the key idea, to be elaborated in the manuscript, concerning the oral (eagerly devouring) object-relational world that gives rise to the Don Juan figure, which is complicated among other things by projection and introjection. The English quotation in brackets is from Obey's play. In the next and final phrase, two more English words are mixed into the German ('rivalry', 'live') as if the author were already envisaging the dictation of the English explanations.

From what period does this page originate? The most obvious supposition is that Klein wrote it shortly after she became familiar with Obey's play. She explains (C.91, images 101–102) that she is referring to Obey's play *Don Juan* that was staged a few years earlier in London by La Compagnie de Quinze. As the play had not been published, she says that she can only refer to the printed synopsis and a few notes that she made at the time. The programme with the printed synopsis is preserved among her documents, and the date of 5 March appears on the page with the cast list, though without a year. I was able to find a later French publication (Obey, 1977, p. 239), which provides the following information.

André Obey (1892–1975) wrote three versions of the play. The first, *Don Juan*, was staged at the London Globe Theatre in 1934, with Pierre Fresnay appearing as Don Juan and Marie-Hélène Daste as Elvire. The theatre and actors correspond to the information in Klein's programme. We can therefore assume that Klein saw this first version on 5 March 1934. For the sake of completeness, the two other versions are mentioned, which she may or may not have known. The second version bore the title *Le Trompeur de Séville* and was shown in 1937 in Porte-Saint-Martin. Essentially for this only the prologue (and this also changed) and the first half of the third act were included from the first version. But Obey was still not satisfied with it and so in 1947 he produced a third version, which is the only one available in print under the title *Don Juan ou L'Homme de Cendres*. Because of the comprehensive revision he made, we cannot use it here to gain a closer impression of the play that Klein saw. We must make do with the synopsis in the programme and Klein's own notes. This page of ideas in German shown in image 79, however, may be some or all of the 'few notes' that she stated she had made 'at the time' (C.91, image 102).

The possibility cannot however be excluded that the page was written close in time to the actual paper, and therefore that when writing it Klein was initially establishing her main thoughts while referring back to some earlier notes. As already noted, the full-length manuscript is also undated, but the time can be relatively clearly determined because of some references contained in it. First, it must have been written after 7 July 1939 because it refers (C.91, image 113) to Paula Heimann's lecture 'On sublimation', which was given on that date (see Hinshelwood, 1997, p. 883 and Chapter 11, p. 191–192 of this volume) at the British Psycho-Analytical Society. Second, it must have been completed before the publication of 'Mourning and its relation to manic-depressive states' at the beginning of 1940 since although this paper was referenced (Klein, 1940) this was only as a lecture at the 15th IPA Congress in Paris in 1938 (C.91, image 99). We know that, when Klein refers to her own published papers, she always gives the publication dates; see for instance C.91, image 18, which gives a reference to Klein (1937) or image 20, which references Klein (1935).

There is an extant correspondence between Klein and James Strachey and Ernest Jones (PP/KLE/A.16) that enables us to restrict the period of time yet further. When the Second World War broke out, Strachey took over the editorship of the *International Journal of Psychoanalysis* from Jones. As Grosskurth (1995, p. 249) reports, Jones appealed in a letter on 28 October 1939 to Klein's 'patriotic duty' to send him something. According to Grosskurth, she immediately sent him a paper about the Don Juan syndrome, which he rejected because it did not conform to their usual standards; this Klein accepted.

If we look at archive file PP/KLE A.16, a letter from Strachey to Klein on 9 November 1939 shows that they had already been endeavouring for some time to obtain from her a contribution to the 'Jones number' of the *International Journal*, to celebrate Ernest Jones' sixtieth birthday. On 15 March 1939 Bibring had invited her to contribute to the issue and had given 1 July as the latest delivery date. Over the summer Strachey had telephoned her twice on this matter and extended the deadline to 1 September and so on. Finally came Strachey's letter to Klein of 28 October, already mentioned by Grosskurth, in which he writes that 7 November is now the last possible date for submitting a paper for the Jones issue. 'I very much hope that you will make a final effort to let me have yours, which I should value most particularly.' On 7 November, Klein sent him the Don Juan manuscript from Cambridge with the following accompanying letter.

Here is the paper at last. I have various points on which to ask your help.

> I shall be most grateful for any suggestions you can make about the English; or about anything which is not clearly enough expressed, or if there are repetitions.
>
> As regards the case history, which I have written at the very last moment,[2] I am not sure whether it could be put as a footnote or inserted in the text, and should be glad for your suggestions about that [. . .]
>
> There are three footnotes which I am afraid I have to trouble you about [. . .]
>
> I feel rather uncertain about the part of the paper from p. 30 to the first line on p. 32, because I had something special in mind but am not sure whether I have made it clear enough.[3]

There had already been some talk of Strachey rejecting the paper. Accordingly, Klein wrote to Jones on 29 November that she was sorry that 'your special number of the Journal' would appear without a contribution from her: 'I want to let you know that my not finishing this paper in time and to my satisfaction is because of the difficulties arising from the outbreak of war.' She said that she had devised the first part and enjoyed writing it before the holidays. The second half entailed some fairly hard work. As a result of war breaking out, however, her entire impulse to write had disappeared. 'Anything I could write seemed so utterly unimportant in comparison to world happenings.' Moreover, she had had to make some important decisions for herself and others, including about her move to Cambridge. It was not until ten days before printing that she had felt in any way able to write again. But she would then have needed a few more weeks. Her only consolation was that the essay would benefit from a revision without any time pressure.

As concerns the date of the conceptual draft of image 79, this might therefore also theoretically have been committed to paper in the weeks after Bibring's request of 15 March 1939. The first few pages of the final manuscript (which cannot be identified as such with certainty because they are probably amplified in images 17–20 and 30–33) would then have been written before the summer holidays, but most of it probably only in response to Strachey's letter of 28 October 1939 with the last, urgent appeal.

What additional context might there be for the project that was, I am suggesting, outlined in our key page of C.91, image 79? Klein's starting-point, insofar as can be gleaned from the text, is clinical experience with melancholics (significantly she turns Freud's *fear of death in melancholia* into the *melancholic's fear of death*). She evidently believed that she was finding an eloquent example of her pertinent experiences, which she was gradually conceptualizing in a new way, in this foray into applied psychoanalysis. Already ten years previously, in her paper 'Infantile anxiety situations reflected in a work of art and in the creative impulse' (Klein, 1929), she had illustrated anxiety situations encountered in her child analyses since 1921 by means of artworks such as Ravel's children's opera *L'Enfant et les sortilège*. And 15 years after our project, in 'On identification' (Klein, 1955), she went on to clarify her concept of projective identification using the example of Julien Green's novel *Si j'étais vous* (cf. Frank, 2007).

We know that in the 1930s Klein was intensely concerned with the psychogenesis of manic-depressive states, with mourning and melancholia (see Klein, 1935, 1940), and developed a further cornerstone of her specific theory of psychic development: the so-called 'depressive position', i.e. the supposition that in every development a 'melancholia in *statu nascendi*' has to be undergone (Klein, 1940, p. 345). The 'melancholic's fear of death' indicated on our page therefore fits precisely with her focus of research at that time. In 1936 Melanie Klein and Joan Riviere gave public lectures in which Klein presented her new observations on the theory of the depressive position. Under the title 'Love, guilt and reparation', these were published in 1937. In the section on 'Difficulties in family relationships', she discusses among other things infidelity and also discusses Don Juan in this context: he is persecuted by the fear of the death of people he loves and therefore of the emergence of depressive feelings against which he has developed his own special form of defence, infidelity:

> By means of this he is proving to himself over and over again that his *one* greatly loved object (originally his mother, whose death he dreaded

> because he felt his love for her to be greedy and destructive), is not after all indispensable since he can always find another woman to whom he has passionate but shallow feelings [. . .] But through his attitude towards women an unconscious compromise finds expression. By deserting and rejecting some women he unconsciously turns away from his mother, saves her from his dangerous desires and frees himself from his painful dependence on her, and by turning to other women and giving them pleasure and love he is in his unconscious mind retaining the loved mother or re-creating her [. . .] In unconscious phantasy he is re-creating or healing his mother by means of sexual gratifications (which he actually gives to other women), for only in one aspect is his sexuality felt to be dangerous; in another aspect it is felt to be curative and to make her happy.
>
> *(Klein, 1937, p. 323)*

Don Juan in the contemporaneous psychoanalytic literature

To be able to evaluate Klein's contribution, we must first form a picture of the state of debate concerning Don Juan at that time in the specialist psychoanalytic world. In my view it is worth distinguishing on the one hand between the literature that mainly deals with Don Juan as a poetic (and musical) figure, and, on the other, statements that are primarily seeking to understand Don Juanism as a clinical phenomenon. These categories can of course overlap.

In the first category, I should start by referring to Otto Rank's monograph *The Don Juan Legend* (Rank, 1975), which was originally published in 1924 by the Internationaler Psychoanalytischer Verlag (*Die Don Juan-Gestalt*). To prepare us for what is to come, Rank begins by sharing with us his experience when listening to Mozart's *Don Giovanni* 'from a psychoanalytic point of view – an attitude that strives to "exclude[s] from consideration the conscious goals of the erotic hero"' (Rank, 1975, p. 38). It is easily noticeable there, yet somewhat surprising, that in Rank's view the plot actually illustrates anything but a sexual adventurer but instead a poor sinner persecuted by misfortune and finally making the Christian journey to hell in accordance with the destiny that befits his social environment. Rank goes on to explain this idea and shows how Leporello can be understood as a split-off part of Don Giovanni and the statue of the commander as the representative of the ideal ego, and so on. Freud's quotation from an aria in Mozart's *Don Giovanni* in a footnote on the 'Schreber case' (Freud, 1911, p. 30) attests how well he knew the opera, however in Freud's published work there are no more specific observations on the Don Juan figure.

The other papers in this group that can be cited do not touch on the Mozart opera with which Rank is concerned but are instead incidental findings or observations. The best-known might here be Ferenczi's (1922) paper on 'The symbolism of the bridge' in which he refers to the legend that Don Juan lit his own cigar on the Devil's across the Guadalquivir River (p. 167). This element mainly serves him as confirmation of his earlier considerations on the unconscious meaning of the bridge, namely its 'phallic, life and death symbolism' (p. 168).

If we turn to my second category, papers predominantly devoted to the clinical phenomenon, we find – insofar I can ascertain – that there are no more detailed published testimonies but countless observations made more or less in passing of which I am presenting only a small selection here. Accordingly, Ferenczi briefly deals in this lecture 'On the nosology of male homosexuality' with Don Juanism, as 'the obsessive and yet never fully satisfied pursuit of continually new heterosexual adventures' (Ferenczi, 1952, p. 316), which he understands under the heading of 'compulsive heterosexuality' as an expression of the repression of same-sex love. Abraham (1922) quotes Don Juan with regard to the frigidity of the prostitute: how Don Juan 'avenges himself on all women for the disappointment which happened to him once on the part of the first woman in his life, and the prostitute avenges herself on every man' (p. 21). Alexander (1930) points out that Don Juan types with their pursuit of ideals never to be attained are only too familiar to the psychoanalyst (p. 299). Referring back to Rank's monograph, Fenichel (1933) also states that Don Juan's behaviour is doubtless based on the Oedipus complex. In the analysis of such patients, however, strong pregenital fixations emerged (p. 565).

Don Juan was discussed more thoroughly, including by Freud, in the Wednesday meetings of the Vienna Psychoanalytic Society, as can be gleaned from their minutes, although these were published only later from 1962 (Nunberg & Federn, 1962–1975) and so were not previously available to analysts who had not taken part. In relation to the Don Juan theme, on 18 November 1908 Fritz Wittels presented a paper on 'Sexual perversity' in which he commented that Don Juan was 'the counterpart of the onanist and therefore identical with him' (Nunberg & Federn, 1962–1975, vol. 2, p. 51). Stekel expresses the view in the discussion of 17 February 1909 that Don Juan is driven by a homosexuality that is never gratified, against which Federn stresses that he sees Don Juan as the person satisfied with every woman who for that very reason goes to another one (p. 142). Freud also states that Stekel's conception is an 'error' (p. 161). The minutes of his contribution continue:

> Poetically, one could construct these conditions approximately in the following manner: the mother is very affectionate and has a great need for love; initially she was conquered gallantly by the father, but later she was neglected by him; he is a stern, cruel, but just man, living somewhere far from wife and child. From the beginning, the mother is very affectionate towards her small son, but she must soon die. The boy then grows up in deprivation ... As the second decisive experience, a girl would have to appear during his earliest years of puberty; this girl makes many advances

> to him, but is suddenly carried off by illness ... Again and again he must conquer what he has lost. Don Juan's father, on his deathbed, confesses to him a paranoiac love for the image of a saint.
>
> *(p. 161)*

Freud refers to this idea again on 1 May 1912 when he considers the 'substitution, by way of the series, for a lost love ideal' (Nunberg & Federn, 1962–1975, vol. 4, p. 98) as the general root of Don Juanism (p. 92). On 21 February 1912 there is also some detailed discussion of Don Juan. Reik presents a paper about 'The parental complex as cultural ferment' and states in this context that Don Juan on the one hand can never find enough and on the other hand never find the one. In the discussion, Rank refers to Ferenczi's above-mentioned lecture in connection with Don Juan as a 'heterosexual[s] by compulsion' (p. 53).

In summary, it can be stated that the psychoanalytic publications of the time repeatedly made reference to the clinical phenomenon of Don Juanism but without any more detailed illustration being given.

Melanie Klein's Don Juan paper

What might have motivated Klein to devote a specific paper to Don Juan? Perhaps something in the production of Obey's play struck such a chord that it generated a creative idea that was then waiting for an opportunity to develop? After all, as Alix Strachey observed as early as 1925, Klein had lots of ideas 'clearly capable of crystallising in her mind. She's got a creative mind, & that's the main thing' (Meisel & Kendrick, 1986, p. 203.) The opportunity to develop this particular idea might have come with Strachey's appeal or Bibring's request –albeit at a time when she could not concern herself with it wholeheartedly. But regardless of what the trigger was for writing her manuscript, the original impetus dated back to years earlier.

I will turn now to the manuscript itself. It begins as follows:

> The Don Juan as we generally picture him is well described by the French author, André Obey, in the following words, referring to the principal character in his play 'Don Juan': At twenty-five years of age he typifies all the ardour, the impetuosity, the fire, the youth, the pride of Spain – he is also representative of human weakness.
>
> *(C.91, image 96)*

Klein goes on to comment that she has observed in her analytic work, as was also confirmed in daily life, that men of the Don Juan type easily become unhappy or even mentally ill when they go through a certain change 'such as falling deeply in love with one woman and striving to remain faithful to her' (C.91, image 97). Her thesis is that by his kind of relationship to women a Don Juan is holding in check specific anxieties that lie at the basis of a depression and so partly safeguarding his mental stability. In her paper, she wants to show the fundamental role that early depressive feelings play in the structure of Don Juan. For reasons of space she can neither describe in detail what internal and external conditions lead to the conflicts of early development turning out in this way nor go into other authors' contributions on the Don Juan problem. But she says she will refer to two theories that have been fully confirmed in clinical practice, namely to Freud's (1912) concept of the separation between the sensual and the tender currents in some men, and to Felix Boehm's (1920) conception of Don Juan as a latent homosexual.[4]

She continues – and I will now quote Klein's own words again directly:

> In order to illustrate my thesis as to the central significance of early depression in the structure of Don Juanism I shall draw upon the play by Obey ... In great contrast to the description just quoted which refers to Don Juan ... at the beginning of the play, Obey later on depicts him as a melancholic. In the words of the [1934 programme] synopsis: 'He is a prey to the constant consciousness of approaching death. His very restlessness is the effect of an intense inner loneliness and of the warfare between his spiritual aspirations, which he is unable to realise, and his uncontrollable desires.' When Don Juan returns after he has had to flee the country because he has killed the Commandeur who was defending his daughter Anna's honour, he is brought to trial, but is set free because Elvire comes forward and offers to marry him. 'For a time Don Juan is as happy with Elvire as it is possible for a man of his restless temperament to be. But the consciousness of approaching death takes possession of him, forcing him to fresh outrages. He seduces Elvire's servant in her own house. The servant commits suicide. Juan now endures the torment of the damned.' We see him crouched on the ground, and Elvire, leaning over him, says, in a low voice full of sympathy, referring to his uncontrollable passions: 'What is it, what is it? Is it an animal inside?' And Don Juan in a whisper says, 'Yes, yes, it is an animal. It feeds on women' ('il mange de la femme'). But Elvire's love cannot save Don Juan. She again forgives him, but he at once betrays her again with a prostitute whom he knew in former years. (The faithfulness to the original object – the mother – which exists in his unconscious mind besides the faithlessness, is indicated by the detail that most of the women Don Juan encounters in the play had already played a part earlier in his life.) While Elvire is busy with the preparations for the wedding, Don Juan is with the prostitute. The guests assembled for the wedding, and Don Juan appears, staggering out of a house. He had, while making love to the woman, placed a dagger on his heart, and in a passionate embrace with her caused the dagger to be driven deep into it.
>
> The greed, jealousy and envy, which are essential features in his nature, are illustrated by his saying to someone in the play, 'Who has got all the

> other women when I satisfy myself with *one* woman only?' If we connect his extreme greed with his constant fear of death, the conclusion presents itself that his greed is reinforced by this fear.
>
> Now his fear, in my view, does not relate to his own death only, but to that of all the women he may want. We know from his own words that women are in danger of destruction, that he is terrified lest the dreaded animal will devour them. Thus he is persecuted by fear that any woman he desires may die at any moment. This fear, however, reinforces his greed, for he must get the most out of them to save what he can for himself. He behaves like someone who expects a famine and hoards up food. I suggest that at bottom he is afraid both of dying from starvation and of being eaten up himself . . .
>
> Another and most important impetus to his greed comes from his identification with the animal inside him which is feeding on women. The animal in his unconscious phantasies wants food . . . The animal, dangerous to women, must also be felt as an internal danger to himself. He has to feed it constantly with the one food it requires, namely women, for otherwise it would turn on him and destroy him from within.
>
> But that is only one aspect of his relation to women. To interpret other more hidden ones I shall now leave the analysis of the play and refer to certain conclusions which I have presented elsewhere.
>
> *(C.91, images 101–108)*

With reference to her 1935 paper, Klein now explains how the baby in the infantile depressive position sees his good internal and external objects as threatened by destruction because he cannot protect them from his own uncontrollable greedy and hateful emotions. And as he attributes his greedy and aggressive impulses to the internal as well as the external object, he also fears corresponding attacks on himself. Klein explains that she wants to limit herself this time to the most fundamental form of the attack – devouring the object, and then continues:

> The destructive, greedy way in which the baby internalizes his loved objects is only one of the sources of danger to them. In the child's feelings further dangers await them within him. In his greed he not only devours the *external* object and destroys it in the process of taking it into himself, but he also devours his *internal* objects, for he feeds on them again and again. His loved objects are furthermore endangered by his internal 'bad' objects, which are quite as greedy and devouring as the individual feels he is himself. Thus greed, fears and sorrow relating to people he loves in the external world are experienced and reinforced in relation to his internalized objects. In addition to all these fears, however, lest its 'good' objects will be destroyed, the ego is itself in the utmost danger of destruction. Fear of starvation, which goes back to the infant's phantasied attacks on

> his mother's breast and whole body (the all-important source of food and goodness being destroyed), may be infinitely reinforced and intensified by the dangers which in his mind threaten his internalized 'good' objects. If these objects perish there is nothing left outside and inside him to protect him against his devouring objects, nothing to keep goodness inside him alive, nothing to *feed* him *within.*
>
> *(C.91, images 109–110)*

In this kind of state, Klein explains, these people cling to external objects, since they are thereby also trying to hold on to their internal good objects, which they experience a persistent fear of losing. This is important in connection with Don Juan and his object hunger (C.91, image 111).

Next Klein illustrates her conclusions with some 'oral material' (omitting the genital references) from the analytic sessions of a five-year-old boy ('A') that took place about one and a half years after the beginning of the treatment. I am limiting my illustration here to a few impressive vignettes (C.91, images 115–117). At times when the boy's anxieties were very acute, the mother would give him a bar of chocolate or ice-cream every day on leaving the waiting room.

> It had become a ritual that he began to eat it while looking down from the play-room at his mother, who waved to him as she left. In one particular hour, he again looked down at her as she was driving away and said, sadly, while eating his chocolate, 'How quickly she is off'. Then, still eating, he looked at me and said, 'What a pretty frock you have, and all right from top to bottom' . . . 'You know, the Bitey'. 'The Bitey' referred to an analytic hour of a year earlier. On that occasion he had attempted in a half playful way to bite my arms and legs. (At that period his urge to bite had become so manifest that he sometimes tried actually to bite his relatives also.) Then he touched my legs, saying that he wanted to see if they were still there. Shortly after that he said in a low and depressed voice, and as though speaking to himself, 'Kill the "Lickie"'. I explained to him, referring to his attempts to bite me and his guilt about this, that he actually meant 'Kill the "Bitey"', an interpretation which impressed him very much. Thereafter he occasionally referred to 'the Bitey' as something understood between us. To come back to the hour when he made the remark about my frock and spoke of 'the Bitie': Eating the chocolate stood for eating me (in the room), his mother (in the street), and therefore he had to reassure himself that she was still alive and could wave to him and that I was still all right 'from top to bottom' – that is to say, not eaten up. (A few days earlier, while eating his chocolate, he had pointed at something he seemed to see on my forehead and said 'You are melting'. I melted – as did the chocolate in his mouth.) After speaking of 'the Bitey' he said, 'Everyone bites everyone', and mentioned all the people at his

> home: 'X. (one maid) eats Y. (another maid) in the kitchen, Y. eats Mummy, Mummy eats Daddy, Daddy eats me, and I eat X.' As he said this he became very anxious. After that he moved about in the room, at first slowly, and also wanted me to move. Then he sat down on the floor and whirled himself round, becoming more and more anxious and excited. Often before, various quick or spasmodic movements and other physical signs of anxiety, in their analytic context, had expressed his feelings and fears about internal processes and happenings relating to his internalized objects. In the present hour he had imagined that the people at his home were eating each other while he was eating the chocolate (standing for me – his remark about my frock), and I had reasons for concluding that he felt they were eating each other inside him. His whirling round expressed, among other things, his attempts to stop the people inside him from eating each other, and was also a physical reaction to his fears of being attacked from within.
>
> *(C.91, images 115–117)*

I am passing over the additional material from this young patient's treatment, which illustrates both his greed and his attempts at reparation, and I will only now quote a closing remark in the case illustration.

> We can now more fully understand A.'s obsession for eating chocolate whilst with me. It was partly to prevent himself from eating me up in phantasy; but also because he had constantly to feed his internal people in order to stop them from devouring each other as well as himself.
>
> *(C.91, image 121)*

Pointing out that the chocolate also represented women (image 122), Klein returns to discussing Don Juan. She develops the argument that the depressive pattern that emerges in the protagonist of Obey's play is latently present in all Don Juans, whatever image they present on the surface. And then she raises the question of the connection between oral anxieties and the typical Don Juan's extraordinary genital potency and masculinity (C.91, image 123). In addition to the various sources of the anxieties that reinforce the oral greed that characterizes his relationships with women, there are some other sources of satisfaction and anxiety in connection with his genital feelings, on to which his oral greed and the related phantasies are very soon transferred (and which in her view play an important role even in the first year of life). She writes:

> If, in the boy's mind, his genital becomes so deeply imbued with oral qualities that it is intensely felt to be a devouring weapon, oral greed, anxiety, sorrow and guilt may dominate his genital relations to women. These are strongly influenced by the fact that his relation to his father also was from the beginning overshadowed by his oral impulses and fear, which

were responsible for the extent to which his father's as well as his own genital soon acquired terrifying qualities. This comes about not simply because he is dominated by sadistic urges and can therefore only conceive of a devouring genital, but also because in his jealousy and hatred of his parents' sexual intercourse he has wished to change his father's penis into an instrument of destruction (devouring animal, and so on). On the strength of his phantasies of having incorporated his father (and mother) he feels constantly endangered and persecuted internally by his father's genital (as well as by the whole father). This devouring father (in Obey's *Don Juan* the animal which feeds on women – in my little patient the foxes) in his mind not only threatens him, the child himself, with destruction but also his internalized loved mother. Since Don Juan has never sufficiently overcome his early depressive anxieties, he is a prey to the fear of loss of this unique and irreplaceable object – his internalized 'good' mother. The dangers which threaten her, however, through his own uncontrollable greed, in which he attacks her internally over and over again as soon as his resentment and grievances are stirred by any external or internal frustration. His despair of being able to protect her against the assaults of the devouring internalized father, are actually the core of the depressive position by which he is dominated. The overwhelming pain and sorrow which he suffers drive him to liberate himself from this slavish dependence on his mother. All these feelings constitute the fear of dependence which is a prominent feature in Don Juan's psychology. The ways in which he fights this fear are characteristic of his particular outcome of development. (Don Juan, as we know, is often aware of his wish to avoid strong emotional ties. His tendency to preserve his independence is one of the motives which he and others would commonly connect with his attitude towards women.)

His fears of harming and destroying his mother, whom he seeks in every woman he desires, by his oral greed and his dangerous genital, the fears of being devoured and punished by her, and by the dangerous penis of the father inside her, are allayed by the peremptory condition Don Juan is tied to in his love life, i.e. that he must not keep to one woman only. The various dangers which threaten himself and his partner are diminished through their being distributed over many women. Thus he is able to feel a woman's body and her genital as attractive and to love her for a time because as soon as his anxieties increase she and her body become 'bad' or injured in his mind, his feelings towards her change, she becomes 'unattractive' and he is already on the search for another woman. The very fact that it is more than one woman he desires and possesses enables him also to deny and disprove the truth that in the depths of his mind his desires, his greed, and the related dangers and anxieties, centre on the loved object only – his actual mother – whom he has internalized and on whom he is so utterly dependent.

[. . .]

> Together with the intense hatred and anxieties about his father's penis as an internal and external persecutor, the boy also feels a great libidinal attraction to it, loves and admires it. This admiration may mainly focus on the sadistic omnipotence of the penis (such boys may develop into asocial or manifestly sadistic individuals or – an entirely different outcome –fail to become potent); or it may, under the influence of an early and very strong feeling of guilt and drive for reparation, lead in the boy's mind to the conception of his father's penis as a most powerful instrument of pleasure and reparation.
>
> I have elsewhere ['*The Psycho-Analysis of Children*', Chapters 8 and 12] footnote in the original manuscript], in my description of the boy's development, expressed my view that male homosexuality is based on the oral sucking position towards his father's penis, which also in the infant boy follows closely on the oral attachment to his mother's breasts. I described there (*op. cit.*) in detail that in manifest homosexuals the libidinal attraction towards the father's genital has been reinforced and used as a means to cover up as well as to counteract and disprove the fears of it. The external penis becomes a panacea by means of which he escapes from the terrifying internalized organ (and father) and – this is decisive for his relations to women – the anxieties about his father's penis are shifted to his mother's body, which in his mind is turned into the receptacle for the 'bad' penis; his mother thus becomes unattractive (unconsciously, 'bad' and terrifying).
>
> In the turn of development, however, which may lead to Don Juanism, the attraction to the father's 'good' penis operates towards the father's penis inside the mother's body, and thus the attraction of her body is enhanced. His anxiety about the 'bad' penis of the father, however, is nevertheless also shifted to his mother's body, and has the effect of making her body and genital more and more 'bad' i.e. 'unattractive' to him as time goes on. Don Juan's attraction to a woman's body can as we already know persist only as long as his anxieties about the inside of her body or her genital are not too strongly aroused. Thus for a time the attraction to the 'good' penis of the father inside her may outbalance his fears of the 'bad' one, and even increase the attraction to her body. On the other hand, this way of focusing his attraction on the penis inside his mother is no doubt only possible if his mother's body itself has retained in the boy's unconscious mind a certain measure of the fundamental goodness.
>
> *(C.91, images 124–131)*

Klein explains this thought in some further depth and goes on to discuss the significance of the idealization: when the external good penis becomes the idealized object for the boy, the pendulum can swing towards homosexuality (C.91, image 133f). Finally, she summarizes as follows:

> His deep anxieties about internal danger-situations are partly counteracted and disproved by his genital potency. The pleasure and satisfaction which

> he himself and his partner derive from the genital act disprove in external relationships the fear both of his own devouring penis and that of his dangerous devouring father inside himself and inside his mother. The distribution of his genital desires and his anxieties among many women, moreover, follows the line of his oral impulses and of the methods by which he avoided and counteracted the results of his oral greed. [. . .] Thus he is driven from one woman to another, seeking to satisfy, cure and restore each in turn by means of his genital, only to rob and injure each in turn once more. He also satisfies his need continually to separate women from other men, since in the original situation he laboured under the constant fear of his father's devouring and destroying his mother in sexual intercourse, and therefore wanted to separate his parents, both in order to save his mother and to get her for himself.
>
> *(C.91, image 135f)*

I hope that by presenting these extracts from file C.91 I have managed to convey an impression of the main line of argument. In my view, Klein vividly works out how Don Juan attempts by his manic acting out to ward off a depressive breakdown, which he then actually suffers at the end of Obey's play in the form of a suicide. Klein (1935) had described a little earlier how in various forms of manic state 'that which is *first of all denied is psychic reality*' and how the ego at the same time 'endeavours ceaselessly to *master and control* all its objects' (italics in original), which is expressed in hyperactivity (Klein, 1935, p. 277). In her Don Juan paper, Klein elaborates the various facets of oral impulses and anxieties and shows how they contaminate the genital plane.

If we now take another look at the conceptual draft presented in the introduction (C.91, image 79), we find it contains everything essential already set out: the oral greed that is projected and potentiated by jealousy, which leads to fear of death; the object hunger and the associated infidelity, in which Don Juan both acts out and wards off his desire; and the ever-threatening melancholia.

'The author's dissatisfaction with it'

The external impetus to undertake writing an article about Don Juan was the invitation Klein received to contribute to a birthday issue for Ernest Jones, which leaves open the question as to what if any identifiable connection there may be between the theme and the person to be honoured. Klein herself makes no comment on this and her biographer Phyllis Grosskurth (1995) does not touch on this question either. She only remarks (p. 236) in relation to the Don Juan passage in the 1937 paper (see above) that Klein was clearly thinking of Emmanuel, Arthur and Klötzel, namely her brother, her husband and her lover. It seems obvious to me that Klein actually had her own deeper reasons for choosing this subject, whether that indirectly suggested by Grosskurth or others in the context of her concern with depression, which is also linked with her son

Hans' fatal accident in 1934. Moreover, the subject was appropriate to a tribute to Jones because of his interest in applied psychoanalysis.

But what may have led Klein, quite apart from the occasion, to undertake to devote a specific article to Don Juan? I think it becomes evident from the manuscript that Elvira's question 'Is it an animal inside?'[5] was central to Klein's interest in Obey's *Don Juan*, with all its associated considerations for her. The 'animal inside' provided an accurate picture of Don Juan's psychodynamics partly determined by oral impulses and anxieties, which explains both his actions and his defence. As far as I can see, this point had not previously been worked out in the same form. Rank (1975) certainly also refers to the fear of being devoured (p. 62ff.) but in another sense. He sees the Stone Guest as a personification of conscience pangs (p. 74) and a derivative of the corpse-demon who is avenging the primal crime. For him the Don Juan phenomenon is actually based on the mother's unattainability (i.e. the pre-natal desire situation and its compensatory substitute, p. 95). Accordingly, he also understands this being devoured as the deepest wish-fulfilment, namely as the return into the mother.

It is already apparent from the conceptual draft that the paper was motivated by a primary clinical interest and this becomes completely clear in the full-length manuscript presented above. Klein deals with the psychology of men of the Don Juan type, emphasizing that a general study even of specific factors is not enough to understand the entire structure of Don Juanism and its many variations (C.91, image 135). One focus is the exposition of the complex oral dynamics, illustrated not least by material from a child analysis. The text gives us a sense of the committed clinician whose elaboration of a genitality charged by oral material is sometimes found helpful to this day. Trevor Lubbe, for instance, used Klein's observations to understand a male hysteric (Lubbe, 2003, p. 1056), to the best of my knowledge the only published reference to the Don Juan paper to this day.

Strachey rejected the manuscript on 9 November 1939 with the following arguments: it was critical first that at this stage he would only have been able to accept a print-ready manuscript, and Klein's paper, as is already clear from her above-quoted accompanying letter, was still nowhere near that point. Besides, it gave Strachey the impression of having been hastily put together – not only in a superficial respect. He did not feel that in the present form it would do justice to her work but very much hoped to be able to publish it later in a revised version. Klein's answer is not available to us but she must have stated that she was straightforwardly in agreement with the rejection because Strachey expresses his relief in a letter of 15 November that she is not annoyed with him. He then amplifies a few points of criticism on the content. His main objection is that Klein has not treated the Don Juan character appropriately. Obey's play, which he has not seen, does not sound as if it paints a typical portrait of what we generally understand by Don Juan (at least on the surface). We would think of the character in Molière or Da Ponte (Mozart). The child's case, which is certainly interesting in itself, had no necessary connection at all with the Don Juan character. And the adult case[6] also revolves around a rather different problem. Altogether the paper seems to lack coherence – adding by way of qualification that he read it rather hastily and his criticism may prove to be unjustified.

On 20 November Klein thanks Strachey for his 'useful comments', without revealing what she thought of them in any more detail. All that is clear is that, contrary to her announcement to Jones in the quoted letter from the end of November, the text was not later published. Evidently Klein did not carry out any further revisions, for reasons unknown. My thoughts on this therefore necessarily remain speculative. A first idea emerges from comparing both the actual publications on applied psychoanalysis (Klein, 1929, 1955) that I have mentioned above. What I think makes these convincing are the many details that Klein had available to illustrate in the one case infantile anxiety situations and in the other case projective identification in their various forms. With Don Juan she 'only' had available the synopsis in the programme and her few notes. There was one essential detail ('the animal inside') that she was able, as we have seen, to address plausibly. Otherwise however she lacked the material to 'go through' the psychodynamics from beginning to end with Obey's protagonist as a possible Don Juan type, as she had done for the other themes in both the articles mentioned.

Now it could be objected that she would not have had to insist specifically on using Obey's *Don Juan* when there were certainly several hundred, if not thousands, of Don Juan plays, essays, libretti and so on available since what was thought to be the first Don Juan drama by Tirso de Molina in 1630. Why not for example use the most famous example, Freud's favourite opera Mozart's *Don Giovanni*? (That was also a thought of Strachey's.) Here too of course we cannot know the answer but I suspect that Obey's play was especially well suited to Klein's purpose because this Don Juan, unlike the other shapings of the material with which I am familiar, commits suicide. Here she found the manifest connection with the melancholia with which she was concerned at that time. In Obey this aspect emerged impressively, whereas in many other versions it is not directly thematized. Surprisingly though Klein does not go further into the feature of suicide, although melancholia plays a key role in her manuscript.

Furthermore, is it perhaps difficult to devote a convincing 'in-depth' study to a figure that also remains fairly blank because of its manic functioning, when there is a great deal that is specifically not intended to go deeper and is repeated any number of times? (It is not for nothing that da Ponte, the librettist for Mozart's opera, chose the stage in Don Juan's life at which something has stopped functioning uninterruptedly.) Does some of the attraction that the material undoubtedly has consist in the participation in a type of manic narcissistic state, which could be a reason for the depressive facets considered by Klein often remaining unexplained? And to what extent is Klein also succumbing to this attraction, despite the view she takes of what is being warded off? My surprise at how little space she has devoted to what Don Juan does with his objects led me to this question. Certainly in her paper there is much discussion of engulfing, devouring and destroying, but the contemptuous, cruel treatment of objects, the arrogance, triumph and so on that along with all charm do also belong to Don Juan do not appear in it. Klein has described all these things in another context. So we read for example in her 1935 paper that the '*disparagement of the object's importance and the contempt for it*' are a characteristic of mania (Klein, 1935, p. 278). But her knowledge did not enter (adequately) into the Don Juan paper.

It may also be because of Klein's later developed concept of projective identification that we find it easier to incorporate this aspect. For example we can see it as an indication that Don Juan fears not only being devoured but also being treated as small and incidental, and recklessly and contemptuously, in the same way as his objects are. It certainly also contains some reference to guilt, but the extent of guilt accumulated by this kind of life goes unconsidered. We know that for Klein at that time everything else was paling in comparison with world events. Is it possible that the threat posed by Hitler's Germany (on the intensity of her concern with this, see Frank (2003) and Chapter 6 of this volume) prevented her from looking more closely at Don Juan's ill-treatment of his objects, so that this aspect was certainly thematized but could not actually be addressed?

Notes

1 An earlier version of this chapter was presented in the original German on 24 February 2007 at the 20th Symposium on 'The History of Psychoanalysis' in Tübingen. It was then published as: Frank (2008) 'Ist es ein Tier im Inneren?' Melanie Kleins unpubliziertes 'Don Juan Paper' (1939). In *Luzifer-Amor*, 41, 120–140.This translation is by Sophie Leighton.

2 This may refer to three pages that are marked a–c (C. 91 images 141–143) and labelled 'case material'. This material concerns a man who has just turned 40 years old and was attached to the figure three in his love relationships, i.e. he could not have sex more than three times with one woman. He had now fallen in love with a woman with whom he wanted to overcome this condition and he did manage to extend the relationship beyond the fatal figure. For external reasons, there was a temporary separation during which the physical attraction disappeared. He wrote to tell the woman that he must separate from her and dated the letter to exactly three months after they had met, although this was actually three months and ten days earlier.

3 In these pages, Klein addresses the problem of aetiology in general: she considers the idea of a specific aetiology of certain pathologies in relation to the complex conditions of the earliest mental conflicts and their solutions. 'The interaction of primary aetiological factors, among which, in my view, the lesser or greater capacity of the early ego to tolerate anxieties plays an important part, has, as we know, a different complexion in every individual. Besides the quantitative factor, the time factor (the moment at which experiences arise and increase or diminish anxieties), the nature of these experiences, the setting in which they are lived through, and other factors – all these are bound to lead to different results in different individuals. This abundant variety of possibilities is still more complex through the effect early defence mechanisms have in influencing the nature of the experiences goes through, which again in turn strengthen some of the defences and weaken others. For instance, strong denial at an early stage of development (which again to a certain extent is influenced by certain external situations) may profoundly affect the relation to people, and thus lead to entirely different results in various individuals.'

4 In this paper, Boehm formulated his view that: '*The size of a person's heterosexual drive* is related to *the size of his monogamous tendency*, as the *size of a person's homosexual drive* is related to *the size of his polygamous tendency*'. Or, in short: 'Heterosex.: monogam. – Homosex.: polygam' (Boehm, 1920, p. 303, translated quotation).
5 The scene concerned appeared in the 1934 version which Klein saw in London, but does not appear in the third version of Obey's play, the only one to have been published.
6 See note 2.

References

Abraham, K. (1922). Manifestations of the female castration complex. *Int. J. Psychoanal.*, *3*, 1–29.

Alexander, F. (1930). The neurotic character. *Int. J. Psychoanal.*, *11*, 292–311.

Boehm, F. (1920). Beiträge zur Psychologie der Homosexualität. I. Homosexualität und Polygamie. (Papers concerning the psychology of homosexuality. I. Homosexuality and polygamy.) *Internat. Zeitschr. Psychoanal.*, *14*, 26–44.

Fenichel, O. (1933). An outline of clinical psychoanalysis – Chapter VII. *Psychoanalytic Quarterly*, *2*, 562–591.

Ferenczi, S. (1922). The symbolism of the bridge. *International Journal of Psychoanalysis*, *3*, 163–168.

Ferenczi, S. (1952). The nosology of male homosexuality. In *First contributions to psycho-analysis*. London: Hogarth Press and the Institute of Psycho-Analysis, pp. 296–318.

Frank, C. (2003). Zu Melanie Kleins zeitgenössischer Bezugnahme auf Hitler und den Zweiten Weltkrieg in ihren Behandlungen. (On Melanie Klein's contemporaneous reference to Hitler and the Second World War in her treatments.) *Psyche*, *57*, 708–728.

Frank, C. (2007). 'Ich bin du' und 'Du bist ich'. Angewandte Psychoanalyse als Untersuchungsfeld für Aspekte der projektiven Identifizierung im Kleinschen Denken. ('I am you' and 'You are me'. Applied psychoanalysis as a field of investigation for aspects of projective identification in Kleinian thought.) In *Projektive Identifizierung. Ein Schlüsselkonzept der psychoanalytischen Therapie.* (Projective identification. A key concept in psychoanalytic therapy.) C. Frank, and H. Weiss (eds), Stuttgart: Klett-Cotta, pp. 65–87.

Freud, S. (1911). Psychoanalytic notes on an autobiographical account of a case of paranoia. In *S.E. 12*. London: Hogarth.

Freud, S. (1912). On the universal tendency to debasement in the sphere of love. In *S.E. 11*. London: Hogarth.

Freud, S. (1923). The ego and the id. In *S.E. 19*. London: Hogarth.

Grosskurth, P. (1995). *Melanie Klein. her world and her work.* Northvale, NJ and London: Jason Aronson.

Hinshelwood, R.D. (1997). The elusive concept of 'internal object' (1934–1943). *International Journal of Psychoanalysis*, *78*, 8777–8897.

Klein, M. (1929). Infantile anxiety situations reflected in a work of art and in the creative impulse. In *Love, guilt and reparation and other works 1921–1945*. London: Virago, 1988, pp. 210–218.

Klein, M. (1935). A contribution to the psychogenesis of manic-depressive states. In *Love, guilt and reparation and other works 1921–1945*. London: Virago, 1988, pp. 262–289.

Klein, M. (1937). Love, guilt and reparation. In *Love, guilt and reparation and other works 1921–1945*. London: Virago, 1988, pp. 306–343.

Klein, M. (1940). Mourning and its relation to manic-depressive states. *International Journal of Psychoanalysis*, *21*, 125–153.

Klein, M. (1955). On identification. In *Envy and gratitude and other works 1946–1963*. London: Vintage, 1977, pp. 141–175.

Lubbe, T. (2003). Diagnosing a male hysteric. *International Journal of Psychoanalysis*, *84*, 1043–1059.

Meisel, P. and Kendrick, W. (1986) (eds). *Bloomsbury/Freud. The letters of James and Alix Strachey 1924–1925*. New York: Basic Books.

Nunberg, H. and Federn, E. (1962–1975) (eds). *Minutes of the Vienna Psychoanalytic Society, Vols. 1–4*. New York: Int. Univ. Press.

Obey, A. (1977). *Don Juan ou l'homme de cendres. Pièce en trois actes et un prologue*. Troyes (La recherche du théâtre perdu).

Rank, O. (1975). *The Don Juan legend*. Translated and edited by D. Winter. Northvale, NJ: Princeton University Press.

9

MELANIE KLEIN AND REPRESSION

An examination of some unpublished notes of 1934[1]

R.D. Hinshelwood

Introduction

Fifteen pages of unpublished Notes were found in the Melanie Klein Archives in file PP/KLE/B.89 dating from early 1934, a crucial moment in Klein's development. She was at this time moving away from child analysis, whilst also rethinking and revising her allegiance to Karl Abraham's theory of the phases of libidinal development. These Notes, entitled 'Early Repression Mechanism', show Klein struggling to develop what became her characteristic theories of the depressive position and the paranoid-schizoid position. Although these Notes are precursors of the paper Klein gave later to the IPA Congress in 1934, they also show the origins of the emphasis she and her followers eventually gave to 'splitting' rather than repression. The Notes give us an insight into the way that she worked clinically at the time. We see Klein's confidence develop as she diverged from the classical theories and technique. Her ideas were based on close attention to the detail of her clinical material, rather than attacking theoretical problems directly. The Notes show her method of struggling to her own conclusions, and they offer us a chance to grasp the roots of the subsequent controversy over Kleinian thought.

The work of Melanie Klein may be divided into two phases. Until 1935, she was basically working within the theoretical framework of Freud and Abraham, though she made many changes in it, some of them inadvertent. After 1935, with the two papers on the depressive position (Klein, 1935, 1940), the paper on the paranoid-schizoid position (Klein, 1946), and *Envy and Gratitude* (Klein, 1957), she developed a new theory of her own (Spillius, 1994, pp. 325–326).

The aim of this chapter is to introduce some significant pages of Notes from the Melanie Klein Archives to be found in file PP/KLE/B.89. A transcription of this file is appended at the end of the chapter and it may also be freely consulted in digital form on the Wellcome Library catalogue (see B.89 images 1–16). My interest was immediately aroused by the title of this file 'Early Repression Mechanism', as Klein makes very few references indeed to repression in the sizeable sum of her published work. In fact she emphasized 'splitting the object' at least as much in her early work, and in her later work she emphasized the mechanism of 'splitting of the ego', together with the extraordinary mechanism she called 'projective identification'. Amongst other things, to understand the differences in usage between splitting and repression would help to clarify the misunderstandings between different schools of psychoanalytic thinking.

On examining the Notes (as I shall refer to file B.89) I could see that they held very considerable further interest and importance. They do not actually carry a date, but circumstantial evidence from the content of the clinical material indicates with some confidence they were written in the early part of 1934. They are not earlier than February 1934, since reference is made to patient T in the 'first half of Feb 1934′ (Section I, page 1 – see Appendix). Later, there is a reference to Goering and Dimitroff (Section II, page 8). Dimitroff was accused of setting fire to the Reichstag in Nazi Germany – in February 1933. He was tried in December 1933 when Goering appeared in the proceedings and harangued the court (surprisingly, Dimitroff was acquitted). All this indicates a date during 1934 and after February that year. This is a very significant date, since Klein's thinking was in an active process of change at that very moment.

Spillius (1994) described a change around 1935, the date of publication of Klein's paper on the depressive position, although presumably the paper took a while to generate. In fact Klein gave it initially at the Lucerne Congress of the International Psychoanalytical Association in August 1934. Petot (1979, 1982) also described two similar phases of change, between 1919–1932, and 1932–1960. The period between 1932 (the publication of *The Psychoanalysis of Children*) and 1934 (the depressive position paper 'A contribution to the psychogenesis of manic-depressive states', published 1935), is crucial in any account of Klein's thought. These Notes are from exactly that moment.

There were three dimensions to Klein's re-conceptualization of her work at this time: firstly her move from working primarily with children to working with adults; secondly her emerging independence from the classical concepts of Freud and Abraham, especially Abraham's libidinal phases of development; and lastly her ambitions moving on from understanding neurotic mechanisms to exploring psychosis. Initially she looked for the very early fixation points and the mechanisms associated with them. That follows Abraham's careful exploration of the fixation points in the sadistic phases of libidinal development (Abraham, 1924).

These Notes give an insight into Klein's struggles to think through her clinical material, and they indicate the beginnings of the ideas that will form the basis of her two great innovations – the depressive position (Klein, 1935) and the paranoid-schizoid position (Klein, 1946). In addition, because the Notes consist of attempts to organize her thoughts about clinical material, they are an unusually transparent window into how she actually worked with patients.

Child and adult psychoanalysis

Nearly all the clinical material in B.89 relates to adult patients; there is one child, 'A', out of the five patients mentioned. Her book, *The Psychoanalysis of Children* (Klein, 1932), had drawn on her substantial clinical material from the early 1920s when she was developing her own method of child analysis, her 'early technique' as she called it.

Klein's method led her to postulate certain amplifications of Freud's theories, and more specific details of infant development in the pre-genital and preverbal phases, using the same method of genetic continuity as Freud in his extrapolation from adults to children. Freud had worked back from adults to children on the basis of genetic continuity; for a closely argued defence of this genetic continuity argument, see Isaacs (1948).

From the early 1930s Klein became much more involved in treating adults. In fact, she had always analysed some adults as well as children, certainly from her time in Berlin (1921–1926). One of the reasons given by Grosskurth (1986, p. 159) for Ernest Jones's invitation to Klein to move to London in 1926 was to analyse his children, but also his wife, Katherine Jones.

The Psychoanalysis of Children (Klein, 1932) had brought about a degree of closure on Klein's work with children. From a theoretical point of view, it was important to test the significance of her findings in the analysis of adults. In 1905, Freud asked his colleagues to report observations of children that would confirm his work with adults. The Little Hans case (Freud, 1909a) was the outcome of that initiative. In effect Klein moved in the opposite direction to Freud.

Klein's book was therefore a thought-out presentation of her method and its results. All through it, she had proclaimed her loyalty to Freud and to her analyst Karl Abraham. These Notes show her continuing to struggle with this loyalty, whilst being pushed towards more original observations of her own.[2]

Klein began to play her full part in psychoanalytic training, and became a training analyst in 1931 when she took her first candidate (Clifford Scott) into analysis. Thus she was moving definitively into adult work as she was completing the text of her book on children.

Technique

Klein's method of working comes across very clearly in the process records she gives in the Notes. We should bear in mind that in her analytic practice with children, she had become extremely observant of the details of the manoeuvring of toys in play. It is striking that in her work with adults there appears to be the same precision in her observation of the patient's thoughts. It is as if they are objects like toys to be manoeuvred safely in relation to each other. In this way, she allowed the patient to convey the internal picture for himself. For instance, one can see the thoughts being dealt with in the way a child might put a doll to bed to sleep. 'Thoughts are put to sleep, i.e. the bad object, excrements, etc' (Section I, page 2). Or in Section II, page 1:

> I did not hear about the paper he was writing until the failure arrived. I was not to be involved into the deeper thoughts connected with this paper and the book, as there were continuous conflicts going on, which were the result of his different internalised objects playing different parts in this production (crime).

The characterization of this as a dramatic production is clear; it corresponds to the narrative structure of children's play. In this case, the drama was about controlling the relation between the thoughts and the analyst. A third example in the Notes:

> A similar instance St who feels continuously hindered in his work by the anxiety that if he has got a good thought it would be taken away by the enemies inside him, who would only interfere when it is worthwhile. So the anxiety increases if it is a good thought. Associations of going up a mountain, leading sheep while he has to control enemies which follow on and which he has to control continuously so that they should not disturb the sheep.
>
> *(Section II, page 1a)*

These objects are evaluated as good and bad, giving rise to an anxiety about keeping the good ones safe. In these examples we see various kinds of relations expressed in a dramatic form; in the three examples the thoughts relate firstly to the self, secondly to the analyst (external object), and thirdly to each other, just as children play in these various ways.

The challenge of psychosis

Klein was keen to understand psychosis. When she moved to Berlin in 1921, it was a time when Abraham (her second analyst) was actively interested in manic-depressive patients. He published his most important work, 'A short account of the development of the libido', based on manic depressive states, in 1924, the year that Melanie Klein was in analysis with him. Klein's high regard for Abraham was a formative influence, and her interest in psychosis probably had that root. A second factor occurred in 1929, when she analysed Dick, an autistic boy (Klein, 1930a; also Chapter 13 of this volume). Dick showed a disorder of the very process of representation and symbol-formation on which play depends – not just a disorder expressed in the dramatic representations of play.

A further factor that stimulated Klein's interest in psychosis was that in the late 1920s until the early 1940s medically trained people, psychiatrists, were beginning to join her circle. Clifford Scott was probably very influential, and

Winnicott was also drawn to Klein, though more because of her child work. Later, Paula Heimann, Herbert Rosenfeld, Hanna Segal and Wilfred Bion were all medically trained and collaborated on her project to analyse schizophrenic patients. Klein's paper to the IPA Congress in 1934 was clearly her first detailed attempt to penetrate the dynamics and aetiology of a major psychosis in her own terms. However she had written a short paper on the psychotherapy of psychosis (Klein, 1930b).

Klein's intention, following the analysis of Dick, appears to have been to develop an understanding of the mind-obliterating mechanisms of schizophrenia. But in 1934, instead of pursuing her original intention, she reverted to her interest in the work of Freud and Abraham on manic-depressive psychosis. The Notes give an insight into that transition.

Klein's emerging independence

In 1926 Klein had also moved from the relatively obscure place she had within Continental psychoanalysis to become a kind of star in the British Psychoanalytical Society, which was relatively distant in geography and language from the heart of psychoanalysis. She had a different relationship with colleagues and assumed a degree of scientific leadership of the Society.[3]

Both in her own thinking and in her professional context, Klein received a major boost to her confidence and reputation. It gave her increased freedom to develop her own ideas; at the same time, distance protected her somewhat from Anna Freud and other Continental analysts. From this point on she claimed the freedom to develop her own ideas. Although she had pursued her independence of thought up to 1932, it was always presented in a discourse that minimized the differences from the classical psychoanalytic authors (Freud and Abraham). After this transitional moment, she abandoned that caution. The Notes display that new freedom, but not yet with a smooth account of original thinking and coherent argument.

In fact the notes are more interesting. They provide an insight into the very process of invention. There is evidence (considered below) that the physical sequence of the Notes was reworked at least once: the pages were re-ordered, then divided into two separate sections, and pages were interpolated (three of them), some of which appear to have been originally intended for an alternative place in the Notes. This process of re-ordering gives the Notes a somewhat fragmented quality and, in particular, a confused sense of purpose. Reconstructing a shape to Klein's thinking, it appears she began the Notes with the intention to display the survival of very antiquated methods of defence, as fixation points to which could be assigned the cause of psychosis. This implies defences which were variants of the classical process of repression, hence her title 'Early Repression Mechanism'. She conceptualized this as a continuum, or dimension, from early mechanisms to late ones. This idea was rooted in the early mechanisms that Freud speculated about in *Inhibitions, Symptoms and Anxiety* (Freud, 1926):

> It may well be that before its sharp cleavage into an ego and an id, and before the formation of a super-ego, the mental apparatus makes use of different methods of defence from those which it employs after it has reached these stages of organization.
>
> *(Freud, 1926, p. 164)*

Freud had described a discontinuity between different defences. For example he distinguished between repression and disavowal in his theorizing of fetishism (Freud, 1927). Already in a paper that depended a good deal on her conclusions from the Dick analysis, Klein also asserted:

> The earliest defence set up by the ego ... in conformity with the degree of sadism, is of a violent character and differs fundamentally from the later mechanism of repression. In relation to the subject's own sadism the defence implies expulsion, whereas in relation to the object it implies destruction.
>
> *(Klein 1930a, p. 232)*

However, by the time of the Notes, Klein had moved her position and given herself the freedom to reconsider the relationship which Freud had mused about. She started the Notes with the idea of a continuity of mechanisms from early (psychotic) to later (repression). As she worked on the Notes, modified, added and re-arranged them, she developed a rather different focus. One of her patients, 'Rt', was occupied by his discovery that he had negative and derogatory attitudes towards his analyst. They were a set of feelings of which he had not been consciously aware, and he had kept in his mind only his positive feelings. In the course, and as a result, of the analysis he did become aware of the negative side to his feelings, and thus ambivalence towards the person he knew as a friendly and helpful person. This shocked the patient, and it attracted Klein's fascinated attention. In order to bring some order to her understanding of the observations, she re-organized the Notes so that her original intention, the dimension of defences, was condensed into the first pages. Then the latter part became an extended description of ambivalent material.

Instead of describing the continuity of defences under the term 'repression', Klein separated them into two sections. In a section headed 'I', she described the earliest defences that varied around the degree and character of sadism and how the patient dealt with (and destroyed) his own thoughts. Section II was then re-organized (not entirely satisfactorily) to deal with the other end of the spectrum, and turned into her new-found interest in ambivalence, so that it became largely an extended clinical discussion of 'Rt''s material.

It is clear Klein was on her way to finding original answers to the problem of psychosis, though she was certainly not there as yet. At the same time, she retained her allegiance to the classical notion of repression, towards Abraham's theories of sadism, and towards the notion of fixation points. Because of her dedication to an approach that left classical theory undisturbed (at least in her own mind), it was a struggle to sort out the conclusions that her material pushed her towards, as it now took her away from the received theories to which she remained loyal.

Klein's struggle involved relinquishing some of the importance of Abraham's notion of the progressive development of the libidinal phases and the character of sadism in each of them. At the same time, it gave her confirmation of the ambivalence both Freud and Abraham saw at the root of manic-depressive illness. Freud had discussed this in relation to mourning and melancholia (Freud, 1917) and Abraham had discussed it in terms of normal mixtures of love and sadism in various proportions in the course of the libidinal phases. She must therefore have been attentive to 'Rt''s shock over his own feelings because it seemed a reflection of those Freud and Abraham described. Because they had found this confluence of impulses in manic depressive illness, this material from Rt moved her away from schizophrenia and away from the intention that I surmised she had after her analysis of Dick, and the 1930 paper (Klein, 1930a, 1930b).

One can say that the later interest in ambivalence combined the ideas of Freud and Abraham on depression with Klein's own unique way of seeing material as the expression of internal struggles. Whereas Freud and Abraham described the conflict of impulses towards objects (and towards the self, in Freud's case) and the pain arising from this conflict, Klein took an interest in the ego's struggle to handle and dissipate the conflictual ambivalence. Thus, Klein described the ego as an agent that was not merely driven by the conflicting impulses in a determinate way, but was the agent that handled and manipulated those impulses.

With her experience of child's play, and her success in unravelling its hidden meanings, Klein described ambivalence in the same characteristic way as 'play' with the internal 'toys', i.e. thoughts. This play separated the contents of the mind so that the good ones could be kept safe. This led to the originality of her contribution, to combine the notions of ambivalence with 'playing' with internal objects. This full theory is not spelled out in her Notes, yet only months later she fully worked it out in the published paper on manic depressive states (Klein, 1935).

Later, Klein did come back to the differentiation of early and late defences, when she described the paranoid-schizoid position (Klein, 1946). However, the later descriptions are in a different vein. Whereas in the Notes she had originally emphasized the continuity of the defences, in 1946 she emphasized the differences. In the Notes she retained the term 'repression' to cover both early and late defences, and used phrases such as 'along the line of'. She seems to have done so in order to stick with Abraham's descriptions of the continuity of development of the libidinal phases. However, in 1946 she explicitly contrasted repression, as a late defence, with 'splitting of the ego' as an early defence; for instance, 'in this early phase splitting, denial and omnipotence play a role similar to that of repression at a later stage of ego-development' (Klein, 1946, p. 7).

For purposes of clarity, we can distinguish two separate contrasts. Klein originally intended to set early defences (evacuation/destruction) in relation to classical repression. In the re-ordered version of the Notes, Klein had come to another contrast. That later contrast was between the early defences on one hand, and ambivalence on the other. In effect, at this point she had begun to work out the distinction between the paranoid-schizoid and the depressive positions.

The Notes: File B.89 'Early repression mechanism'

These 15 pages are typewritten, with a number of alterations inserted. They are notes and are not in polished English. Klein had in fact learned English just prior to settling in England and had lived there for only eight years.

Klein obviously worked over her Notes in the course of writing them, added pages (numbered 1a, 2a, etc), and re-ordered and renumbered the pages into two sections. I have reconstructed the final result in the Appendix. My organization is not certain, and other researchers might make a different one. It consists of Section I with two pages, and Section II with 13 pages; the last page is actually typed on the reverse of the fourteenth page. As I have described, the re-ordering suggested that she started off her Notes with one intention but moved subsequently to another one. This presents the reader with some degree of lack of clarity and confusion, and to my mind betrays the struggles involved in coming to her new formulations. Despite that, the material in these Notes allows some important conclusions.

In the Appendix to this chapter is transcribed the relevant part of file B.89 as faithfully to the original as possible. In my comments I shall refer to this text. Readers who wish to see a digitized version of the original manuscript may consult the Wellcome Library documents online (https://wellcomelibrary.org; see the Editor's Introduction, p. xv of this book, for how to do this).

Klein's method was to give relevant pieces of clinical material, often very short, with interpolated theoretical understanding. At the start, her selection of material and the way she understood it led to her sequencing the material according to the phases of libidinal development. Each mechanism was assigned to one or other of the sub-phases which Abraham (1924) had characterized with a different degree and character of sadism: the early and later oral phases and the early and late anal phases.

Starting with the early or deeper end of the dimension, which she associated with psychosis, Klein observed this clinical material from 'A', a child patient:

> A having tried to fix up the bits of the internalised dangerous penis on a string, announcing that the bad man (his penis) should be kept in bed – prison – when anxiety increases, denies all the dangers and pretends everything is sleeping in him. Reminded of former material, where he faced the dangerous objects by burning and breaking them up, sincerely says: this is not true, – does not think this.

> Thoughts are put to sleep like everything else was supposed to sleep, i.e. the bad object, excrements, etc. This mechanism would occur at a very early stage on the line of a psychotic defence [. . .] the thoughts were identified with the internalised eaten bits of the dangerous objects. As the bits could not be kept in order, the thoughts had to be denied – put to sleep.
>
> *(Section I, pages 1 and 2)*

Here 'A' fails to deal with a bad and dangerous internal state. So, more desperately, the contents are made to sleep or are burnt and destroyed. The contents lose their energy and in effect die. They are obliterated. She continued to regard this as a variant of repression: 'This mechanism of repression ought to follow on quite closely on to the early internalisation process' (Section I, page 2). By early internalization Klein means the oral phase, and thus the process is to deal with the oral-sadistic impulse to bite into bits. Klein also described evacuative processes:

> T. having spoken of fog as a poisoning bad thing – equated with his bad breath, excrements and bad words, which exhaust me (note T. material first half of Feb 1934), showing his cigarette case being empty, cleaning it from outside and inside, says: – that what he thought before has nothing to do with today's thoughts he always has a thought only when it is just needed. – Material shows that thoughts are equated to bad excrement and objects, and are not kept inside his mind.
>
> *(Section I, page 1)*

As Klein says later, 'the thoughts were to be evacuated like the fog' (Section I, page 2). Evacuation from the mind is distinguished, together with the destruction of thoughts, from the other end of the dimension that approximates more to classical repression, 'separating the different objects inside' (Section II, page 1). Instead of obliterating the contents of mind, or evacuating them, the person separates them and keeps them apart:

> St who feels continuously hindered in his work by the anxiety that if he has got a good thought it would be taken away by enemies inside him, who would only interfere when it was worthwhile. So the anxiety increases if it is a good thought. Associations of going up a mountain, leading sheep while he has to control enemies which follow on and which he has to control continuously so that they should not disturb the sheep. Then he might still fall back from the top if he meets an enemy, but could be helped if he meets a friend.
>
> *(Section II, page 1a)*

In this material, the patient describes how he has to keep things apart in his mind so that good things, good thoughts, are not interfered with or disturbed.

This internal separation is driven by a constant anxiety that if it fails then some disturbance will happen to him. The patient, Klein indicated, is describing a separation of thoughts, and this is the subjective account of what analysts call repression. There is an internal *separation* of contents, good from bad (sheep from enemies). If repression breaks down, i.e. separation of thoughts fails, he anticipates becoming disturbed.

A few pages into Section II, Klein summarized the ways in which the mechanisms vary:

> The mechanism – instance R. – of disconnecting oneself from the thoughts and actions of the internalised object, is a very early one and on the line of defence through denial of the psychic reality. The mechanism of hiding and changing thoughts because of being afraid of internalised object finding them out, – instance Rt. – seems a little later on the line of plotting and attacking objects with internal weapons, or making them fight each other, which would go along with the earlier anal-sadistic stage. Instance S. seems more connected with disconnecting things inside him, separating the objects, connecting more with the second anal-sadistic stage.
>
> Here the idea would be to get away, to dissociate oneself from certain thoughts equated to faeces, attributed to the objects as their productions. Along with this the necessity to keep the good objects apart from the bad objects and their thoughts.
>
> *(Section II, pages 2a, 2)*

I should note here that in the way I have reconstructed the Notes, pages 1a and 2a come after page 1; and page 2 follows on from page 2a. To add to the confusion there is another page numbered 2a (and originally numbered 4a), but crossed through. I have placed it after Section II, page 2 (itself originally numbered page 4, but crossed out and renumbered as page 2). These added pages have been included where their content makes most sense in my judgement. Even though it appears to break up sentences at times, I have tried to follow the continuity of thought.

At this point (Section II, the second paragraph of page 2), Klein started her discussion of some extended material from the patient 'Rt'.

Relational ambivalence

'Rt' has positive flattering thoughts about the analyst, her theories and what he expects of his analysis with her. However the patient reports a dream which sets her thinking further about the separation of thoughts, keeping the good from the bad:

> Prof. L. [added in Klein's handwriting *surgeon knows nothing about analysis*] analyses him in front of students (suspicions about me that might give him away but actually says – would not mind if I would use his material).
>
> *(Section II, page 2)*

Implicitly there are mixed feelings here – both a suspicion of the analyst, plus an extreme co-cooperativeness. The dream brought associations:

> Rt had read my book and deeply impressed that I lead certain fundamental things further. This implies to him that I will be more able to cure him than anybody else [. . .]
>
> I am compared with the physician from whom I know from former associations that he does not think very highly of him, just as of somebody who can neatly or correctly carry out an operation, like he is careful about his appearance, but not really good in diagnosis and who was repeatedly blamed by his seniors and not very well judged by his students. Following associations show that [Dr] G. and [Dr] I. did not realise at all his illness, while I am quite right with what he feels to be my diagnosis. He is amazed to find that he actually, with one part of his mind, compared me with the unimportant physician who cannot diagnose well, and the other two men with good diagnosticians, while he knew that he has a triumphant feeling of having misled them. He says he must have thought so, but he cannot understand how he could, because he has just recently felt that I am the only one to help him.
>
> *(Section II, pages 2–3)*

The patient's ambivalence is described in further associations:

> Prof. C. – good diagnostician, the physician Dr H.I. – bad diagnostician but neat and accurate – standing for me (Patient dislikes Dr H. I. thoroughly). He always puts himself in the foreground, his importance and so on. – This alludes to the fact that the patient recently discovered in his analysis that I go further in analysis of melancholia than Freud and Abraham. Here too the patient is amazed to find that while he admires this and is grateful for it, he at the same time in other layer of his mind belittles me, is sarcastic and so on.
>
> *(Section II, page 2a)*

Klein is represented in the dream by two contrasting figures, Prof. C. and Dr H.I. The patient views them in opposing ways, admiring or belittling. This separation of the object into good and bad manifestations as 'Rt' did with his analyst, was called 'splitting of the object' by Klein in her work with children. These alternating perceptions of the important (primary) figures, the good breast versus the bad breast, for example, were features of the play she described in *The Psychoanalysis of Children* (Klein, 1932). However the internalized versions of these opposing figures became important concepts at this time.

In June 1933, Strachey read a paper to the British Psychoanalytical Society on mutative interpretation about these distorting perceptions based on internal figures, and about their modification (Strachey, 1934). A footnote to the published paper says 'Portions of this paper were read at a meeting on June 13, 1933' (Strachey, 1934, p. 127n), so the development of the idea of internal objects was clearly in the air at this time. It is not clear what relations Strachey's paper on internalized figures making up the superego had to Klein's developing idea of internal objects. The timing of their contributions is significant, but one can only speculate on what discussion there was between them.

From this point onwards, Klein's interest was no longer in the mechanisms by which the patient maintains a safe internal state; in this case 'Rt' separated opposing ideas; he was both impressed with Klein, and the same time ironic and sarcastic. Instead her interest turned to the patient's 'amazed' state of mind when he realized his very mixed feelings. In other words, she was interested in the moments when the repression was lifted and a fuller appreciation of the internal state became apparent to the patient. When Klein described to the patient how his mind was dealing with the opposing currents of feelings, he gave not just confirmatory associations, but a very graphic picture of the dangerous internal situation which the patient contemplated:

> When I suggested to him this concealing and deceiving way is going on in his own mind, (from all the material just described), how he has to keep apart thoughts and objects, he, while listening to me thinks of an article he read: – A trainer who managed to have in one cage lions and tigers. Most dangerous. One lion bit a tigress in the throat, – she died. One young lion was made not to feel superior, was made to feel meek, by his brothers being put into the same cage, who, when he started fighting, ill-treated and wounded him thoroughly.
>
> *(Section II, page 4)*

This dangerous and potentially murderous situation, pictured in terms of the lions and tigers, comes in a communication about the fears of dangers within the internal world of mental objects and relations. Internal mental objects can be wounded and die. Klein was at this moment precisely indicating the situation at the centre of the depressive position that she would describe explicitly a few months later.

Klein's attempts to use the psychotic-neurotic dimension do not disappear altogether; she simply seemed more drawn to 'Rt''s amazement at his own ambivalence, and the threats to the representations in his own mind that result. Her loyalty to Abraham's thinking on the libidinal sub-phases also remains, but it too was diminishing as her own new conceptions emerged. This evidence of the development of her thinking during 1934 suggests we are witnessing the moment when the idea of the depressive position began emerging in her mind. To Freud's and Abraham's theories on the ambivalent confluence of love and aggression in depression, she added the ambivalence towards the thoughts and representations within the person's own mind – ambivalence towards the *internal* objects.

The historical context of the Notes

Klein's Notes are of considerable interest for a number of reasons. They date from a period of transition in her career. She was also in the midst of a personal crisis at that time. They demonstrate her ambition to solve the riddle of psychosis. They antedate by a few months her first paper on the depressive position. They also offer a particularly clear window onto the carry-over of clinical technique Klein used in her work with children.

Klein's personal crisis

The years 1933–1934 were ones of considerable personal adversity on several counts. It seemed that this reached a peak in mid-1934. Klein had always been prone to spells of depression, including postnatally in 1904 (after the birth of Melitta, her daughter), in 1907 (after the birth of Hans) and in 1914 (after the birth of Erich). The last of these had led her into analytic treatment during the First World War.

After her unhappy marriage had ended in 1920 Klein had a deeply romantic affair with Chezkel Zvi Klötzel from 1925, but this ended in 1933 when Klötzel emigrated to Palestine. This was an unhappy affair not only because her longings were not fully reciprocated, but also because Klein moved to London in 1926 (Grosskurth, 1986).

That sad ending coincided with the beginning of an entrenched and bitter opposition to her work by her daughter Melitta Schmideberg, an analyst herself. Because of these reversals, Klein sought further psychoanalytic help from January to July 1934 with Sylvia Payne (Grosskurth, 1986). Thus she worked on her Notes in this context of a personal crisis. Typical of Klein, she coped with a crisis by throwing herself into her work. Then in April 1934, her son Hans was killed in a climbing accident, resulting in a period of bereavement and depression, which must have made the 'Rt' material in the Notes especially relevant. Her efforts to continue working produced the paper on the depressive position in August that year. Thus a period of unhappiness followed by a period of intense mourning was a background to her work.[4] It is not uncommon for a death to stimulate creative work but in Klein's case it actually moulded her work as well, by making her revisit Freud's (1917) classic study of mourning, and Abraham's developments of it.

The depressive position (1934)

The depressive position paper was read in August 1934 following this traumatic period. It took from Klein's earlier child work the observation and experience of internal objects, which adult patients manipulate in the way a child manipulates physical toys. However, the paper also drew on the two central ideas in the Notes: early defence mechanisms and emotional ambivalence.

In that published paper Klein (1935) stressed the internal situation, the damage to the psychic representations which are felt as actual objects within the self related to in ambivalent ways. She described the depressive position arriving in early infancy as a change in relation to the object:

> For the ego, when it becomes fully identified with the object, does not abandon its early defence-mechanisms ... the annihilation and expulsion of the object ... initiate the depressive position. If this be so it confirms my concept of the genetic connection between paranoia and melancholia.
>
> *(Klein, 1935, p. 265)*

The hostile relations with objects evolve in continuity, she says, towards the fear of internal bad objects that threaten internal good ones. Or, as she succinctly put it:

> The dread of persecution, which was at first felt on the ego's account, now relates to the good object as well and from now on the preservation of the good object is regarded as synonymous with the survival of the ego.
>
> *(Klein 1935, p. 264)*

Klein also described here the important consequences of 'identifying' with representations, the good objects, inside the ego. The newness of her idea is stated thus: 'With this change in the relation to the object, new anxiety contents make their appearance, and a change takes place in the mechanisms of defence' (p. 264). The central thrust of her paper is to make the contrast before and after this change in the relation with objects; in effect, from what she calls paranoia to a relationship of sad concern for the object. That emphasis stands out in the material that 'Rt' gave her, such as his 'amazing' suspicion whilst admiring his analyst.

Klein constantly made reference to the similarity between the depressive position and paranoia, and how the first evolves out of the second. She gives an honourable nod to Abraham's distinction between the two conditions. With these considerations, the paper strikes a much more theoretical tone than the Notes, which stick so closely to the struggle a patient conducts with his own thoughts and feelings, leading to aggression, expulsion, repair and ambivalence.

Klein turned in the 1935 paper to the defence mechanisms in the depressive position. She drew on the idea in the Notes of 'blotting out' or 'putting thoughts to sleep'. In the paper however, it became 'scotomization, the *denial of psychic reality*', as 'one of the earliest methods of defence' (p. 262). As in the Notes, she attributed this to the impulses of the early anal phase. The paper contrasted the ego's destruction of its objects in the phase prior to the depressive position (called at the time the 'paranoid position' (Klein, 1932)) with the depressive emphasis on protecting and saving the object if it is felt to be good (Klein, 1935). Similarly there is a contrast in the Notes between early mechanisms when thoughts are obliterated or evacuated, and later repression.

The idea of repair comes in strongly in the 1935 paper. Klein mentions 'anxiety how to put the bits together in the right way and at the right time' (p. 269). In the Notes 'A' is a child who, failing to put the bits back together again (reparation), then resorted to an earlier mechanism – putting thoughts to sleep. There are two extended pieces of clinical material in the 1935 paper. The first refers to internal objects; tapeworms inside the patient's abdomen which represent his parents. They give rise to anxiety about destructive parents, and also about attacking and spoiling them and their intercourse. This case emphasizes the internal world of objects. The dreams in the second case are more specifically about the patient's aggression and then pity, especially towards the father and his penis. None of this material is from the Notes, and she never used the clinical material from 'Rt' in published papers.

Klein's technique

Klein's technique comes through clearly in these Notes. The practice of psychoanalysis had evolved uncertainly in a number of directions. Around the time that Klein was in analysis with him, during and immediately after the First World War, Ferenczi was beginning to move in his own direction. He had experimented in various ways; one particularly egalitarian experiment gave rise to the kind of co-work principle which Balint later promoted (Balint & Balint, 1939). One can certainly be impressed with the emotional closeness and fellow-feeling that appeared to exist between Klein and her patients too, something which emerges in these Notes.[5]

When Klein went to Berlin in 1921 she was no doubt influenced by Abraham's technique as he practised it in 1924 when Klein was in analysis with him. It is likely (though not certain) that he, like Ferenczi, was reaching towards a greater use of the treatment situation, but in a different way. He gave greater emphasis to the process, especially as this was informed by patients' phantasies. This would have connected with Klein's work with children where she observed phantasy played out with objects which illustrated the child's struggles with its own impulses and feelings.

Transference

Whilst Abraham (1924) described the way in which patients in phantasy manoeuvred the representations of objects inside themselves, Klein followed the way patients manoeuvred their feelings, wishes and thoughts with the same interior concreteness. For Klein internal objects were the feelings and thoughts, as well as the internal representations, of primary and external objects. This gave the transference a special quality in these Notes. The feelings for the analyst were also objects which needed manipulating. Thus thoughts and feelings are internal objects. They have to be handled in the setting but connect with the concrete experiences of relations elsewhere.

This emphasis on transference is clear also in Klein's recently published lectures on technique (Steiner, 2017). The objects struggled with are the feelings right now; the transference is no longer the struggle with the analyst as the representation of another person from the patient's past (or even present). At the same time the treatment relationship is occupied with the thoughts and feelings about the analyst as an external figure too, one who can be a friend who could help with the internal situation or maybe someone who hinders the struggle.

At this stage the help the analyst could offer is not clear. It could be to assist with the mechanism of separation (defensively), or it could be to manage the internal situation in a less defensive way. It is likely that Klein had not at that stage thought this through. In fact the analyst as an unwitting helper in the defensive organization of the patient is only recently being understood in Kleinian terms (Joseph, 1989; Steiner, 1997; Hargreaves & Varchevker, 2004).

Structure and content

Because Klein was attentive to the patient's struggles with his own ego functioning and its products (his good and bad feelings and wishes) she gained a quite original purchase on the way the mind operates upon itself. The awareness of good or dangerous ways of relating leads to mental activity, which actually creates mental structure, either the separation of thoughts, or their evacuation. The idea that some self-reflective activity can receive awareness of the structure of the mind was described by Freud (1911) and called 'endopsychic perception'. As many have noted, it is implicit in dream censorship. Abraham went a stage further in which he recognized in his patients' dreams and delusions an omnipotence of fantasy, in which intentional mental activity – projection and introjection – results in actual effects on the mind.

The possibility that endopsychic perception is an awareness of the structure of the mind, or can lead to changing it, has received considerable scepticism. In his paper on internal objects, Sandler (1990, expanded in Sandler & Sandler, 1998) specifically asserted that the structure of the mind is not part of that experiential world. He distinguished 'between the experiential content of a mental representation – the perceptual and ideational content – and the structural organization behind the content, an organization that lies outside the realm of conscious and unconscious experience' (Sandler, 1990, p. 869).

The Notes in fact provide a powerful counter-example that thoughts are intentionally separated in a process that creates the repression barrier. That description comes from the *patient*'s mind, not the analyst's.

Nowhere in her published work does Klein illustrate how the minds of her patients operated upon their own functions, as she does in these Notes. Repression as separation of thoughts is a product of unconscious phantasy, for instance, in the material about the sheep going up a hill and the need to keep enemies away (Section II, page 1a). The separation of the contents, especially the products of the ego, creates the structure of conscious and unconscious.[6] Thus, instead of the mental structure of conscious and unconscious being there for the purpose of repression, Klein's approach implies that the structure is the outcome of these processes.[7]

Later developments

Klein was only beginning to explore these internal processes that underlie the splitting of the object, processes to which she had given great attention to in the 1920s. The mind as the agent in manoeuvring its thoughts for the purposes of safety led to the development of another concept, 'unconscious phantasy'. Klein, Susan Isaacs and others came to understand its importance in the course of the Controversial Discussions in 1943 (Isaacs, 1948; King & Steiner, 1991).

During the 1940s some of Klein's students, with her encouragement, began to work with psychotic, schizophrenic patients. The upshot of this was her own paper on schizoid mechanisms (Klein, 1946). There she described the fundamental mechanisms of 'splitting of the ego',[8] which obliterated parts of the ego and its functions by projection into the external objects, 'As far as the ego is concerned the excessive splitting off and expelling into the outer world of parts of itself considerably weaken it' (Klein, 1946, p. 8). In the Notes she had described an evacuative process, for example when the man empties his cigarette case (Section I, page 1), which corresponds to 'projective identification', a term she adopted in 1946 to describe exactly that kind of evacuation. As Forrester has pointed out (unpublished communication), others used the term previously, for example, Brierley (1945); see also Scott (1998). Thus, the processes Klein described as nearly psychotic at the beginning of her Notes were not abandoned forever. As she said at the beginning of the 1946 paper, her interest in these schizoid processes dates from 'even before clarifying my views on the depressive position' (Klein, 1946, p. 1). She may well here have had her 1934 Notes in mind.

The very concrete mode of manipulating thoughts links back to Freud's notion of the omnipotence of fantasy in the Rat Man case (Freud, 1909b). However, it also seems to presage concrete 'symbolic equation', which Segal (1957) described. It appears to link also Bion's idea of thoughts in search of a thinker (Bion, 1970). These links hint that Klein's particular way of seeing clinical material was probably still in use when Segal and Bion were in analysis with Klein in the 1940s, and where they absorbed her technical approach so that it later influenced their new theories.

In the immediate aftermath of this personally difficult period Klein wrote her depressive position paper, but perhaps not surprisingly there followed a relatively fallow period. However the Archives preserve many notes from 1936–38 recording detailed material of depressive features of many patients, many entitled 'Mourning and melancholia'. These supplied her with the material for her second paper on the depressive position given in 1938 and published in 1940.

Repression and splitting: continuity of defence

In 1932, in Chapter IX of *The Psychoanalysis of Children*, Klein took up Freud's (1926) speculation that there were kinds of defences specifically aimed at dealing with aggressive impulses. Klein was interested in this clear-cut distinction between genital and pre-genital defences, because it connected with her own observations of young children. However, at the outset of writing her Notes she changed tack and emphasized the continuity, calling them simply 'early repressive mechanisms'. Her investigation certainly exposed contrasts that exist between the early (evacuative) mechanisms and the late (separating) mechanisms, but the title is obviously intended to convey and stress the continuity between the early and late forms. When writing the depressive position paper, she referred to her concept of genetic continuity between paranoia and melancholia. Then in 1946 she changed again, returning to the stress on discontinuity; the mechanisms, processes and experiences of the paranoid-schizoid position are described as quite distinct from those of the depressive position.

This is a vacillating course of development of the ideas of repression and splitting. We are left wondering about the motives and strategy for these changes. Possibly Klein never really noticed such changes of theoretical structures. Very likely they were of little interest to her, as they had little relevance as she listened in to the practical efforts that patients made to struggle with themselves. Perhaps this is expressed in a different way of looking at the issue which she implied later. She talked in more fluid terms in *Envy and Gratitude* of 'the fluctuations in the process of integration' (Klein, 1957, p. 227). Here reflecting on some case material she said: 'I had no doubt that he was still splitting off a part of his personality, but the *repression* of greedy and destructive impulses had become more noticeable' (p. 227). There is the sense that in practice the patient will fluctuate from time to time between using one type of defence or another. This is in fact what she described with patient 'A', the child in the Notes. When the child could not repair the bits, he reverted to a more primitive defence, putting the pieces to sleep.

Though splitting and repression are different defences, there is another kind of continuum between them, a time line. Particularly important is the moment when Klein's originality assumed more confidence and authority, enabling us to understand how new terminology evolved, and old terminology bifurcated into different meanings. The way, for instance, the terms 'splitting' and 'repression' are used in contemporary psychoanalysis is not simply a wayward deviance. Klein showed in the Notes how phenomena in her actual work were pushing her thoughts in a particular direction. Freud's much more restricted term 'splitting' arose out of considering very different patients, fetishists.

Differences such as that between repression and splitting are not just arbitrary. They are the product of the combined forces, of evidence and speculation at the precise moment when the terms began to diverge.

Acknowledgements

I would like to acknowledge the very helpful discussions with the late Elizabeth Spillius and with Joe Aguayo, who generously gave me their views, their time and further information. The Wellcome Library has been as always extremely willing and helpful over finding and photocopying material from the archives. And I am grateful to the Melanie Klein Trust, not only for the permission to use this material, but also their care of an archive that is so valuable for the history of British psychoanalysis.

Notes

1 An earlier version of this chapter was published in: Hinshelwood (2006). Melanie Klein and repression: An examination of some unpublished notes of 1934. *Psychoanalysis and History* 8(1), 5–42.

2 Aguayo (2000) also makes this point: 'Although Klein profusely cited Freud's pioneering work on locating the pre-latency origins of the neuroses in the Wolf Man case in her paper at Würzburg in 1924, at the First Conference of German Psychoanalysts, these copious references were reduced to one footnote by the time she published the Erna case in her book on child analysis in 1932. For all that, Klein still felt compelled to represent herself as a staunch and loyal Freudian' (Aguayo, 2000, p. 747).

3 See, for instance, Aguayo's (2000) account of the patronage offered Klein by Ernest Jones and the British Psychoanalytical Society. He contrasts that with the remarkable antagonism to Klein's work in Vienna and Berlin from 1925 onwards. The need in Vienna, he speculated, was to find a loyal enough successor to Freud once the diagnosis of his cancer in 1923 had been made. What is less clearly enunciated is why Jones should have offered such a degree of professional (and personal) patronage, in direct conflict with Freud and Continental psychoanalysts. One possibility (Hinshelwood, 1997) is that Jones's complex character needed an acolyte to enact his own independence of thought whilst he could simultaneously indulge his almost abject loyalty to Freud.

4 No-one develops theories without a considerable input of personal factors, as we know from Freud's account of dreams (Freud, 1900). Lussier (2000) has looked also at the factors impinging on Freud when he wrote: 'Mourning and melancholia' (Freud, 1917); whilst I tried to contextualize Klein's idea of internal objects in terms of personal, organizational and social factors (Hinshelwood, 1997).

5 Ferenczi also began his collaboration with Rank on active technique around this time (Rank & Ferenczi, 1924). Using the treatment relationship in a very non-analytic and rather manipulative and didactic way which harked back to the suggestive techniques that Freud had so decisively dismissed (Freud, 1912–1913), Klein seems to have been much less influenced in that development, probably by the influence of Abraham.

6 In contrast, Freud's view of repression is that it 'is [not] present from the very beginning, and that it cannot arise until a sharp cleavage has occurred between conscious and unconscious mental activity' (Freud, 1915, p. 147), thus the cleavage is prior to the onset of repressive mechanisms. He goes on to imply that earlier mechanisms operate before repression and would seem to be implicated in causing the cleavage. A fuller treatment elsewhere of how Klein's conception of 'repression' relates to Freud's definition is needed.

7 The contrast with Freud's views is striking. In his paper on repression (Freud, 1915) he gives several views of the central feature of repression: 'the essence of repression

lies simply in turning something away, and keeping it at a distance from the conscious' (p. 147); 'as a rule it creates a substitutive formation' (p. 154); and 'the mechanisms of repression have one thing in common: a withdrawal of the cathexis of energy' (pp. 154–155). These are quite different from what Klein makes of her material. It is as if she was not very cognizant of Freud's exposition.

8 Freud had used the term 'splitting of the ego' for a pathological manifestation of a division of the ego only in 1940 in his posthumous paper (Freud, 1940), however it had been used to refer to the normal 'grade' in the ego that Freud had discussed as early as 1921. Searl (1932), however, did refer to a pathological form of this in depersonalization.

References

Abraham, K. (1924). A short study of the development of the libido, viewed in the light of mental disorders. In *Selected Papers*. London: Hogarth.

Aguayo, J. (2000). Patronage in the dispute over child analysis between Melanie Klein and Anna Freud 1927–1932. *Int. J. Psycho-Anal., 81*, 733–752.

Balint, M. and Balint, A. (1939). On transference and counter-transference. *Int. J. Psycho-Anal., 20*, 223–230.

Bion, W.R. (1970). *Attention and interpretation*. London: Tavistock.

Brierley, M. (1945). Further notes on the implications of psycho-analysis: Metapsychology and personology. *Int. J. Psycho-Anal., 26*, 89–114.

Freud, A. (1926). *Enfühirng in die Technik der Kinderanalyse*. Vienna: Internazional Psycho-analyse Verlag.

Freud, S. (1900). The interpretation of dreams. In *The standard edition of the complete psychological works of Sigmund Freud*, vols. *3*, *4*. London: Hogarth Press.

Freud, S. (1905). Fragment of an analysis of a case of hysteria. In *The standard edition of the complete psychological works of Sigmund Freud*, vol. 7. London: Hogarth Press.

Freud, S. (1909a). Analysis of a phobia in a five-year-old boy. In *The standard edition of the complete psychological works of Sigmund Freud*, vol. *10*. London: Hogarth Press.

Freud, S. (1909b). Notes upon a case of obsessional neurosis. In *The standard edition of the complete psychological works of Sigmund Freud*, vol. *10*. London: Hogarth Press.

Freud, S. (1911). Psychoanalytic notes on an autobiographical account of a case of paranoia. In *The standard edition of the complete psychological works of Sigmund Freud*, vol. 12. London: Hogarth Press.

Freud, S. (1912–1913). Recommendations to physicians practising psychoanalysis. In *The standard edition of the complete psychological works of Sigmund Freud*, vol. *12*. London: Hogarth Press.

Freud, S. (1915). Repression. In *The standard edition of the complete psychological works of Sigmund Freud*, vol. *14*. London: Hogarth Press.

Freud, S. (1917). Mourning and melancholia. In *The standard edition of the complete psychological works of Sigmund Freud*, vol. *14*. London: Hogarth Press.

Freud, S. (1926). Inhibitions, symptoms and anxiety. In *The standard edition of the complete psychological works of Sigmund Freud*, vol. *14*. London: Hogarth Press.

Freud, S. (1927). Fetishisms. In *The standard edition of the complete psychological works of Sigmund Freud*, vol. *21*. London: Hogarth Press.

Freud, S. (1940 [1938]). Splitting of the ego in the process of defence. In *The standard edition of the complete psychological works of Sigmund Freud*, vol. *23*. London: Hogarth Press, pp. 275–278.

Grosskurth, P. (1986). *Melanie Klein: Her world and her work*. London: Hodder & Stoughton.

Hargreaves, E. and Varchevker, A. (2004). *In pursuit of psychic change*. London: Routledge.

Hinshelwood, R.D. (1997). The elusive concept of 'internal objects' and the origins of the Klein group 1934–1943. *Int. J. Psycho-Anal., 78*, 877–897.
Hinshelwood, R.D. (2006). Melanie Klein and repression: An examination of some unpublished notes of 1934. *Psychoanal. Hist., 8(1)*, 5–42.
Isaacs, S. (1948). On the nature and function of phantasy. *Int. J. Psycho-Anal, 29*, 73–97. Republished in M. Klein, P. Heimann, S. Isaacs and J. Riviere, *Developments in psycho-analysis*. London: Hogarth.
Joseph, B. (1989). *Psychic equilibrium and psychic change*. London: Routledge.
King, P. and Steiner, R. (1991). *The Freud–Klein controversies 1941–1945*. London: Routledge.
Klein, M. (1930a). The importance of symbol-formation in the development of the ego. In *The writings of Melanie Klein*, vol. *1*. London: Hogarth Press.
Klein, M. (1930b). The psychotherapy of psychosis. In *The writings of Melanie Klein*, vol. *1*. London: Hogarth Press.
Klein, M. (1932). The psychoanalysis of children. In *The writings of Melanie Klein*, vol. *2*. London: Hogarth Press.
Klein, M. (1935). A contribution to the psychogenesis of manic-depressive states. In *The writings of Melanie Klein*, vol. *1*. London: Hogarth Press.
Klein, M. (1940). Mourning and its relation to manic depressive states. In *The writings of Melanie Klein*, vol. *1*. London: Hogarth Press.
Klein, M. (1946). Notes on some schizoid mechanisms. In *The writings of Melanie Klein*, vol. *3*. London: Hogarth Press.
Klein, M. (1957). Envy and gratitude. In *The writings of Melanie Klein*, vol. *3*. London: Hogarth Press.
Lussier, M. (2000). Mourning and melancholia: The genesis of a text and a concept. *Int. J. Psycho-Anal., 81*, 667–686.
Paris, M.L. (2000). Mourning and melancholia. *Int. J. Psycho-Anal., 81*, 667–686.
Petot, J-M. (1979) *Melanie Klein: Premières découvertes et premier système 1919–1932*. Paris: Bordas.
Petot, J-M. (1982) *Melanie Klein: Le moi et le bon objet 1932–1960*. Paris: Bordas.
Rank, O. and Ferenczi, S. (1924) *Entwicklungsziele der Psychoanalyse*. Vienna: Inter-nazional Psychoanalyse Verlag. (*The development of psycho-analysis*. New York: Nervous and Mental Disease Publishing Company, 1925).
Sandler, J. (1990). On internal object relations. *Journal of the American Psychoanalytical Association, 38*, 859–880.
Sandler, J. and Sandler, A-M. (1998). *Internal objects revisited*. London: Karnac.
Scott, C. (1998). Memories and reflections. In *Psychoanalysis and the zest for living*. Binghampton: ESF Publishers.
Searl, M.N. (1932). A note on depersonalization. *Int. J. Psycho-Anal., 13*, 329–347.
Segal, H. (1957). Notes on symbol formation. *Int. J. Psycho-Anal., 37*, 339–343.
Spillius, E.B. (1994). Developments in Kleinian thought: Overview and personal view. *Psychoanal. Inq., 14*, 324–364.
Steiner, J. (2017). *Lectures on technique by Melanie Klein. Edited with a critical review by John Steiner*. London: Routledge.
Steiner, J. (1997). *Psychic retreats: Pathological organizations in psychotic, neurotic, and borderline patients*. London: Routledge.
Strachey, J. (1934). The nature of the therapeutic action of psycho-analysis. *Int. J. Psycho-Anal., 15*, 127–159.

Appendix: Melanie Klein's 1934 notes on the 'early repression mechanism'. Melanie Klein Archives PP/KLE/B.89

These Notes were typed double spaced on lined octavo sheets. The text is reproduced in Courier New, similar to the type face Klein used. There are a number of alterations that she made to the text. Some words are crossed out, which are included in this version but with a strike-through line. Typed insertions between lines or in the margins simply added, but insertions in pen are placed in italics. Some comments of mine are added in square brackets. There are a number of errors in Klein's typing, which I have left. The material can be found online via the Wellcome Library catalogue and constitutes images 1–16 of B.89.

Elizabeth Spillius has commented in a personal communication that Child A is 'Dick' (see Chapter 13 of this volume), 8 years old at the time of these Notes. Although she had not found any other notes on 'Rt' and 'St' in the Archive, there were more on 'R' and she thought that there may actually be two patients referred to as 'R'.

1.

I Early Repression Mechanism

I. On the line of blotting out ~~things~~ thoughts like doing away with bad things. *suspended animation* Instance: T. having spoken of fog as a poisoning and bad thing – equated with his bad breath, excrements and bad words, which exhaust me, (note *T.* material ~~at the beginning of February~~ first half of Feb. 1934), showing his cigarette case being empty, cleaning it from outside and inside, says:- that what he ~~said~~ thought before has nothing to do with today's thoughts he always has a thought only when it is just needed. – Material shows that thoughts are equated to bad excrements and objects, and are not to be kept inside his mind, as well as the former inside his body.

Instance: A. having tried to fix up the bits of the internalised dangerous penis on a string, announcing that the bad man (his penis) should be kept in bed – prison – when anxiety increases, denies all the dangers and pretends everything is sleeping in him. Reminded of former material, where he faced the dangerous objects by burning and breaking them up, sincerely says: this is not true, – does not think this.

2.

I Early Repression Mechanism. (cntd.)

~~I~~Thoughts are put to sleep like everything else was supposed to sleep, i.e. the bad object, excrements etc.

This Mechanism would occur at a very early stage on the line of a psychotic defence. It goes along on the line of a psychotic defence against the internalised danger.

In the instance A. the thoughts were identified with the eaten bits of the dangerous/internalised objects. As the bits could not be kept in order, ~~the thoughts had to be driven out.~~ the thoughts had to be denied – put to sleep. This mechanism of repression ought to follow on quite closely on to the early internalisation process. The denial of the internalised bits (instance A) would, perhaps, be an earlier repression mechanism than the one of instance T. where the thoughts were to be evacuated like the fog, because the latter seems more connected with ejection.

~~3.~~ 1.

Early Repression Mechanism.

II. On the line of separating the different objects inside, and to keep the good – external – object away from them. Instance R., Several weeks in analysis I did not hear about the paper he was writing until the failure arrived. I was not to be involved into the deeper thoughts connected with this paper and the book, as there were continuous conflicts going on, which were the result of his different internalised objects playing different parts in this production (crime). Ideal:- the secretary who would just work at some part where she would just follow out his orders without interfering with the essential part of his book. In the analytic situation – me – the secretary, who would put right some superficial part of his mind, but not get involved with the bad object. At this time association while he is difficating and reading – that he felt quite detached of the diffication process, it was as if the lodgers ought to settle this between themselves, – the faeces being their products.

~~Early Repression Mechanism (cont. II).~~

II. Early Repression Mechanism

~~8.~~ 1a

~~more with the second anal sadistic stage.~~

A similar instance *St* who feels continuously hindered in his work by the anxiety that if he has got a good thought it would be taken away by the enemies inside him, who would only interfere when it is worth while. So the anxiety increases if it is a good thought. Associations of going up a mountain, leading sheep while he has to control enemies which follow on and which he has to control continuously so that they should not disturb the sheep. Then he might still fall back from the top if he meets an enemy, but could be helped if he meets a friend.

[The text on this page was cut from another page and stuck onto this one.]

II Early Repression Mechanism (~~cont. II).~~

~~7.~~ 2a.

The Sheep represented his thoughts and his strain at working, the anxiety he feels to produce, impatience about this, which he expresses that he has not enough confidence in himself to let the thoughts simply mature in him, but must bring them out to light quickly. All this is felt as a struggle, strain and slavery. In his case blotting out of thoughts, forgetting, not thinking in analysis of things which had actually happened, are very striking. Definite connection with the objects disappearing because of being eaten up. The mechanism – instance R. – of disconnecting oneself from the thoughts and actions of the internalised object, is a very early one and on the line of defence through denial of the psychic reality. The mechanism of hiding and changing thoughts because of being afraid of the internalised object finding them out, – instance Rt. – seems a little later on the line of plotting and attacking objects with internal weapons, or making them fight each other, which would go along with the earlier anal-sadistic stage.

Instance S. seems more connected with disconnecting things inside him, separating the objects, connecting more with the second anal-sadistic stage.

Early Repression Mechanism (cont. II).

~~4.~~ 2.

Here the idea would be to get away, to dissociate oneself from certain thoughts equated to faeces, attributed to the objects as their productions. Along with this the necessity to keep the good objects apart from the bad objects and their thoughts. –

~~This mechanism would be a later one than mechanism I as it is connected~~

Instance: Rt.T. (NB strike Rt.T. through) *Rt* had read my book and deeply impressed that I lead certain fundamental things further. This implies to him that I will be more able to cure him than anybody else. *Dr* G. and *Dr I.* appear in associations. Those associations came to the following dream:- Prof. L. [Handwritten margin note indicated to appear here] *surgeon knows nothing about analysis*

analyses him in front of students (suspicions about me that might give him away), but actually says – would not mind if I would use material). (see p.4a). [Page 4a was subsequently renumbered 2a, which follows on in my reconstruction.]

analyses him in front of students (suspicions about me that might give him away), but actually says – would not mind if I would use material)

as the better diagnosticians, while I am compared with the physician from whom I know from former associations that he does not think very highly of him, just as of somebody who can neatly or correctly carry out an operation, like he is careful about his appearance, but not really good in diagnosis and

Early Repression Mechanism (cont. II)

~~4a~~. 2a.

In dream patient says repeatedly, like a child asking for his doll:- I want my lost object (laughs when telling this) *feels Irony* –. Had recently read Abraham and Freud about Melancholia, but obviously ironical about it. Associations:- doll has got sawdust instead of blood inside, is not a live object. *really horrified of dead objects irony cover* Then follow associations Prof.C. – good diagnostician, the physician Dr. H.I. – bad diagnostician but neat and accurate – standing for me. (Patient dislike Dr. H.I. thoroughly, *He* always puts himself in the foreground, his importance, and so on. – This alludes to the fact that patient recently discovered in his analysis that I go further in analysis of melancholia than Freud and Abrahm. Here too the patient is amazed to find that while he admires this and is grateful for it, heat the same time in other layer of his mind belittles me, is sarcastic and so on.

[This page referring to the dream of 'Rt' on page 2 was clearly written later. However, even though the text at the bottom of page 2 continues on page 3, page 2a's proper significance is clearly between them.]

Early Repression Mechanism (Cont. II)

~~5.~~ 3.

who was repeatedly blamed by his seniors and not very well judged by the students. Following associations show that he actually thinks that G. and I. did not realise at all his illness, while I am quite right whith what he feels to be my diagnosis. He is amazed to find that he actually, with one part of his mind, compared me with the unimportant physician who cannot diagnose well, and the other two men with good diagnosticians, while he knows that he has a triumphant feeling of having misled them. He says he must have thought so, but he cannot understand how he could, because he had just recently felt that I am the only one to help him. His associations show that in belittling me he follows the little man inside him in his early history – the father – who made mother bad though making her pregnant. Here associations about bloody sanitary towels and mother being injured and dirty. But there seems some triumph that he sees through and knows much better than father that the good mother would be helpful and better than father. He must not let father – the little man inside him –

~~6.~~ 4.

Early Repression Mechanism (Cont. II)

know that he believes in mother helping him and keeping mother for himself because father, brothers and sisters would get jealous and would want to take her away from him. Here number of people – Dr. K., his brother, his wife, etc., whom he feels guilty about that they don't get analysed by me. His astonishment is based on the fact that here one part of his mind is deceiving the other one. In order to keep certain thoughts hidden away, or

even quite changed for this purpose, in order to let the bad internal object not know.

When I suggested to him this concealing and deceiving way is going on in his own mind, (from all the material just described), how he has to keep apart thoughts and objects, he, while listening to me – thinks of an article he read:- A trainer who managed to have in one cage lions and tigers. Most dangerous. One lion bit a tigress in the throat, – she died. One young lion was made not to feel superior, was made meek, by his brothers being put into the same cage, who, when he started fighting, illtreated and wounded him thoroughly.

[The part of this page above the line was torn from another page and stuck on this one, with the lower text added.]

~~7.~~ 5.

Early Repression Mechanism (cont. II)

Next association – a patient he saw in an asylum who saw himself surrounded by lions. Psychologist I., who lectured to the students, explained that this man saw the day before a picture of a lion in a newspaper and feels they are real. Patient laughs about the silly interpretation. Patient interprets that he feels identified with the mad person with the lions and that the lion cage and the whole story about the trainer he thought of while I was interpreting the ways of his mind – represents his inside with lions and tigers as objects and difficulty to keep them *and thoughts* apart. I interpret:- *H*is triumph – that psychologist I. – standing for me – does not understand about psychosis. This alludes to my diagnosis I gave him some time ago (when pressed forit by him, I said that he is not psychotic, has, it is true, melancholic and paranoid trends but enough normality and capacity of co-operation to ~~be~~ get cured.) (His deepest anxiety since childhood is to go mad). Patient was *then* reassured, but not very much. Now these associations about psychologist I. show that he thinks I do not understand his psychosis.

~~8~~. 6.

Early Repression Mechanism (cont. II)

Now the triumph is that he knows he is psychotic, and I don't. – Patient is amazed to find that this could be a triumph. Interpretation:- psychosis stands for the lions and tigers inside him. The triumph is based on denial of psychic*al* realities – they can kill each other inside him – he does not mind, – proves that he is better than little man inside him, leaves responsibility *for all destructions* to him.

Association:- remembers that at Zoo *as a child* sexually very excited when lions fought each other in cage. Memory *regular masturbation phantasie* of Mrs. B. fighting on top of his mother with her. ~~This was another phantasy of sexual excitement~~. This leads to the sexual thrill at cinema (age between 8

& 10) when love stories were on, dangers, where people on screen seemed to him quite real. The thrill of the harm which could happen in love stories – lion cage and so on – is the tension of the danger hapenning to parent in intercourse. Sadistic phantasies and anxiety connected with them. These dangerous fighting animals – parents in intercourse inside him, at the same time his madnessand psychosis.

~~9~~. 7.

Early Repression Mechanism (cont. II)

I suggest that those phantasies still cause the disturbance in sexuality. He agrees that *he is phantasying intercourse* ~~it is~~ still quite on the line of masturbation phantasies, forgetting the object.

After week-end report; had been with people he got to know at wife's friends' house. Amazed about the change in his attitude. Usually most critical and dogmatic, inclined to argue with other people's views. Different things *he* didn't like *much* but did not mind them; not inclined to discussion; compares it with one week ago when deeply depressed after an afternoon which passed with an American doctor whom he thoroughly disliked, argued with him. Association showed that he disliked this man so much because of different things reminding him of his father and ways which patient thoroughly fights in himself. – Yesterday entirely different attitude. Patient says the first time he remembers having been at ease and really enjoyed new people's company. Asks how this is connected with material? – I suggest that his bad relation to his father, which led to

~~10~~ 8.

Early Repression Mechanism (cont. II)

arguing in a dogmatic way, while he hated those dogmatic ways very much (hate against father and identified with him against his will) became internalised. Could have got rid of the external father, but not of little man inside him, and this whole strain of coping with internal objects, in concealing thoughts (material of the last few pages). – Analysis of this material makes better relation with external objects possible. While patient listens has the following association. – Last night talk about Gen.Goering, somebody suggested that he takes drugs. Pat. Doubted it, – might have tendencies to do so. – I interpret:- that Gen.Goering came up when I interpreted about difficulties to get on with internal little man. Little man defends against big and dangerous man – Goering. That is why all the time took little notice of the whole Nazi business, denied danger and denied yesterday that he takes drugs – is mad. Pat.: he called Goering a rat in connection with Dimitroff. The way D. was shouted down in court reminded him of himself as a little boy shouted down by father. Felt quite identified with D. Awful to think

~~11.~~ 9

Early Repression Mechanism (cont. II)

that they now might keep him so long, and probably dope him, so that he is broken down when they let him go. – I interpret:- his denial Goering dopes himself connected with his anxiety D. – himself – being doped by internalised Goering. Then Pat.: would be the prisoner of Goering inside him as dependant/on and delivered out to what the internal object does. His irony against people like Dr.J., *Dr.*G., etc. defence against deeper anxiety of lions, tigers and Goerings. – Pat. remarks:- Bernard Shaw very ironical but obviously gets pleasure out of his sadism. – When I agree*d* to the primary irony in ~~sarcasm~~ sadism Pat. objects to my pronunciation of sadism. I interpret:- that this objections comes after I have shown so frightening things in his inside I became frightening internal object myself and fight about and with words stands for other, more dangerous fights.

[Reverse of page 9]

Illuminating material for co-relation between external and internal object.

Material for paranoic anxiety and defences on deceiving and plotting lines.

10

MELANIE KLEIN AND COUNTERTRANSFERENCE[1]

A note on some archival material.

R.D. Hinshelwood

Introduction

Five pages of notes on countertransference from 1953 are to be found in the Melanie Klein Archive in file PP/KLE/D.29.[2] Klein also discusses her views on this subject in file C.72. Because of the paucity of references to countertransference in Klein's published writings these Notes fill in our knowledge. Her views were provoked by the work her students were doing in their experimental analyses of schizophrenic patients. Apocryphal stories suggest that Klein remained aligned with Freud's view of countertransference as simply interference. The Notes confirm that, whilst there is some truth in that, she did have a more sophisticated and nuanced view of the unconscious relations between analyst and analysand.

In the four collected volumes of Melanie Klein's writings, there is precisely one indexed reference to countertransference. It is generally assumed that this apparent neglect means that Klein followed Freud's condemnation without much question. For Freud, the analyst's countertransference arises 'as a result of a patient's influence on his unconscious feelings' (Freud, 1910, p. 144), and he adds the warning that 'no psychoanalyst goes further than his own complexes and internal resistances permit' (p. 145). Countertransference, Freud believes, is a limiting factor in an analyst's effectiveness, due to the analyst's own neurotic traits.[3] In one of his papers on technique, Freud (1915) described how erotic transference love always threatens a corresponding countertransference love, which must be resisted. Since sexual libido is the underlying problem in neurosis, erotism is bound to surface as a transference, and therefore as a countertransference problem for the analyst. The countertransference is solely the analyst's problem.

Countertransference and the Klein group

By 1950, however, countertransference came to be described as a potential instrument usable to understand transference (Annie Reich, 1951; Winnicott, 1949; Racker, 1957 and others). One of Klein's most sturdy supporters, Paula Heimann (1950), had joined this group of revisionists. Heimann eventually left the Klein group in 1955, but a distance had grown up between them from 1953, resulting partly from Heimann's countertransference paper of 1950. Interestingly, Heimann (1960) had second thoughts ten years later, and was somewhat concerned at the wild analysis her original paper had apparently invited and condoned. Those second thoughts therefore seemed to echo Klein's misgivings.

Other Kleinians too were attracted to this new view of countertransference. Rosenfeld described countertransference 'as a kind of sensitive "receiving set"' (Rosenfeld, 1952, p. 116). Bion (1954), as we shall see in his first paper on his work with schizophrenia, described the specific processes by which his patient affected his mind. Money-Kyrle (1956) in his quiet way set out a thoroughly Kleinian framework based on primitive processes, projection and introjection, which formed the foundation of the countertransference process in the analytic setting. He coined the term 'normal countertransference' in direct contrast to Freud's definition of the countertransference as the expression of the analyst's complexes and inner resistances.

Rosenfeld had worked very closely with Klein for some years on the analysis of schizophrenic patients. Bion, who was in analysis with Klein until 1953, had also been working with three schizophrenic patients, but had not published anything about psychosis until the paper at the 1953 London Congress of the International Psychoanalytical Association (Bion, 1954). It is not clear if he had discussed this work with Klein prior to finishing his analysis. However, some Notes in the Archives indicate that she had seen a copy of Bion's paper prior to the Congress. In a personal communication, Bion's widow, Francesca Bion, conveyed that there is no archival indication of when, in 1953, Bion finished his analysis with Klein; whether it was before or after this 1953 Congress.

Klein's paper in 1946 on schizoid phenomena benefited from Clifford Scott's analysis of schizophrenic patients in the 1930s, and Rosenfeld's patient who was the basis of his membership paper in 1947. Rosenfeld read a paper at the IPA Congress in 1949, in Zurich (Rosenfeld, 1950), and Segal gave her first paper to the British Society in 1949 (Segal, 1950).

It is worth mentioning that there are differences between the approach that Kleinians take to countertransference and the approach that analysts from the Independent group and more recent American schools of psychoanalysis take. Kleinians are interested in the intrapsychic elements and processes, whilst other groups explore the authentic interpersonal encounter, influenced perhaps by Balint (Balint & Balint, 1939) and Ferenczi.

Elizabeth Spillius (1992) argued that Klein remained simply critical of the use of countertransference as it evolved after 1950, on grounds that were similar to Freud's; and she claimed: '[Melanie Klein] thought that such extension would open the door to claims by analysts that their own deficiencies were caused by their patients' (Spillius 1992, p. 61). Spillius (1983) quoted an apocryphal story from an unpublished paper of Segal's (1982) as she summarized Klein's view:

> She appears to have felt that both ideas, both a wider concept of countertransference and the idea of projective identification, could easily be misused – as shown in the now classic story about a young analyst who told her he felt confused and therefore interpreted to his patient that the patient had projected confusion into him, to which Melanie Klein replied, 'No, dear, you are confused'.
>
> *(Spillius, 1983, p. 326)*

This endorses the classical view of countertransference as the analyst's problem. The impression is that Klein remained disinterested and more or less dismissive of these developments. However, since Klein's closest supporters and students had such a strong interest in the new view of countertransference, it seems unlikely that she can have been completely indifferent. Klein normally kept a tight control over the views of her close collaborators. If she really did endorse Freud's view that countertransference was nothing more than the analyst's pathology, how was it that her followers such as Rosenfeld, Money-Kyrle, and Bion felt the freedom to develop a view of countertransference that was quite out of accord with Klein's own views?

Two sets of archival material suggest that Klein may have taken more of an interest in countertransference during the 1950s. First is a seminar Klein gave for some newly qualified analysts in 1958 (See Spillius, 2007 and Steiner, 2017, based on the archive file C.72). This 'discussion with young colleagues' became heated, but Spillius summarized it fairly: One can but sympathize with both parties in this discussion. The young analysts were espousing the wider view of countertransference that was beginning to become generally accepted in modern Kleinian thinking. But Klein was 'right' too: she did not want analysts to be carried away by their transference to the patient and to regard this aspect of their own character as valid data about the patient (Spillius, 2007, p. 80).

The second archive file is a couple of sets of Notes on Countertransference in connection with the London Congress of the International Psychoanalytic Association, to be found at the beginning of file D.29. I shall consider these latter Notes in some detail, and they are reproduced as an Appendix to this chapter. These comments on countertransference do not completely confirm Melanie Klein's simple rejection of the countertransference.

The 1953 symposium

By the early 1950s, a number of Klein's students had been working with schizophrenic patients, following on from Klein's paper on schizoid mechanisms (Klein, 1946). In 1953, the International Psychoanalytical Congress came to London. It was a moment when interest in the psychoanalysis of schizophrenia was at its height in Britain. There were two symposia on psychosis to which Klein's students contributed. One was on 'The Psychology of Schizophrenia' to which Bion gave a paper ('Notes on the theory of schizophrenia'); and the other was on 'The Therapy of Schizophrenia', to which Rosenfeld contributed ('Considerations regarding the psycho-analytic approach to acute and chronic schizophrenia'). Klein's Notes in D.29 concern her contribution to the discussion of the first of these symposia, the one to which Bion gave his paper. Bion's paper is the first in his series on schizophrenia published between 1954 and 1959, and later collected as *Second Thoughts* (Bion, 1967). At the core of that paper is Bion's interest in words.

> Language is employed by the schizophrenic in three ways: as a mode of action, as a method of communication, and as a mode of thought. He will show a preference for action on occasions when other patients would realize that what was required was thought; thus, he will want to go over to a piano to take out the movement to understand why someone is playing the piano.
>
> *(Bion, 1954, p. 113)*

Bion is conveying that the schizophrenic patient investigates the analyst's mind in the same dismantling way as the piano, and as if it is as concrete as the piano. One of his most telling examples of this intrusive dismantling is the following:

> The patient comes into the room, shakes me warmly by the hand, and looking piercingly into my eyes says, 'I think the sessions are not for a long while but stop me ever going out.' I know from previous experience that this patient has a grievance that the sessions are too few and that they interfere with his free time. He intended to split me by making me give two opposite interpretations at once, and this was shown by his next association when he said, 'How does the lift know what to do when I press two buttons at once?'
>
> *(Bion, 1954, pp. 113–114)*

This exemplifies how words are actions on someone else's mind, and how they inflict a particular state of mind on the analyst. Bion implied it is not just the patient's mind that is split; the mind of the analyst treating a schizophrenic patient is also under pressure to split. So, Bion indicated, there is a particular kind of countertransference in which the analyst feels his mind is interfered with. In consequence, he asserted that: 'Countertransference has to play an important part in the analysis of the schizophrenic' (Bion, 1954, p. 113). It is this countertransference interference that Melanie Klein pointed to in the comments she made in her discussion (see D.29 in Appendix).

One of Bion's later papers was 'Differentiation of the psychotic from the non-psychotic personalities', in which he gives clinical evidence of the co-existence of two parts of the personality, one psychotic and one non psychotic. In fact, he read this paper to the British Psychoanalytical Society in 1956, and it was published in 1957. However, Moritz Katan's paper to the London Congress in 1953 (Katan, 1954) was on this topic, 'The importance of the non-psychotic part of the personality in schizophrenia', and three years earlier than Bion's. Bion never refers to Katan's work in any of his papers on schizophrenia.

It is hard not to conclude that Bion got his idea of the divided personality from being on the same panel of the 1953 Congress mentioned above when Katan's paper was read (by Ralph Greenson). In fact, Klein picked up Katan's point briefly in her discussion, 'I fully agree with Dr Katan, who stresses the importance of keeping in mind, in the analysis of schizophrenics, the sane part of their personalities.'

Speculatively, one could wonder if, after the Congress, Klein and Bion discussed Katan's idea in depth and Bion set to work eventually to produce his 1957 paper.

It is worth however noting the differences between Katan's conception and Bion's. Katan followed Freud's analysis of fetishism, in which two parts of the ego use different defences, repression and disavowal, the latter being potentially psychotic. Katan thought that in schizophrenia the two parts operated oedipal and pre-oedipal defences. His model was that the patient has a sane part, which is tackling oedipal problems, whilst there exists another part, the psychotic part, which is pre-oedipal and in fact denies oedipal issues altogether.

The Notes in D.29

The Notes (see Appendix) consist of two documents in archive file D.29 concerned with the discussion at the symposium to which Bion gave his paper. These comprise five well-typed pages in all. In fact, they are two separate versions of Klein's comments; one version was prepared beforehand and entitled 'Intended contribution to congress discussion' (the word 'intended' is inserted in handwriting, presumably added later). A second, somewhat expanded and to some extent rephrased version, seems to have been typed up afterwards and was a recollection of what she had said entitled 'Remarks in congress discussion on countertransference, 1953'.

From the beginning of her 'intended contribution' Klein had in mind to discuss countertransference. She started, 'I want to say a few words about countertransference.' She went on to point to negative and hostile attitudes in the patient which initiate difficult countertransference feelings of rejection. She described two specific countertransference reactions that result:

> Firstly, the analyst may attempt to 'reinforce the positive transference by methods such as reassurance' and secondly, she said that, in recent years, 'the analyst is on the lookout for negative feelings only and under-rating the complex fact that both love and hatred will express themselves in the transference situation', so that 'we could say that the too- vigilant analyst has found a way of dealing with anxieties by excessively tackling the hostile feelings in the patient.
>
> *(D.29 image 8)*

One way or another, either by sweetly reassuring, or by more muscular interpretation, the analyst effects a separation of the currents of both love and hate in the transference and countertransference. Klein is clear that this is a collusion between analyst and patient. It is not, as Freud would have had it, solely the analyst's doing.

Klein then turned with some sympathy to countertransference with schizophrenic patients. She fully described the particular intrusive and schismatic effect on the analyst: 'the patient's violent processes of splitting the analyst and pushing into him parts of his self and of his impulses – a process which I have named projective identification – has a most strenuous effect on the analyst' (D.29 image 8).

In support of this, Klein specifically referred to Bion's vignette in which his patient split the analyst's mind by demanding how two opposite buttons can be pressed at the same time. She must have read Bion's draft and the vignette beforehand, in order to refer to it in her 'intended contribution'. She went on to stress the importance of understanding these projective processes:

> The point I wish to emphasise is that only by studying the processes of projective identification in their roots in the first few months of life, as well as their implications, that the analyst can cope in himself with this particular countertransference difficulty.
>
> *(D.29 image 8)*

Klein is clearly claiming that the countertransference is rooted in the patient's psychodynamics; she is not claiming that the experience comes from the unanalysed neurosis of the analyst. So, countertransference for Klein is more than Freud's judgement that it is the analyst's complexes and internal resistances.

The splitting of the analyst's mind is specifically a reaction to the encounter with a schizophrenic patient. Klein, it seems, is pointing to a specificity here about the patient's use of the analyst's mind. To be sure, she does not make an explicit claim about the specificity, nor that it can be informative in any particular case; and she still describes this as disturbance the analyst should cope with. However, the recognition of a specific interaction occurring generally with all analysts means that the countertransference can also stem from the patient, and the patient's pathology, and is not solely from the analyst's neurosis. It is a reaction brought out in the analyst by the patient, and would in our contemporary terms be regarded as an enactment. Klein is describing a complex psychic enactment involving the intrusive transfer (projective identification) of parts of the patient's mind and experiences.

Remarks on countertransference

Presumably, when Klein came actually to make her remarks at the Congress, she adapted what she intended to say, probably having heard the papers of other contributors to the symposium as well as Bion's. As a result, she makes a new off-the-cuff point. The importance of that point may have been the reason for typing out what she had said as a separate set of notes. The new point is to observe the emphasis placed on libido by generations of psychoanalysts. She speculated that this emphasis and the neglect of hostility resulted from a general countertransference that occurs in all analysts:

> The fact that the predominance given to libido in psycho-analytic thought was maintained for so long and that only recently the importance of aggression is being fully evaluated, has had something to do, I believe, with the counter-transference of analysts. By giving fuller attention to libido, they also gave fuller attention to the positive transference and in this way saved themselves from the effects of negative transference, that is, from having hatred and hostile feelings by the patient directed at them.
>
> *(D.29 image 1)*

Klein is venturing bravely across contentious territory. In criticizing the single-minded emphasis on positive impulses (libido), she implicitly takes issue with Freud's paper on transference love (Freud, 1915). She implies that transference love and a countertransference response do not arise, as Freud says, from the libidinal problem, but from the joint problem analyst and patient have with hostility. Perhaps she was not fully aware of the implications of this off-the-cuff remark, as she tried to strengthen her point about the negative countertransference. Rhetorically, she was merely taking a step towards her main point about the countertransference in schizophrenia, which was in her 'Intended Contribution' text. However, the point she actually made is more emphatic than in the 'Intended Contribution':

> In addition to all this, there is a point I wish to stress – the particular processes of the schizophrenic of splitting his own ego and the analysis of projective identification, a term I coined to denote the tendency to split parts of the self and to put them into the other person, stir in the analyst very strong countertransference feelings of a negative kind.
>
> *(D.29 image 1, continued in image 3)*

Klein is pointing here to a specific psychodynamic process in which the analyst's resulting experience is not simply from his complexes, but is directed by the patient's characteristic defences of splitting and projective identification.

I am suggesting that the points in these two texts show Klein confirming a view of countertransference as a product of projective processes, as later Kleinians have fully exploited. She remained more alert to the misunderstandings to which these projective intrusions of the schizophrenic patient give rise than to their communicative quality.[4] Quoting from C. 72 (Spillius, 2007, Steiner, 2017) Klein said:

> I have been called counter-countertransference. Now, it isn't so. You know of course that the patient is bound to stir certain feelings in the analyst and that this varies according to the patient's attitude, according to the patient, though there are of course feelings at work in the analyst which he has to be aware of.
>
> *(Steiner, 2017, p. 103)*

This acknowledged the patient's role in the analyst's feelings, and the analyst's potentially specific response is accorded to the patient; but Klein did not go so far as to acknowledge the possibility of using these countertransference feelings as information about a specific patient. She added, 'I have never found that the countertransference has helped me to understand my patient better .... I have found it helped me to understand myself better' (Steiner, 2017, p. 103).

Klein moved here from the general acknowledgement of the specificity of countertransference, to a personal caution. However, it seems to me an exaggeration to say Klein was simply against the new developments, and it cannot be claimed she followed Freud's position exactly that countertransference is the analyst's pathology. We can see her attempting to carve out an intermediate position; which might explain how, in the early 1950s, Klein's followers felt they might be allowed a freedom to develop the notion of countertransference, and particularly to ground it in projective mechanisms.

The published comment on countertransference

Klein's point that analysts can collude with patients in developing a cosy relationship, and thereby split off aggression from both parties, is the substance of her one published comment on countertransference. In 1957, in *Envy and Gratitude*,[5] Klein wrote:

> Even the patient's co-operation, which allows for an analysis of very deep layers of the mind, of destructive impulses, and of persecutory anxiety, may up to a point be influenced by the urge to satisfy the analyst and to be loved by him. The analyst who is aware of this will analyse the infantile roots of such wishes; otherwise, in identification with his patient the early

> need for reassurance may strongly influence his countertransference and therefore his technique.
>
> *(Klein, 1957, p. 226)*

Klein discussed this kind of lapse in her own technique in session 65 of Richard (Klein, 1963, p. 326), where she follows the impact of her reassurance on the splitting of the patriotic and not foreign Mrs K from the suspect Mrs K.

This short comment confirms the view that, unlike Freud's paper advising that all analysts will have their own neurotic problems with erotic love, Klein is here saying again that the analyst's trouble comes from the patient's specific splitting. The patient's intention is to create either a reassuring analyst or a hostile one. The analyst may or may not accept one or other of these invitations. The situation however arises, in Klein's estimation, from the patient's intention to cause a splitting. The analyst may or may not be vulnerable to that invitation; countertransference is not a simple expression of the analyst's neurosis.

Conclusion: Melanie Klein and Paula Heimann

Klein's position on countertransference is clear enough in these Notes. It would seem fair to say that Klein did not altogether regard countertransference as pathology, just that it could lead to loss of insight, especially in cases where there is a great deal of hostility in the transference. A question arises then about Klein's reticence in writing about countertransference, especially as it led, during her life-time, to a partial misunderstanding of her views. Why did she not publish more of the views she expressed in these Notes? It was not that she decided they were wrong, since she did mention them briefly four years later in *Envy and Gratitude* (Klein, 1957).

One speculative answer is that she wished to avoid a public disagreement with Paula Heimann. When Klein wrote the Notes in 1953, there had been a considerable history to their relationship and Klein was greatly indebted to Heimann's fierce defence of Kleinian views during the Controversial Discussions (see King & Steiner, 1991). Klein had been interested in psychosis since before her book on children was published in 1932. In 1934 she was actively considering the primitive defence mechanisms (see Hinshelwood, 2006). She published her first paper on manic-depressive states in 1935. In January that year, 1935, Paula Heimann started her analysis with Klein. Heimann was medically trained and with some experience of psychiatry. She read a paper for her membership of the British Psychoanalytical Society in 1939, on a patient with delusional experiences about being occupied by demons. The paper was given in part in order to state a Kleinian position on internal objects. It was also a response to a paper given by Anna Freud, the first paper Anna Freud gave to the scientific meetings of the British Psychoanalytical Society (see Hinshelwood, 1997).

Heimann's thesis was that the psychotic features of this case derived from a violent form of internalization. The paper was not published until 1942, and not long afterwards was superseded by Klein's paper on schizoid processes (Klein, 1946) where Klein particularly emphasized projective processes in schizoid states.

In 1949 Heimann wrote the paper on countertransference for the IPA Congress in Zürich, though Klein apparently advised her not to. Heimann did not take that advice, and read her paper to the Congress, publishing it in 1950 (Heimann, 1950). There ensued a period in which Klein and Heimann moved apart. Grosskurth (1986) described it as a 'serious disagreement' (p. 378). It may have been so, but the disagreement, Grosskurth conveyed, was a personal one as much as a scientific conceptual one. If in fact it had a strong personal quality, this would explain the fact that, when published in 1950, the paper contained no reference to Klein at all. Tonnesman (1989) also said that Heimann had longstanding criticisms of Klein's theories and techniques. These are not made public in the 1950 paper, and Klein may have felt it best not to make her criticisms of Heimann public either. She did not go as far as Heimann in arguing for the countertransference as part of the technical tool-kit. Whereas Heimann was radical in her testimony to countertransference, by 1960 she had become more cautious (Heimann, 1960). She seemed to have moved closer to Klein's own cautious concern, and there could have been some *rapprochement* between them on this point. However, Melanie Klein died in that year, 1960.

The Notes in D.29 are of interest if Klein's position on countertransference was somewhere between Freud's and the contemporary one. Even if my claim is incorrect, the Notes still give us an insight into a topic Klein was very reticent to write about, which has led to speculations about her views, evidenced only by apocryphal stories. The Notes are a brief but substantive resource to study her actual views, and to accept that Klein did think there were important things to say about countertransference and to contribute to understanding its effects on the development of psychoanalytic technique itself.

Notes

1 An earlier version of this chapter was published as Hinshelwood (2008) 'Melanie Klein and countertransference'.
2 In Hinshelwood's (2008) original journal paper this is mistakenly referred to as file D.31.
3 These views on countertransference were one of the strong reasons for the development of a training programme for psychoanalysts in the 1920s including a personal analysis of the trainee. At first it was called a 'control' analysis, precisely because it was intended to be an analysis of the trainee's reactions to his patients, and thus assist in controlling his own neurotic interference with the patient's material. It was perhaps one of the reasons for revising the view of countertransference, that by the 1940s a generation of psychoanalysts had been trained who had had their own personal analysis, and they were still having feelings about their patients. Countertransference seemed to be here to stay and therefore it pointed to a more human encounter in the psychoanalytic setting being inevitable, and therefore in need of study, not just condemnation and eradication.

4 Note also that in her enthusiasm to make her contribution known Klein is claiming she coined the term 'projective identification'. In fact, she did not. It had already been used by in 1945 by Marjorie Brierley; and apparently in 1925 by Edoardo Weiss, according to Spillius (2007).
5 There is a history to this text. It was originally given as a paper in July 1955 to the IPA Congress in Geneva, but not published. Subsequently an enlarged version was given to the British Psychoanalytical Society in early 1956, and published much later in Mitchell (1986). Klein further worked on her text to produce a short book in 1957. The remark quoted about the effect of envy on countertransference did not appear until 1957, in the book-length version.

References

Balint, M. and Balint, A. (1939). On transference and countertransference. *Int. J. Psycho-Anal., 20*, 223–230.
Bion, W.R. (1951). The imaginary twin. In W.R. Bion, *Second thoughts*. New York: Jason Aronson, 1967.
Bion, W.R. (1954). Notes on the theory of schizophrenia. *Int. J. Psycho-Anal., 35*, 113–118. Reprinted in W.R. Bion, *Second thoughts*. New York: Jason Aronson, 1967.
Bion, W.R. (1957). Differentiation of the psychotic from the non-psychotic personalities. *Int. J. Psycho-Anal., 38*, 266–275. Reprinted in W.R. Bion, *Second thoughts*. New York: Jason Aronson, 1967.
Bion, W.R. (1967). *Second thoughts*. New York: Jason Aronson.
Brierley, M. (1951). Further notes on the implications of psychoanalysis: metapsychology and personology. *Int. J. Psycho-Anal., 26*, 89–114.
Freud, S. (1910). The future prospects of psychoanalytic therapy. *The standard edition of the complete psychological works of Sigmund Freud*, vol. *11*. London: Hogarth, pp. 139–152.
Freud, S. (1915). Observations on transference love. *The standard edition* vol. *12*. London: Hogarth, pp. 157–171.
Grosskurth, P. (1986). *Melanie Klein: Her life and work*. London: Hodder & Stoughton.
Heimann, P. (1942). A contribution to the problem of sublimation and its relation to processes of internalization. *Int. J. Psycho-Anal., 23*, 8–17. Reprinted in P. Heimann, *About children and children-no-longer*. London: Hogarth, 1989.
Heimann, P. (1950). On countertransference. *Int. J. Psycho-Anal., 31*, 81–84. Reprinted in P. Heimann, *About children and children-no-longer*. London: Hogarth, 1989.
Heimann, P. (1960). Countertransference. *Brit. J. Med. Psychol., 33*, 9–15. Reprinted in P. Heimann, *About children and children-no-longer*. London: Hogarth, 1989.
Hinshelwood, R.D. (1997). The elusive concept of 'Internal Objects' (1934–1943): Its role in the formation of the Klein group. *Int. J. Psycho-Anal., 78*, 877–897.
Hinshelwood, R.D. (2006). Melanie Klein and repression. *Psychoanalysis and History, 8(1)*, 5–42.
Hinshelwood, R.D. (2008). Melanie Klein and countertransference: A historical note. *Psychoanalysis and History, 10*, 95–113.
Katan, M. (1954). The importance of the non-psychotic part of the personality in schizophrenia. *Int. J. Psycho-Anal., 35*, 119–128.
King, P. and Steiner, R. (eds) (1991). *The Freud–Klein controversies 1941–1945*. London and New York: Routledge.
Klein, M. (1935). A contribution to the psychogenesis of manic-depressive states. *Int. J. Psycho-Anal., 16*, 145–174. In *The writings of Melanie Klein*, vol. *1*. London: Hogarth.

Klein, M. (1946). Notes on some schizoid mechanisms. *Int. J. Psycho-Anal., 27*, 99–110. In *The writings of Melanie Klein*, vol. *1*. London: Hogarth.
Klein, M. (1957). Envy and gratitude. In *The writings of Melanie Klein*, vol. *1*. London: Hogarth.
Klein, M. (1963). Narrative of a child analysis. In *The writings of Melanie Klein*, vol. *4*. London: Hogarth.
Mitchell, J. (1986). *Selected writings of Melanie Klein*. London: Penguin.
Money-Kyrle, R. (1956). Normal countertransference and some of its deviations. *Int. J. Psycho-Anal., 37*, 360–366. Reprinted in R. Money-Kyrle, *The collected papers of Roger Money-Kyrle*. Strath Tay: Clunie Press, 1978.
Racker, H. (1957). The meanings and uses of countertransference. *Psychoanal. Q., 26*, 303–357.
Reich, A. (1951). On countertransference. *Int. J. Psycho-Anal., 32*, 25–31.
Rosenfeld, H. (1947). Analysis of a schizophrenic state with depersonalization. *Int. J. Psycho-Anal., 28*, 130–139. Reprinted in H. Rosenfeld, *Psychotic states*. London: Hogarth, 1965.
Rosenfeld, H. (1950). Note on the psychopathology of confusional states in chronic schizophrenias. *Int. J. Psycho-Anal., 31*, 132–137. Reprinted in H. Rosenfeld, *Psychotic states*. London: Hogarth, 1965.
Rosenfeld, H. (1952). Transference-phenomena and transference-analysis in an acute catatonic schizophrenic patient. *Int. J. Psycho-Anal., 33*, 457–464. Reprinted in H. Rosenfeld, *Psychotic states*. London: Hogarth, 1965.
Segal, H. (1950). Some aspects of the analysis of a schizophrenic. *Int. J. Psycho-Anal., 31*, 268–278. Reprinted in H. Segal, *The work of Hanna Segal*. New York: Jason Aronson, 1981.
Segal, H. (1982). *Melanie Klein*. Unpublished paper.
Spillius, E. (1983). Some developments from the work of Melanie Klein. *Int. J. Psycho-Anal., 64*, 321–332.
Spillius, E. (1992). Clinical experiences of projective identification. In R. Anderson, *Clinical lectures on Klein and Bion*. London: Routledge.
Spillius, E. (2007). *Encounters with Melanie Klein*. London: Routledge.
Steiner, J. (ed.) (2017). *Lectures on technique by Melanie Klein*. London: Routledge.
Tonnesman, M. (1989) Editor's introduction. In P. Heimann, *About children and children-no-longer*. London: Hogarth.
Winnicott, D. (1949). Hate in the countertransference. *Int. J. Psycho-Anal., 30*, 69–74. Reprinted in D. Winnicott, *Through paediatrics to psychoanalysis*. London: Tavistock, 1958.

Appendix: Two manuscripts of Melanie Klein on countertransference and schizophrenia

In the Melanie Klein Archives there are two manuscripts which Klein wrote for the 1953 Congress of the IPA in London, both in archive file D.29. One of these manuscripts was typed, probably by her secretary, as the comments she intended to make in the discussion to a session on 'The Psychology of Schizophrenia'. The other is typed less well and therefore possibly by Klein, after the discussion, and represents her recollections of the slightly fuller remarks that she did make in the discussion. In the digitized archive the pages of each manuscript have become separated, so that the 'intended contribution' appears in image 8 followed by image 7 and the three pages constituting the 'remarks' are separated by two domestic items.

All italicized text in these Notes was added in handwriting.

Intended Contribution to Congress Discussion (D. 29 images 8 and 7)

I want to say a few words about counter-transference. Negative attitudes in the patient, hostility and hatred have, I think, always been a great difficulty for the analyst and have influenced the tendency to reinforce the positive transference by methods such as reassurance. In passing I may add that in more recent years we can also observe the opposite tendency in the analyst, which also does not do justice to the situation, and that is his being on the look-out for negative feelings only and under-rating the complex fact that both love and hatred will express themselves in the transference situation. Since I am touching on the topic of counter transference, we could say that the too vigilant analyst has found a way of dealing with anxieties by excessively tackling the hostile feelings in the patient.

To turn now to the schizophrenic. Counter-transference in the case of schizophrenics has particular difficulties. The patient's attitude of non-cooperativeness behind which a deep negative and hostile attitude is operative, but particularly the patient's violent processes of splitting the analyst and pushing into him parts of his self and of his impulses – a process which I have named projective identification – has a most strenuous effect on the analyst. Dr. Bion has illustrated the way in which his patient split him by the instance of the two opposite buttons which the patient wanted to press in the lift. Such processes are apt to make the analyst tired, sleepy, and stir up strong resistance against the work in him. The point I wish to emphasise is that only by studying the processes of projective identification in their roots in the first few months of life, as well as their implications, that the analyst can cope in himself with this particular counter-transference difficulty.

The facts which I have mentioned have had a profound influence on the development of psycho-analytic knowledge and technique. Since the countertransference in the cases of schizophrenia – and I wish particularly to stress the chronic schizophrenic – produce such difficulties in the analyst, this has vitally influenced the attitude of analysts towards these patients. There has always been – notwithstanding the scientific interest – a tendency in the analyst to reassure the patient, to bring about a positive transference and create a situation which would not impose on himself such strenuous demands. The effect of that tendency was, I believe, to hold up the development of psychoanalytic knowledge and therapy as far as schizophrenia is concerned. Since we have come to see more clearly that the understanding of psychosis also throws light on the mental life of less ill patients, it is of greatest value to explore as deeply as we are able the fixation points of schizophrenia.

Remarks in Congress discussion on Countertransference, 1953 (D.29 images 1, 3 and 5)

I shall make a few remarks about countertransference. The fact that the predominance given to libido in psycho-analytic thought was maintained for so long and that only recently the importance of aggression is being fully evalued, has had something to do, I believe, with the countertransference of analysts. By giving fuller attention to libido, they also gave fuller attention to the positive transference and in this way saved themselves from the effects of negative transference, that is, from having hatred and hostile feelings by the patient directed at them. In passing, I would say that, more recently, one can observe that some analysts give undue attention to the negative transference, that is to say, they do not allow sufficiently for the mixture of love and hatred which, alternatively or simultaneously, will show itself in the transference. This, too, I would connect with the counter-transference, for to concentrate on the negative feelings of the patient only is also, I think, a way of overcoming the anxieties aroused by the hostility of the patient.

To turn now to the schizophrenic patients, the fear of his hostility in some cases where he is actually dangerous is no doubt an influence on the countertransference of the analyst, even where precautions are taken. With schizophrenic patients who are not dangerous, but who direct their silent, nonco-operative and deeply hostile attitude towards the analyst, his countertransference is inclined to be a negative one. In addition to all this, there is a point I wish to stress – the particular processes of the schizophrenic of splitting his own ego and the analysis of projective identification, a term I coined to denote the tendency to split parts of the self and to put them into the other person, stir in the analyst very strong countertransference feelings of a negative kind. He may get tired, he may wish to go to sleep, he feels assailed by the patient intruding into him and may fight against this intrusion. In my view, this fact, more than any other, is the reason why, in such situations, analysts have always been inclined to alter the situation by reassuring the patient, by trying to bring about a positive transference, by not touching on the deepest anxieties of the patient, etc. I think that it is only by knowing more of these processes, derived from the ~~paranoid schizoid~~ infantile that analysts can cope with the counter-transference.

I wish to draw a conclusion from this. I believe that the understanding of the psychopathology of schizophrenia and the therapy have been very much held up by counter-transference feelings of the analysts, notwithstanding their scientific interest in the study of schizophrenia.

The work of some of my colleagues has shown that, by taking full account of both the negative and the positive transference, and by tracing it back to its earliest sources, a promising therapy of schizophrenia is possible. I believe that only by going back to these earliest processes, the patient is enabled to achieve greater synthesis and integration, with his splitting processes diminished, and that he acquires a greater capacity to introject good objects ~~all of which~~ underlies the process of the cure of schizophrenia.

I fully agree with Dr Katan, who stresses the importance of keeping in mind, in the analysis of schizophrenics, the sane part of their personalities. I always thought it important to take into account, when analysing even very young children, that part of their ego which has already developed, and not only consider the primitive and earliest processes, but I believe that, if the attention paid to the sane part of the schizophrenic is too much stressed and accordingly the analysis of the psychotic part underrated, the prospects of the cure will suffer.

Dr Hartman has again mentioned his concept of neutralization. I described, many years ago, the processes underlying neutralization in the terms of the mitigation of hatred by love, of aggression by libido. In doing so, I had very much in mind that the analyst has to go back to the earliest stages of development, whereby the mitigation of hatred by love becomes possible, and also suggested that such changes at bottom imply changes in the fusion between the life and death instinct.

Also reference to Dr Bion, saying he intimated importance of sane part by stressing necessity of 'mature' interpretations.

11

THE ELUSIVE CONCEPT OF INTERNAL OBJECTS (1934–1943)

Its role in the formation of the Klein Group[1]

R.D. Hinshelwood

Introduction

Here I trace a debate about the concept of 'internal objects' that took place between 1937 and 1943 at a time when a group of British analysts was forming around Melanie Klein. Using archival and other material, I show how the debate is set within a complex of personal, group and organizational dynamics. The history of the British Psycho-Analytical Society at this time exemplifies Bion's notion of group schism. The events in the Society's history demonstrate defensive aspects of the interaction between the opposed groups, which support members against various anxieties. These include the stress of the work of analysis, but also in this instance the particular anxieties deriving from the collapse of psychoanalysis in Europe, the state of war, and the death of Freud shortly after he came to London. This psychoanalytic anxiety/defence model clarifies some aspects of the debate about internal objects, and demonstrates the way in which anxieties and defences become organized around a scientific debate in a scientific society.

The concept of the 'internal object' is little debated now in the British Psycho-Analytical Society. However, it was not always so. From 1934 to 1943 the concept was discussed on many occasions, with 1939 the focal year. This scientific development interacts with two important historical events; the arrival of the Freud family in London and the beginning of the development of the Klein group. Both would have profound effects on the dynamics of the British Society.

The Society was established in 1919 and by 1926, when it had consolidated itself, a dramatic clash had occurred between Melanie Klein in London and Anna Freud in Vienna over their different forms of child analysis. This rivalry endured and was a feature of the correspondence between Ernest Jones and Sigmund Freud (Steiner, 1985; Paskauskas, 1993).

Klein's book *The Psycho-Analysis of Children* appeared in 1932 to great acclaim in Britain (Klein, 1932). It was a landmark for her and for the British Society. No psychoanalyst in Britain had previously made a contribution of such strength and quality. There were continual references to this book by British analysts. Future members of the non-aligned, independent group (e.g. Brierley, 1934; Karin Stephen, 1934, and later Payne, 1937) were as respectful as her own followers (Riviere, 1936a, 1936b; Scott, 1947). Even future detractors were complimentary (Glover, 1933; Schmideberg, 1934). Notably, Anna Freud's book *Four Lectures on Child Analysis*, published in German in 1927 (A. Freud, 1927), was not translated and published in England by the Hogarth Press as might have been expected, and in fact did not appear until 1948, after she had moved to London (A. Freud, 1948a); although a US edition in English was published in 1928 in New York (A. Freud, 1928).

By 1934 the British Society had achieved a considerable degree of internal harmony and was particularly proud of its own scientific achievements, particularly Melanie Klein's work with children. She was a figurehead who promised to put the British Society 'on the map' of scientific psychoanalysis, to complement Ernest Jones's role as organizer and chief politician within the movement.

At this time conflict had remained focused between London and Vienna (Steiner, 1989). With Federn and Anna Freud, Jones organized the so-called Exchange Lectures (1935–1936), a series of lectures between the London and Viennese Societies, in order to deal with the enduring conflict between them. For details of these lectures see Jones (1935), Waelder (1937) and Riviere (1936b). The series was not successful in developing mutual understanding, although as position papers each is very informative. The lack of success must have been due partly to the preoccupation in Vienna with something else – the progressive collapse of psychoanalysis in Germany.

By contrast with the confidence evident in 1934, by 1944, the Society had declined into two warring camps. Open dissent and often ad hominem criticism between distinct groups emerged within the British Society. Rivalry with Vienna was no longer across the breadth of the continent of Europe but had become heated controversy within the Society itself. Freud was dead and Jones had retired from active participation in Society affairs, so their friendship and need of each other no longer mediated the quarrel. Without the damping effect of geographical distance, the quality of scientific debate became seriously, and permanently, affected. Only a degree of political agreement was eventually patched up after the ferocious Controversial Discussions in 1943–44 (King & Steiner, 1991). The outcome of the internal war led directly to the strict and enduring tripartite structure of training that has marked the life of the British Psycho-Analytical Society ever since.

The period from 1934–1943 was one of change that prepared the ground (or battle-ground) for the Controversial Scientific Discussions. How did this change from early harmony to outright war come about?

The depressive position

Hanna Segal commented as follows:

> Up to the time when Mrs Klein read in the Society her paper on the psychogenesis of the manic-depressive states, one could not speak of a distinctive Kleinian school. There was rather an English school of psychoanalysis, diverging somewhat from the Viennese and Berlin schools ... This, however, began to change in 1935 when she introduced the concept of the depressive position.
>
> *(Segal, 1979, p. 77)*

That paper, 'A contribution to the psychogenesis of manic-depressive states' (Klein, 1935), was a watershed, describing processes of internalization that are directly derived from the Freud/Abraham theory of manic-depressive psychosis in which Freud had developed the theory of the superego as internalized parents.

Following Abraham, Klein suggested that internalization is the main process by which the whole of the personality develops. Objects taken in create an internal world of object relationships. Such objects are integral to the sense of self but are at the same time experienced as separate and quite concrete objects within the body. She carefully exemplified this idea with clinical material in that paper:

> The patient complained about different physical troubles and then went on to say what medicines he had taken – enumerating what he had done for his chest, his throat, his nose, his ears, his intestines, etc. It sounded rather as if he were nursing these parts of his body and his organs. He went on to speak about his concern for some young people under his care (he is a teacher) and then about the worry he was feeling for some members of his family. It became quite clear that the different organs he was trying to cure were identified with his internalized brothers and sisters.
>
> *(Klein, 1935, p. 275)*

Klein's addition to the Freud/Abraham theory was that loss of the external object resonates internally as an insecurity of the internal object. The object's fate inside the person is crucial to the whole mental state and symptomatology. Klein was describing something quite different from, and more concrete than, 'presentation', as Freud described, or 'representation' as we might say today.

The paper, read at the International Congress in August 1934, caused unease in Vienna. But when Klein read it later to the British Psycho-Analytical Society in January 1935, interest began in earnest. Though very perplexed by this kind of description, the members of the British Society really wanted to know what Klein meant.

Internal objects

In modern psychoanalysis the depressive position is important as a development of whole object relationships out of earlier part-object ones. However, when the paper was first presented, a different element was stressed: this idea of 'internal objects'. The scientific meetings of the Society had very varied topics, but the most common between 1935 and 1942 was on the internal object (see list below).

Seven papers were presented to the British Psycho-Analytical Society on this theme, and the continual return to the topic shows how difficult it was to grasp. The respect, even awe, with which Klein's paper was received in 1935 was not however the only response. Such acclaim could also turn sour. An unpleasant emotional reaction emerged into the life of the Society.

First and most forceful was Klein's daughter, Melitta Schmideberg. She had recently (1934) gone to Glover for a further psychoanalysis (Grosskurth, 1986). Soon he too was involved in disputes that rather quickly became distasteful ad hominem attacks upon Klein. These attacks became persistent, and such strong animosity was painful for Society members to witness.

The arrival of the Freud family

Freud escaped Vienna in 1938, arriving in London on 6 June. Illness prevented him taking part in British Psycho-Analytical Society life but Anna Freud regularly attended scientific meetings from as early as 29 June 1938. She found a Society in a quite extraordinary condition, at the crest of a confidence about its emerging scientific concepts, though its members were often in confusion, and sometimes in spiteful dissent, about the actual concepts themselves. Psychoanalysis in Europe had succumbed catastrophically to the political invasions. Freud wrote on the occasion of the twenty-fifth anniversary of the founding of the London Psychoanalytic Society in London: 'the events of recent years have so ordained that London has become chief venue and centre of the psychoanalytic movement' (letter to Jones, 7 March 1939; Paskauskas, 1993 p. 769).

The British Psycho-Analytical Society found itself surviving in a Europe in which nearly all psychoanalysis had been obliterated. Its sense of mission in rescuing Freud and his family reflected also a mission to preserve psychoanalysis itself. However, it was in difficulties. The rivalry hitherto conducted across the continent was now on its doorstep.

Papers on internalization and internal objects 1937–1942

1937 Fuchs read 'On introjection' to the Society and published it that year (Fuchs, 1937).

1938 Adrian Stephen read 'Transference and counter-transference in superego modification' to the Society, published in 1947 as 'The super-ego and the internal object' (Stephen, 1947).

1938 Isaacs read 'Temper tantrums in early childhood and their relation to internal objects' to the Society, published in 1940 (Isaacs, 1940).
1939 Brierley published 'A prefatory note on "internalized objects" and depression' (Brierley, 1939).
1939 Heimann read 'A contribution to the problem of sublimation and its relation to processes of internalization', published in 1942 (Heimann, 1942).
1938 Klein read her paper to the Paris Conference, 'Mourning and its relation to manic depressive states', read it to the British Psycho-Analytical Society in October, published in 1940 (Klein, 1940).
1940 Matte-Blanco read 'On introjection and the processes of psychic metabolism', published in 1941 (Matte-Blanco, 1941).
1941 Alix Strachey published 'A note on the use of the word "internal"' (Strachey, 1941)
1942 Brierley read 'Internal objects and theory' to the Society, published the same year (Brierley, 1942).
1939 Rickman read 'The nature of an internal object' (unpublished).
1941 Schmideberg read '"Introjected object": a terminological issue or a clinical problem' (unpublished).

Early confrontation

Events quickened after the Freuds' arrival London, with the Kleinians particularly threatened. Soon after Anna Freud's arrival, in October 1938, Melanie Klein gave her second paper on the depressive position 'Mourning and its relation to manic-depressive states', and two months later, Susan Isaacs gave a paper entitled 'Temper tantrums in early childhood and their relation to internal objects'. Her exposition, with detailed and vivid clinical illustration, was an attempt to clarify the concept of internal objects to the Society still uncertain about the idea. The paper does not break new ground and was clearly intended to provide instances of the relation to inner objects and the dimension of interiority that the depressive position stressed. Her paper mainly offered evidence from child analysis. Isaacs gave the detailed case of a 3½-year-old boy. She concentrated on the phantasies of taking in 'the place where he puts objects or takes them from is quite as important as the particular object he is using' (Isaacs, 1940, p. 283).

Isaacs quoted a 4-year-old girl's phantasy of a desperate attempt to control through internalization: she nearly choked herself in swallowing her brother's whistle, and told her nurse: 'I didn't like the noise it made, and so I hid it in myself' (p. 293).

> [F]rom the beginning of his analysis ... [the boy] showed an absorbing interest in the insides of things, drawers, cupboards, boxes, the gas fire, electric fire, etc. For instance, he found he could lift off a portion of the front of the gas fire, and look at its inside parts ... one day he pointed to

> what he called 'the crack', across the head of a large screw inside this part of the fire, saying: 'I don't like that'... [He is] preoccupied with the fact that this 'crack' is inside.
>
> *(p. 283)*

Isaacs chose temper tantrums, an intense behavioural disturbance out of key with the objective social environment, because it suggested a preoccupation with an internal state. She was concerned not with 'the general theory of internal objects, but with the way in which an understanding of the various phantasies connected with internal objects serves to illuminate the phenomena of temper tantrums' (p. 282).

Isaacs emphasized phantasies. Clearly they played a key part in the way she understood the material of child analysis. The case was complex and she described it in a dense fashion. It did not successfully clear the fog of misunderstanding. In a footnote to the published version she candidly comments that the paper she read was 'far too condensed and not well balanced, taking for granted many points that needed further explication in order to show their connections' (p. 285n). Even in the extended version, as published, it is still dense and reads today as if she is jumping steps in her argument.

So, Anna Freud was confronted within six months of arriving in Britain by the Society's fascination with internal objects, in two very detailed and dense expositions. One was Klein's second paper on the depressive position, and the other was Isaacs', illustrating a rigorously applied Kleinian child technique. How would she introduce the classical Viennese point of view to the British Society? The crucial moment came in the summer of 1939.

The sublimation debate

Anna Freud did not speak in the discussion following Isaacs' paper in December 1938 and she did not give a paper herself to the Society for another six months. But when she did it was on her own terms. If she had been provoked by the Kleinian papers she seems to have responded especially to Isaacs' emphasis on phantasy, because when she did present her first paper it was on sublimation (entitled 'Sexuality and sublimation'). It is not known what Anna Freud said on that occasion as her paper was never published. Young-Bruehl commented as follows about Anna Freud's customary method of giving her papers without a text:

> The 1939 paper on 'Sexuality and sublimation' that you mention was never published; it may not even have been an actual paper, as Anna Freud most often delivered her lectures from notes of an outline, and only wrote things out later. But she did – after much delay – work up what seems to be the material for that lecture for several popular papers in non-psychoanalytic publications.
>
> *(Young-Bruehl, personal letter of 29 August 1989)*

Young-Bruehl mentioned in her letter to me 'Sex in childhood' (A. Freud, 1944a), 'Difficulties of sex enlightenment' (A. Freud, 1944b), and 'Sublimation as a factor in upbringing' (A. Freud, 1948b). But those papers, for non-psychoanalytic readers, do not really engage with Kleinian views. However, from these 'popular papers' it is likely that what she said in 1939 connected with the fundamental work on sublimation which Freud and Anna Freud herself did nearly two decades previously (Freud, 1919; A. Freud, 1923). In that original work Sigmund Freud had reported a number of cases of fantasies of beating. One case in particular impressed him as an example of the process of sublimation where erotic fantasies had evolved into day-dreams and creativity: 'an elaborate superstructure of day-dreams . . . had grown up over the masochistic beating-phantasy. The function of this superstructure was to make possible a feeling of satisfied excitation, even though the masturbatory act was abstained from' (Freud, 1919 p. 190).

Freud emphasized the process of desexualization and the developmental steps towards conscious day-dreaming in which fantasy activity becomes independent of sexuality.

It is convincingly argued by Anna Freud's biographer Young-Bruehl (1988, p. 103) that in her 1923 paper on sublimation the only psychoanalysis that Anna Freud was in a position to write about was her own; and her patient was the same one as Freud's; that is, herself. That adolescent girl patient had written down, as Freud's patient did, large numbers of what she called 'nice stories'. Anna Freud's 1923 paper distinguished failed from successful sublimation:

> While the phantasies of beating thus represent a return of the repressed [sexual phantasies], the nice stories on the other hand represent a sublimation of it. The beating fantasies constitute a gratification for the directly sexual tendencies, the nice stories for those which Freud describes as 'inhibited in their aim'.
>
> *(A. Freud, 1923, pp. 152–153)*

It is therefore aim-inhibited libido, thus desexualized, that becomes these day-dreams or fantasies.

My hypothesis at this stage is that as Freud's collaborator on sublimation in 1922, Anna Freud aimed her paper in 1939 at reiterating this classical theory of sublimation and fantasy life to the British Society. If that first paper to the Society, on 30 June 1939, was on this topic, then she would have taken up Isaacs' theme of phantasies (of internal objects) by asserting the classical view of sublimation and fantasies and connecting it with the development of the inner world of the personality. Here, as in so much of her life, she acted as her father's most loyal disciple.

There is no direct confirmation of my claim that the 1939 paper did respond to Isaacs' paper. However there is indirect, circumstantial evidence for my view from other historical sources. Later we will see that there is further evidence from the Melanie Klein Archives that suggests this; and it also makes clear that

Anna Freud did prepare a written paper beforehand, contrary to Elisabeth Young-Bruehl's surmise. As there is no surviving copy of this manuscript, we are left with the question: why did Anna Freud not publish her paper? One possibility is that the Kleinian responses to her paper made her want to reconsider it and to recast her argument, to convince them, to correct them, or possibly to eradicate any loopholes in her own theoretical position. Much discussion on phantasy did in fact come out between the two groups in 1943 (see King & Steiner, 1991).

One piece of evidence that Anna Freud was responding to the Kleinian papers comes from the minutes of the Scientific Meetings of the Society. These show that Klein's supporter Paula Heimann also gave a paper on sublimation, on 7 July, only one week after Anna Freud's paper. As scientific meetings in the British Psycho-Analytical Society were in those days, as today, fortnightly, the fact that only a week intervened between these two leads to the tempting suggestion that they were planned as a symposium between the Viennese group and the early Klein group.

There are other possible reasons that the date of the scientific meeting was changed. Minutes record that the meeting on 30 June to which Anna Freud gave her paper was a joint one, in London, with the French Society, and the date seems to have been adjusted for the visitors (delayed by a week). There is perhaps an entirely innocent explanation for the proximity in time between the two meetings. However, for the Kleinians, a quick response to the international meeting, at least to the British analysts, may have been important.

If these papers were in fact planned formally or informally as a symposium then it was a moment poised between the Exchange Lectures of 1935–1936 and the later Scientific Discussions of 1943–1944; and largely obscured by them. It makes us more intrigued by Anna Freud's paper.

Heimann's paper was called 'A contribution to the problem of sublimation and its relation to processes of internalisation' (Heimann, 1942). Like Susan Isaacs, her intention was to explore 'unconscious phantasies related to internalised objects' (Heimann, 1942, p. 8). Explicitly, she wanted to extend the Kleinian theory of internal objects by linking it with sublimation. The patient, a woman artist, felt herself to be 'inhabited by devils. These devils ... roamed about inside her, caused her physical pain and illnesses, inhibited her in all her activities, especially in painting, and compelled her to do things she did not want to do' (p. 9). The problem to which she alludes in the title concerns the 'element of internal freedom and independence which I consider to be an essential condition for successful sublimation' (p. 15).

The purpose of Heimann's paper is to describe processes by which an internalized object becomes part of the ego; or, alternatively, if things go wrong, the internalized object becomes an alien entity experienced in a 'not-me' fashion, like devils, but actually still located within the self and the body. For this artist certain internal objects – the devils – inhibited her capacity to paint, and therefore her sublimatory activity. The conclusion is this: anxiety inhibits sublimation.

Heimann's thesis contests Anna Freud's position and the contrast is stark. On the one hand (Heimann) anxiety, arising from unconscious phantasies such as persecutory internal objects, results in inhibition and then the expression of symptoms; on the other hand (Anna Freud) anxiety, from obstructed libido, results in inhibition and then sublimation as (desexualized) fantasies. It is possible to make these chains of causal relations compatible (see Appendix I), but the conditions of the time led the participants to stress the differences.

In a letter concerning this point in an earlier draft of this chapter, Anne-Marie Sandler wrote: 'What I find so interesting in your paper is that it illustrates so clearly the difficulty we have in our society to understand each other because different groups use the same terms to indicate very different concepts' (personal communication dated 8 January 1996).

The Kleinian view of sublimation and its relations to internal objects and phantasies is a completely new and original development.

The study group

Heimann's 1942 paper is written with confidence and authority. It lacks the didactic quality of Isaacs' and is consequently more persuasive. And that may be because, quite possibly, it is a joint effort. The paper was Paula Heimann's membership paper, which means certainly that it was carefully vetted by Melanie Klein.

Melanie Klein had felt very threatened by Anna Freud coming to settle in London (Grosskurth, 1986). She criticized Jones for inviting the Freuds. She felt her own work, which had slowly gained credibility amongst British analysts, would be in jeopardy. To protect Melanie Klein's views a group of those who were especially interested formed a study group. It was called 'The Internal Objects Group', according to Clifford Scott, and was meeting by April 1939 but had clearly been mooted before. Isaacs described the purpose of this study group in a letter to Clifford Scott dated 13 January 1939 (Grosskurth, 1986) only a month or so after her paper had tried but failed to elucidate the concept. She wrote:

> we don't make it easy for the Viennese to understand our views, and ... one ought to give much more attention to the educational side of our work – to find ways of putting things which will get rid of intellectual obstacles at least.
>
> *(Isaacs quoted in Grosskurth, 1986, p. 244)*

The original idea of an Internal Objects Group is attributed (by Grosskurth) to Eva Rosenfeld, and the members were, it seems, variable. Scott recollected: 'Heimann, Isaacs (and sometimes, I think, her husband), Rickman, Riviere, myself and perhaps Evans met irregularly (every few weeks) for a time and circulated notes. Klein rarely came' (Scott, personal letter of 30 May 1989).

The comment about Melanie Klein's absence is a surprise, but nor does Scott mention Eva Rosenfeld. The uncertainty about the exact membership of this group and its fairly brief duration indicate that this may have been part of a very fluid situation at this point in 1939. In 1941, when Melanie Klein was living and working in Pitlochry in Scotland, she was still suggesting (in a letter to Winnicott, then an important member of Klein's circle) that discussion groups should be formed (Grosskurth, 1986 p. 261). We might conjecture that the study group remained informal and variable to avoid notice since, if it was too visible, it might be seen politically to risk a schism within the Society and an expulsion of Melanie Klein and her group.

What does seem clear is that after Susan Isaacs' paper, Klein and her close colleagues recognized that the concept of 'internal objects' needed urgently to be understood better and discussed further. Part of file PP/KLE/D.16 from the Melanie Klein Archive, reproduced in Appendix II, deals explicitly with internal objects. Klein wrote:

> The psychoanalysis of young children, which allows a very precise, clear, specific concrete picture of the unconscious conceptions of the mind, led me to use a term which has not proved acceptable and clear enough to a number of my colleagues. It is the term 'internal objects' or 'inner objects' and 'good' and 'bad' objects.
>
> *(D.16 image 24)*

This manuscript is undated but the notes were typed and probably intended for a presentation to just such a group as the Internal Objects Group. The heading to the manuscript is 'Notes re terms "internal objects", "inner objects", etc., "good" and "bad" objects etc.'. The text includes a very specific description of what she meant by an internal object, and how it contrasts with the classical concept of the superego. It is worth quoting:

> My reason for preferring this term to the classic definition, that of 'an object installed in the ego' is that the term 'inner object' is more specific since it exactly expresses what the child's unconscious, and for that matter the adult's in deep layers, feels about it. In these layers it is not felt to be part of the mind in the sense, as we have learnt to understand it, of the super-ego being the parents' voices inside one's mind. This is the concept we find in the higher strata of the unconscious. In the deeper layers, however, it is felt to be a physical being, or rather a multitude of beings, which with all their activities, friendly and hostile, lodge inside one's body, particularly inside the abdomen, a conception to which physiological processes and sensations of all kinds, in the past and in the present, have contributed.
>
> *(D.16 image 24 and 26)*

This summarizes the quality Klein had tried to describe in her 1935 paper, of the patient who conceived of his internal objects as his family of brothers and sisters. She emphasized the extreme concreteness of the internal objects.

Another set of notes from the archive, an extract from C.68, and also reproduced in Appendix 11, is also relevant. It is entitled 'Notes about character formation and inner relationships with reference to castration complex; Study Circle Feb 11, 1942'. Here are ideas about character which are more explicit than in any of Klein's published work. There are 20 pages which appear to be the basis for an unfinished paper. They include a detailed examination of insincerity as a character organization of impulses, defences and object relations. This is reminiscent of contemporary Kleinian understanding of the severe borderline character (Joseph, 1989; Steiner, 1993).

The heading 'Study Circle Feb. 11, 1942' is to be noted. The situation which produced a small and inconsistent group, or groups, in 1939, had evolved into one where a formal 'study circle' was addressing both scientific topics and also perhaps organizing for the political situation within the Society, which was coming to a head. Melanie Klein examined here the relation between internal objects and character. For instance:

> Consider instances I gave in the discussion following Scott's suggestions re a finger which the patient hallucinated when it had been removed by operation. What did this imply in internal relations? I suggested that, when hallucinated, it definitely implies an internal object, but it may be a person who is restored. Here I referred to the fact that external relations and external objects or situations are not simply to be translated into internal ones, or the other way around, but that they have a nature of their own, do not simply coincide, that they are always interrelated. In Scott's case in which the patient hallucinated the finger which had been lost there, it afterwards appeared from Scott's report that the patient spoke about his mother wishing him to be there when she was dying, and that seems to confirm that the lost finger could quite well have stood for the internalised mother.
>
> *(C.68 images 28–29)*

The internal mother, alive and revived, is not just a replica or representation of the external mother who is dying. The independent life of the internal object, a live mother and a live finger, contrasts with the reality. This very concrete hallucination is a specific indicator of the inner life, as distinct from the external one.

Character development

The relation between internal objects and character formation has been important since the settled debate about the tripartite structure of personality that was brought into the British Psycho-Analytical Society by the Viennese unsettled the

Kleinians. For Melanie Klein the precursors of the superego (in what she called the 'deeper layers of the unconscious') were being organized from birth. Her theories of character development in the late 1930s were in terms of the internal objects that literally form character, a topic Susan Isaacs' paper had touched on. Later her views on character development rested more on the notion of projective identification as a means by which the internal world of objects and self are dealt with.

Another remarkable relic in the Melanie Klein Archives is a typed out version of what was entitled, 'Intended response to Anna Freud's paper on sublimation' (C.92). So, it is a response to the missing paper of Anna Freud's that I speculated about earlier. In this case Anna Freud's paper must have been written out and circulated, at least to Melanie Klein to prepare her views. The fact of Melanie Klein's prior knowledge of the paper contradicts Young-Bruehl's surmise mentioned earlier.

Klein might well have taken considerable care in preparing her response. Anna Freud was not only the central figure in the challenge to Melanie Klein's position within the British Society – Anna Freud's paper and Melanie Klein's response would be in front of the visiting French Society as well as her colleagues in London.

I shall refer to only one of several claims Melanie Klein made in her responding comments. She begins in this way: 'I have been very interested in the particular aspect of character-formation and sublimation which Anna Freud has presented tonight' (C.92 image 2).

Anna Freud's paper on sublimation seems therefore to have centred on the claim that sublimation was the grounding of the development of character. Klein made a very powerful counter-claim to Anna Freud's: 'the anxiety stirred up by these unconscious phantasies is the cause of the inhibition of those very sublimations which are promoted by the masturbation phantasies' (C.92 image 10–11).

In essence Melanie Klein claimed that the activity of phantasy caused the inhibition of sexuality; Anna Freud claimed, classically, that the activity of fantasy was a result of the inhibition of sexuality. Melanie Klein's response, reiterating Susan Isaacs' stress six months previously on the anxious unconscious phantasies, leads us to suppose that Anna Freud, in her paper, was dealing with the nature and function of f/phantasy. It would appear that f/phantasy is therefore the crucial contention between Anna Freud and Melanie Klein. Unconscious phantasy and conscious fantasy are at the opposite ends of a chain of causal relations (see the diagram in Appendix I), but this appeared to be insufficiently recognized in this and subsequent debates. The rather obvious nature of the difference between them makes it strange that there was not a proper recognition of it; and this in turn suggests complex forces from outside the domain of scientific debate. These forces are, I suggest, at the group dynamic level, and in particular the anxiety that the vying groups in the British Society engendered in each other. Perhaps the unconscious phantasies about each other, and the emergence of sophisticated scientific debate between them, are themselves an example of the chain of causal events that are involved in sublimation.

Even though the Klein group was focused on internal objects, the concept of 'unconscious phantasy' had now come to the fore. Despite the ambiguity, phantasy/fantasy acted as a common thread in this series of contributions:

Isaacs introduced the phantasies about internal objects (Dec. 1938);
Anna Freud re-stated the classical position on fantasy and sublimation (June 1939);
Melanie Klein responded with her contrasting position on the role and effects of phantasy (June 1939); and
Paula Heimann contributed a case study of a patient with an inhibition of her sublimatory activity resulting from concrete phantasies of internal objects (July 1939).

If we take this series as a true reconstruction, it appears as a co-ordinated sequence of Kleinian contributions and does suggest that there was a good deal of collaboration behind the scenes. Therefore, the surviving evidence of the Internal Object Group heralds the beginnings of an organization into a group.

The debate I have reconstructed, between December 1938 and July 1939, was then sadly interrupted by Freud's death in September 1939. The Second World War rapidly followed and many psychoanalysts were dispersed outside London.

This reconstructed narrative concerns a certain scientific activity within the British Society. It is clear that there were extraneous forces acting on this debate not of a purely scientific or academic kind. I shall now attempt to discuss how these various forces and their influences might begin to be disentangled.

Discussion

Biography, organizations and history not only shape intellectual activity and development, but can themselves be organized by intellectual activity. In this chapter I have shown how the concept of the internal object has its own history, which quite clearly demonstrates the focal role of an intellectual idea around which many personal and group dynamics and anxieties revolve.

Defence and anxiety in the organization

This is a case study in a certain form of institutional dynamic i.e. the splitting into separate groups identified consciously by contrasting professional and scientific positions. Bion described a group splitting or schism as he called it:

> The defence that schism affords against the development-threatening idea can be seen in the operation of the schismatic groups, ostensibly opposed but in fact promoting the same end. One group adheres to the dependent group ... popularizes established ideas by denuding them ... The

> reciprocal group, supposedly supporting the new idea, becomes so exacting in its demands that it ceases to recruit itself. Thus both groups avoid the painful bringing together of the primitive and sophisticated that is the essence of the developmental conflict.
>
> *(Bion, 1961, p. 159)*

This seems to cover the circumstances, and indeed perhaps Bion had the state of the British Psycho-Analytical Society in mind when he wrote it originally in 1952. The debates and group formations in the British Society could have been dealing with just the tension he described between a commitment to innovation on one hand, and a reverence to the past on the other. In Bion's terms, the development of the Klein group is a venture, perhaps reckless, to push forward regardless of the rest of the Society. For instance, in a letter to Ernest Jones in 1941, Melanie Klein reflects on the problems of presenting her work to the rest of the Society:

> I am not despairing and if I have fifteen or twenty more years left to work I should be able to accomplish my task. But I realize how difficult it is and what powers of presentation would be needed to give evidence for the truth and importance of these findings.
>
> *(quoted in Grosskurth, 1986, p. 283)*

On the other hand, Anna Freud's work looked back in a persisting dedication to the work of her father. Young-Bruehl is explicit about this:

> Her labour of checking and revising all of her father's maps of psychic life was not original in the sense that it revealed a mapless territory. But it provided her with a survey-making or synthetic sense that was without equal in her generation.
>
> *(Young-Bruehl, 1988, p. 461)*

This is not to suggest that the individuals themselves were particularly prone to intrapsychic splitting. Melanie Klein and Anna Freud were clearly very different people, and thus their relationships with psychoanalysis were very different. Equally their relationships with children, and with being a child (daughter), were also very different. Following from these differences they developed different forms of child analysis and different conclusions about child development. However, within their group context they came to represent a deep schism. On the basis of character differences they become polarized into opposites.

In fact, their differences may have been previously exploited by Ernest Jones and Sigmund Freud to carry their own rivalry. The dissent of the British had been controlled by the enduring loyalty that Jones and Freud had for each other. At the same time the quarrel between these two women seems to express something for Freud and Jones too. Jones had lived out a rivalry, though one that was intermingled in a complex way with an extreme loyalty to Freud. We might consider therefore that, by displacing his rivalry on to a quarrel between this protégée and Freud's, Jones could maintain his customary tactful adulation of Freud. The uncomplicated rivalry between Anna Freud and Melanie Klein allowed Jones and Freud an uncomplicated loyalty.

When personal issues are depersonalized in the group schism, it makes us suspicious of a defensiveness operating at the level of the group and organization. Menzies (1960) described how ordinarily mature individuals can come to function in a setting in which they are induced to operate with a level of defensive splitting that is much below their level of personal maturity. In this way character differences are made into intensely felt opposites. As Steiner points out:

> The militarization and polarization of differences between groups and between members of groups themselves ... can lead to an endless paranoid 'ping pong' of accusations. Groups, even when composed of psychoanalysts, have inevitably unconscious, unresolved components ... Sometimes even psychoanalytic groups are defending themselves from primitive anxieties using primitive mechanisms of defence based on excessive idealization and denigration.
>
> *(Steiner, 1991, p. 918)*

Group schisms involve individuals pushing each other apart. In the historical instance reported in this paper the Kleinian group initially shared their conclusions about internal objects with the rest of the Society. But eventually the intricate discussion work seems to have pressed ahead, urgently, outside the Society as a whole. As a result others in the Society were left behind.

Despite the intention to 'give much more attention to the educational side of the work', the development of exclusively formed, and increasingly private, meetings, study groups and seminars led to separate scientific activity. Diverging scientific conclusions separated the groups into further mutual antagonism. Once division between the two groups was set, an inevitable falling away from each other to draw up battle lines became inevitable. The very difficulty of the concept of the internal object supported the mutual exclusiveness of the two groups.

The move from public to private debate linked with personal rivalries to form a defensive group dynamic. In particular, during the lead-up to the Controversial Discussions in 1943 a to-and-fro process of mutual influence between Anna Freud's group and Melanie Klein's appeared as follows: the Scientific Committee had asked for a Kleinian paper on 'The role of introjection and projection of objects in the early years of development' to start the discussion off on internalization and internal objects; however, Susan Isaacs' first paper was on 'The nature and function of phantasy' (Isaacs, 1948), developing the points Melanie Klein had made about unconscious phantasy in her response to Anna Freud in 1939. It would appear that the 'sublimation debate' with Anna Freud in 1939 had influenced the Kleinians. It would also appear that the contradictory notions of phantasy that were only half appreciated then led the Kleinians to attempt to further establish and, as it were, 'prove' their point about unconscious phantasy.

Thus between 1939 and 1943 the Kleinians had driven Anna Freud back to her classical work on fantasy, and she in turn had driven the Klein group beyond internal objects and towards more fundamental work on unconscious phantasy.

We can see not just the linear search for a greater and greater approximation to a truth. Instead the development of each group's set of ideas and values was influenced by, and penetrated, those of the others. A degree of mutual influencing went on. Thus the two groups were dialectically dependent on each other.

Schisms operate as an organizational defensiveness against specific anxieties, whereby organizations not only provide opportunities to work collectively, but also 'social defences', ways in which the anxieties of members are collusively and imperceptibly addressed (Eisold, 1994, p. 787). Psychoanalytic institutions bear the mark of the anxieties inherent in being a psychoanalyst. They offer protection for personal anxieties by coordinating behaviour that Eisold catalogued as:

Firstly, the nature of the work;
Secondly, the nature of psychoanalytic institutions; and
Finally, the characteristic relationship with psychoanalysis itself.

Eisold argued, in line with Bion's view, that schisms within psychoanalytic organizations are social defences occasioned by the tensions in the work. So, common anxieties in the work can form coordinated responses, including institutional schism. The stress of being a psychoanalyst is evident, though the toll it takes on the functioning of psychoanalytic institutions is not so familiar.

The conditions described here would have led many psychoanalytical societies to divide into two separate Societies. That this did not eventually happen is remarkable (Hinshelwood, 1995). There were powerful forces within the British Psycho-Analytical Society that led to the members deciding to stick together come what may. Thus the schismatic process was in this case distorted. The Society did not divide into two, but eventually the training course did, run by a single training committee (King & Steiner, 1991). The anxieties that tend to lead to schism in this case were deeply complicated by anxieties about schism itself, and the meaning of schism in the context of the time. I want to mention these added anxieties briefly. But first it needs to be mentioned that the group dynamics within the Society threw up a third group that came to be known eventually as the Middle Group (later as the Independents), who operated as a kind of 'buffer zone'.

The Middle Group embodied a determination to mediate the interminable further scientific and organizational debate and dispute. In effect this began with a written debate on psychoanalytic technique in 1943 (see King & Steiner, 1991) and culminated in the unwritten 'gentlemen's agreement' in 1946. This agreement between the Klein Group and Anna Freud's Group was brokered with great skill by the Middle Group and, in particular, Sylvia Payne, who became President of the Society in 1944. I shall not describe the scientific and particularly the organizational efforts of the Middle Group in detail as these are outside the time period of this chapter.

Freud's death

The anxieties affecting the British Psycho-Analytical Society at this time were augmented from outside the professional and scientific work by firstly the War and the fate of psychoanalysis in Europe, and secondly the individual and collective mourning of Freud's death in these circumstances. These profoundly important and shattering events must, I claim, have driven the British Society and its members to stick together at all costs.

The whole of Britain was enormously insecure, at war, and at great risk of invasion by Germany. By 1940 many European Societies and analysts had been lost, so that the importance of the survival of the British Society for the whole of psychoanalysis was enormous. Because American psychoanalysis was still given second-rate status by Europeans (Gay, 1988), the British Society represented the survival of psychoanalysis itself, having as it were swallowed the whole body of psychoanalysis. Britain's lonely stand against Nazism and Germany from 1939–1941 struck a chord with the British Psycho-Analytical Society. Its special mission to embody the survival of psychoanalysis must have been severely shaken when, very shortly after his arrival in Britain, Freud died in September 1939. Having lost Europe, the psychoanalytic world now lost Freud.

Little has been written of the effect Freud's death had on the psychoanalytic movement. Baudry (1994) did mention 'the large impact on the psychoanalytic movement of the death of Freud ... In all likelihood, this event interfered with the group's identificatory processes and ego-ideal formation' (Baudry, 1994, p. 368). Though brief, it is a reference to the collective mourning processes that must have gone on. Only a fortnight after Freud's death the minutes of the meeting of the British Society (8 October 1939) record that Jones had, so soon, proposed a 'permanent memorial' to Freud in the form of a biography and an English translation of the *Collected Works*. Jones took on the 'official' biography and James Strachey headed a sub-committee to organize the translation. Both projects lasted decades.

The immediate attempt collectively to relinquish Freud himself and to recathect psychoanalysis happened at that point in time when psychoanalysis, like Britain, was possibly on the verge of collapse. There was no shortage of potential psychoanalytic debate at hand. Many analysts had left London, the medical people often into the forces. The refugee members of the Society were however required by the government to stay in London and they were therefore a significant part of the Society until late 1941 when analysts who were not in the army began to return and reform the Society in an atmosphere of pervading insecurity. This led individuals to redirect their cathexes towards something else, not the scientific debate of differences but towards the condition of the Society itself, to protect it from harm and schism. The Society kept extraordinarily meticulous records of the discussions of its committees and meetings (King & Steiner, 1991). The planned debates on the scientific controversies, when they came in 1943, were then in the context of the survival, or schism, of the Psycho-Analytical Society itself.

The specific background of immense anxiety, insecurity and loss created a fraught defensiveness in the organization itself. It led to a less complete cathexis of psychoanalysis than there might have been. Instead, schismatic icons were created for adulation, either by reverting to Freud himself or by the promotion of Melanie Klein. These were mediated by scientific debate across an increasing divide over the future of psychoanalysis.

Conclusions

Scientific debate and the progress of knowledge are irretrievably entangled with the complex of personal, group and organizational dynamics. To establish their identity as a group, the individuals of the emergent Klein followers, in 1939, found the puzzling concept of the internal object a suitable axis of debate. It was available as a prior persistent field of investigation in the Society, ready to be mobilized for its elusive quality as the whole British Society struggled, through defensive dynamics and structures, to cope with its emotional burden – the death of psychoanalysis abroad, and the 'dead Freud' within.

As the climax of controversy resolved, and the groups institutionalized their split, the scientific concept that focused the psychodynamic forces dropped out of interest. Instead the Society undertook a non-scientific task, to embody the survival of psychoanalysis itself. Through its surface debates on scientific issues, the need to survive was expressed and the creation of the three groups was an institutionalization of the process the Society found to ensure the survival of psychoanalysis in the early 1940s. The intense and eventually traumatizing debates about the concepts of unconscious phantasy in general and of the unconscious phantasy of internal objects in particular have hardly been revisited and there is little debate now in the British Society about the concept of 'internal objects'.

There are now analysts who use the term 'internal object' in the way that Melanie Klein originally meant it. There are those who regard the term as a rather eccentric way of talking about the internal representation of external reality (Sandler, 1990). And there are others who do not understand or use the term at all. The groups and the personal psychodynamics are organized around other issues now. The concept of the internal object remains an important feature of the Kleinian view of primitive processes. But it is equally important for its historical role in initiating the shape the British Society has taken in the last 50 years.

Note

1 An earlier version of this chapter was published as Hinshelwood (1997), 'The elusive concept of internal objects (1934–1943): Its role in the formation of the Klein Group'. *International Journal of Psychoanalysis*, 78, 877–897.

References

Baudry, F. (1994). Revisiting the Freud–Klein controversies fifty years later. *Int. J. Psychoanal.*, *75*, 367–374.

Bion, W.R. (1961). *Experiences in groups*. London: Tavistock.

Brierley, M. (1934). Present tendencies in psycho-analysis. *Brit. J. Med. Psychol.*, *14*, 211–229.

Brierley, M. (1939). A prefatory note on 'internalized objects' and depression. *Int. J. Psychoanal.*, *20*, 241–245.

Brierley, M. (1942). 'Internal objects' and theory. *Int. J. Psychoanal.*, *23*, 107–112.

Eisold, K. (1994). The intolerance of diversity in psycho-analytic institutions. *Int. J. Psychoanal.*, *75*, 785–800.

Freud, A. (1923). The relation of beating fantasies to a day-dream. *Int. J. Psychoanal.*, *4*, 89–102.

Freud, A. (1927). *Einführung in die Technik der Kinderanalyse*. Vienna: Internationaler psychoanalytischer Verlag.

Freud, A. (1928). *Introduction to the technique of child analysis*. New York: Nervous and Mental Disease Publishing Company; and as parts I and II of (1946) *The psycho-analytic treatment of children*.

Freud, A. (1944a). Sex in childhood. *Health Education*, *2*, 2–6.

Freud, A. (1944b). Difficulties of sex enlightenment. *Health Education*, *2*, 81–85.

Freud, A. (1946). *The psycho-analytic treatment of children*. London: Imago.

Freud, A. (1948a). *Four lectures on child analysis*. London: Hogarth.

Freud, A. (1948b). Sublimation as a factor in upbringing. *Health Education*, *2*, 25–29.

Freud, S. (1919). 'A child is being beaten': a contribution to the study of the origin of sexual perversions. *Standard edition of the complete works of Sigmund Freud* vol. *17*. London: Hogarth.

Fuchs, S.H. (1937). On introjection. *Int. J. Psychoanal.*, *18*, 269–294.

Gay, P. (1988). *Freud: A life for our time*. New York: Norton.

Glover, E. (1933). Review of the psycho-analysis of children. *Int. J. Psychoanal.*, *14*, 119–129.

Grosskurth, P. (1986). *Melanie Klein: Her world and her work*. London: Hodder and Stoughton.

Heimann, P. (1942). A contribution to the problem of sublimation and its relation to processes of internalization. *Int. J. Psychoanal.*, *23*, 8–17.

Hinshelwood, R.D. (1995). Der Mythos vom britischen Kompromi (The myth of the British compromise). In *Spaltungen in der Geschichte*, ed. L. Hermans. Tübingen: Diskord, pp. 250–265.

Homans, P. (1989). *The ability to mourn*. Chicago: Chicago Univ. Press.

Isaacs, S. (1940). Temper tantrums in early childhood in their relation to internal objects. *Int. J. Psychoanal.*, *21*, 280–293.

Isaacs, S. (1948). The nature and function of phantasy. *Int. J. Psychoanal.*, *29*, 73–97; reprinted (1952) in *Developments in psycho-analysis*, by M. Klein et al., London: Hogarth, pp. 67–121.

Jones, E. (1935). Early female sexuality. *Int. J. Psychoanal.*, *16*, 263–273.

Jones, E. (1940). Obituary: Sigmund Freud. *Int. J. Psychoanal.*, *21*, 2–26.

Jones, E. (1957). *The life and work of Sigmund Freud*, vol. *3*. London: Hogarth.

Joseph, B. (1989). *Psychic equilibrium and psychic change*. London and New York: Routledge.

King, P. and Steiner, R. (eds) (1991). *The Freud–Klein controversies: 1941–1945*. London and New York: Routledge.

Klein, M. (1932). *The psycho-analysis of children*. London: Hogarth.

Klein, M. (1935). A contribution to the genesis of manic-depressive states. *Int. J. Psychoanal.*, *16*, 145–174; reprinted (1975), *The writings of Melanie Klein*, vol. *1*: Love, guilt and reparation. London: Hogarth, pp. 262–289.

Klein, M. (1940). Mourning and its relation to manic-depressive states. *Int. J. Psychoanal.*, *21*, 125–153; reprinted (1975), *The writings of Melanie Klein*, vol. *1*: Love, guilt and reparation. London: Hogarth, pp. 344–369.

Matte-Blanco, I. (1941). On introjection and the processes of psychic metabolism. *Int. J. Psychoanal.*, *22*, 17–36.

Menzies, I. (1960). A case study in the functioning of a social system as a defence against anxiety. *Human Relations*, *11*, 95–121.

Paskauskas, A. (1993). *The complete correspondence of Sigmund Freud and Ernest Jones, 1908–1939*. Harvard: Belknap.

Payne, S. (1937). Post-war activities and the advance of psychotherapy. *Brit. J. Med. Psychol.*, *16*, 1–15.

Rickman, J. (1939). *The nature of an internal object* (unpublished).

Riviere, J. (1936a). A contribution to the analysis of negative therapeutic reaction. *Int. J. Psychoanal.*, *17*, 304–320.

Riviere, J. (1936b). On the genesis of psychical conflict in earliest infancy. *Int. J. Psychoanal.*, *17*, 395–422.

Sandler, J. (1990). On internal object relations. *J. Am. Psychoanal. Assoc.*, *38*, 859–880.

Schmideberg, M. (1934). The play analysis of a three-year-old girl. *Int. J. Psychoanal.*, *15*, 245–264.

Schmideberg, M. (1941). *'Introjected object': A terminological issue or a clinical problem* (unpublished).

Scott, C. (1947). On the intense affects encountered in treating a severe manic-depressive disorder. *Int. J. Psychoanal.*, *28*, 139–145.

Segal, H. (1979). *Klein*. London: Fontana.

Steiner, J. (1993). *Psychic retreats*. London and New York: Routledge.

Steiner, R. (1985). Some thoughts about tradition and change arising from an examination of the British Psycho-Analytical Society's Controversial Discussions, 1943–1944. *Int. J. Psychoanal.*, *12*, 27–71.

Steiner, R. (1989). 'It is a new kind of diaspora. . .'. *Int. J. Psychoanal.*, *16*, 35–78.

Steiner, R. (1991). Editorial comments. In *The Freud–Klein controversies: 1941–1945*, King, P. and Steiner, R., eds. London: Routledge, pp. 914–919.

Stephen, A. (1947). The super-ego and other internal objects. *Int. J. Psychoanal.*, *28*, 114–117.

Stephen, K. (1934). Introjection and projection, guilt and rage. *Brit. J. Med. Psychol.*, *14*, 316–331.

Strachey, A. (1941). A note on the use of the word 'internal'. *Int. J. Psychoanal.*, *22*, 37–43.

Waelder, R. (1937). The problem of the genesis of psychical conflict in earliest infancy. *Int. J. Psychoanal.*, *18*, 406–473.

Young-Bruehl, E. (1988). *Anna Freud: A biography*. London: Macmillan.

Appendix I: Theories of sublimation

If we set out the chains of causal relations proposed by Anna Freud (1923) and by Paula Heimann (1942), we can see that they overlap in a significant way:

TABLE 11.1

	Anna Freud	*Paula Heimann*
1		Phantasies (unconscious)
2	Anxiety	Anxiety
3	Inhibition	Inhibition
4	Sublimation	Symptoms
5	Fantasies (conscious)	

Step four indicates different paths – one towards a healthy sublimation in Anna Freud's account (though in the abnormal condition it would lead to masturbation phantasies and activity) and the other towards psychopathology and symptoms. In other words it is a comparison between health and illness. But more than this, the diagram demonstrates that the place of fantasy (phantasy) is quite different: unconscious phantasies appear at the beginning of this chain in one version, whilst conscious fantasies are the eventual product of the other chain. This points towards the nature of unconscious phantasy and conscious fantasy being quite different.

Appendix II: Extracts from some of Melanie Klein's notes in the Klein Archives

PP/KLE/D.16 extract

Notes re terms 'internal objects', 'inner objects' etc., 'good' and 'bad' objects etc.

The psychoanalysis of young children, which allows a very precise, clear, specific concrete picture of the unconscious conceptions of the mind, led me to use a term which has not proved acceptable and clear enough to a number of my colleagues. It is the term 'internal objects' or 'inner objects' and 'good' and 'bad' objects. My reason for preferring this term to the classic definition, that of 'an object installed in the ego' is that the term 'inner object' is more specific since it exactly expresses what the child's unconscious, and for that matter the adult's in deep layers, feels about it. In these layers it is not felt to be part of the mind in the sense, as we have learnt to understand it, of the superego being the parents' voices inside one's mind. This is the concept we find in the higher strata of the unconscious. In the deeper layers, however, it is felt to be a physical being, or rather a multitude of beings, which with all their activities, friendly and hostile, lodge inside one's body, particularly inside the abdomen, a conception to which physiological processes and sensations of all kinds, in the past and in the present, have contributed. I may add a word about the technical aspect of the use of such a term. In my experience the more concretely, the more specifically, I should say vividly if this did not have a flavour of dramatization which is unnecessary, we can convey to the patient the content of the unconscious phantasies we see in action, the more effective our interpretation will be. It is therefore, when we meet with these phantasies of an internal world populated by beings which are partly a reflection of external beings, but through their being internal acquire qualities of their own, to express this in the ways the patient feels it; and that is in my experience, 'inner objects' and 'good' and 'bad' objects or rather all the gradations of good and bad (D.16 images 24, 26–27).

PP/KLE/C.68 extract

Notes about character formation and inner relationships with reference to castration complex; Study Circle Feb 11, 1942

Flexibility and mobility through establishing securely the strong points inside.

Thus originally in external relationships, the parents and adults to whom the child can look up for security and help etc. from whom he gets his standards if these are securely installed, then the bad objects can be tolerated, or rather dealt with by means other than denial. Flexibility includes that these radical strongholds can be replaced by others, by principles, etc. The giving out and taking in, the whole question of communication within and with the outer world – all this was contained in the analogy with the mobile warfare, in A's case, and in the adult case referred to. Heimann pointed out that these strongholds, if they are securely established, would also mean assimilated. As an interesting point: apparently when those particular objects are not so strongly established (also in R's case the light blue mummie), then the goodness or belief in good objects may be disturbed and easily fade away or break down. On the other hand, the strong division into good and bad which seems necessary to establish these strong points may in itself be a source of much difficulty. Some compromise and balance between these various possibilities. To be stressed more than in the notes is [. . .] that the two primary ethical laws I referred to, particularly the second one, are also fundamental for character formation. [Author's note: Earlier in C.68 the following 'laws' were described: thou shalt not kill = thou shalt not kill the loved object; thou shalt save from destruction – the loved object – and from your own aggression.]

The particular aspect of internal relationships in so far as aggression is bound to lead to suspicious, cunning and secretive methods, has the effect in cases in which aggression is so much turned inwards, of influencing character formation in an unfavourable way, the point being that external relationships, though they may coincide with internal ones, have a quite different character.

Consider instances I gave in the discussion following Scott's suggestions re a finger which the patient hallucinated when it had been removed by operation. What did this imply in internal relations? I suggested that, when hallucinated, it definitely implies an internal object, but it may be a person who is restored. Here I referred to the fact that external relations and external objects or situations are not simply to be translated into internal ones, or the other way around, but that they have a nature of their own, do not simply coincide, that they are always interrelated. In Scott's case in which the patient hallucinated the finger which had been lost there, it afterwards appeared from Scott's report that the patient spoke about his mother wishing him to be there when she was dying, and that seems to confirm that the lost finger could quite well have stood for the internalised mother. My point here is to stress that internal and external relationships even when closely interrelated are not identical, and that the inner world is always different, and bound to be by the whole nature of the internal as compared with the external one. Therefore to good and evil when the internal relations so strongly predominate, the relation to external objects must be deserted and character influenced by that (C.68 images 27–29).

PP/KLE/C.92 in full

Intended contribution to Anna Freud's paper on sublimation

I have been very interested in the particular aspect of character-formation and sublimation which Anna Freud has presented tonight. I would like to add one or two points which seem to complete the picture.

Anna Freud has spoken of the fate of masturbation phantasies in the latency period. Since at this stage the forces of the ego, among them the intellect, are strongly exerted in repressing instinctual urges and mastering anxieties, the flow of unconscious processes is, as we know, impeded, and there are difficulties in the way of gauging the dynamic forces behind the rather static formations which the mind presents. To understand fully, therefore, the formations which can be observed in the latency period, and which have been discussed tonight it is most helpful to consider the earlier stages in which all these developments are in the making, and to study the unconscious as well as the conscious mind of the young pre-latency child.

In analysing the masturbation phantasies of children between 2 and 4–5 years of age, we find them to be a most complex phenomenon and a clue for the understanding of the whole of the child's sexuality, his phantasies in general and his emotional life. The analysis of his unconscious masturbation phantasies enables us to get to the roots of his conflicts, his anxieties and his feelings of guilt, which – and this is a point I want to stress – are caused by his aggressive impulses and phantasies which are fused with his libidinal satisfactions. It is his sadism which gives rise to feelings of guilt and anxieties from various sources, in particular to the anxieties of having destroyed or of destroying his parents. In his masturbation phantasies which centre around his parents sexual gratifications, and which therefore are loaded with jealousy, greed and hatred because he feels excluded from their gratification, in an omnipotent way he injures or destroys them. I think we are all familiar with these phantasies, which have been discussed so much in former years in this Society, and I am now referring to them only briefly. In these sadistic unconscious phantasies, primarily linked with masturbation, he attacks his parents directly in the ways sadism can devise. Indirectly in omnipotent phantasy, the child makes his parents destroy each other, and therefore experiences deep anxieties lest at any time when he does not see his parents they may be performing sexual intercourse and endangering each other. These attacks, these feelings of guilt, are at the bottom of the child's struggle against his masturbation phantasies. Anxiety and guilt, however, though they inhibit sexual activities in many children and lead to a very severe repression of their phantasies, in other children they stimulate sexual activities, and in any case increase fixations. I have found in every case of obsessional masturbation which I have analysed that this obsession is never due to one factor only, that is to say the strength or the excess of instinctual urges, but to the complicated interaction of various factors, to which I have just referred. It is important to bear in mind that the feelings of guilt and the fears of having injured one parent or both parents through the sadistic phantasy, drive the child to repeat the masturbatory act over and over again, partly as a means of testing the dangerousness of his destructive phantasies and finding out whether they have taken, or are going to take, effect, partly in order to restore the parents by the same act which had injured them. The various factors which bring about obsessional masturbation, however, according to my experience and that of many of us, are also to some extent operative in non-obsessional masturbation. Instinctual urges and libidinal desires are, as we know, always bound up with aggressive ones, and therefore they always arouse some guilt and fears. Guilt gives rise to the wish to make reparation, and all these elements enter into the masturbation phantasies and increase libidinal fixations. Whether or not the guilt and anxiety will lead to this inhibition of masturbatory activities (or for that matter of sexuality in later life) or will stimulate them depends upon a certain optimum of the various factors interacting; but in any case guilt and anxiety are, to varying degree, integral elements in sexual anxieties and sexual phantasies.

They are however no less important for the development of sublimation and of the ego as a whole.

I don't think we can fully understand sublimation and the interaction between sexual and ego development, at any stage of the child's development, without giving full due to the anxiety and guilt arising from the masturbation phantasies and from unconscious phantasies in general. The drive to reparation which is activated by guilt and sorrow many of us have found to be a fundamental factor in sublimation as well as in sexual development, and it enters into the whole of development of character and formation of the ego.

The part masturbation phantasies play both in the sexuality of the child and in his sublimation is a topic which absorbed my own interest very early on in my work and my conclusions at that time were that the child's masturbation phantasies stimulate and increase all his play activities, intellectual and other interests by vesting these with sexual pleasure; furthermore that the anxiety stirred up by these unconscious phantasies is the cause of the inhibition of those very sublimations which are promoted by the masturbation phantasies. These early conclusions still hold good, but they have been amplified as our work on aggression, anxiety, guilt and depression has progressed. I cannot now go into the elaborate ways in which anxiety and guilt, which can inhibit sublimations, are on the other hand most essential in stimulating and furthering them. My main point was to stress the central part anxiety and guilt play in the development of the ego and character formation, and in those various disorders and inhibitions which Miss Freud described and discussed tonight.

12

KLEIN'S FURTHER THOUGHTS ON LONELINESS[1]

Jane Milton

Introduction

Writing in the notes to Melanie Klein's collected works, Edna O'Shaughnessy (1984) comments on Klein's (1963) final paper 'On the sense of loneliness' thus:

> It must be remembered that Melanie Klein had not offered this paper for publication before she died – the present version was published posthumously after some slight editorial work – presumably because she did not consider it ready, and indeed it would have benefited from further work; it seems in places incomplete and its thought is not altogether resolved.
>
> *(O'Shaughnessy, 1984, p. 336)*

In the archive there are four different versions of the loneliness paper, to be found in the sections marked PP/KLE/C.27 and C.28. One is marked 'Given to the Society of Psycho-Analysts, Wednesday 17 February 1960'. Another is headed 'Congress paper' and probably referred to the Copenhagen congress of 1959. A third is headed 'revised version for America'. This referred to a planned visit to the Institute of Pennsylvania Hospital in Philadelphia, in November 1960. Sadly Klein died before this on 22 September 1960 at the age of 78. I think I have identified the version (C.27 part 2) that O'Shaughnessy and her colleagues edited for publication. This part of the archive can be viewed online by entering the Wellcome Library catalogue and putting into the search box the word 'digklein' followed by the file number C.27, C.28 or C.29.

What becomes clear from additional archival material particularly in section C.29 is that Klein was indeed not ready to publish the paper and instead intended to expand it into a 'book' on loneliness, by which she probably meant a monograph.

In this chapter I will first remind readers in outline of the published version of the paper. I will then show some of the new material Klein was collecting for her 'book on loneliness'. The material is fascinating and sometimes moving, and speaks for itself; I am not attempting to theorize it. One striking aspect is that besides jotting down her own thoughts as they arose, Klein was collecting comments and opinions from colleagues for use in her book. In the archive are two letters from Wilfred Bion and one from Elliott Jaques. Klein also makes notes of suggestions from Hanna Segal and Herbert Rosenfeld, and some notes on Winnicott's 1958 paper 'On the capacity to be alone'.

Brief outline of the published paper: 'On the sense of loneliness'

The paper is admired as one of Klein's important late works. However as O'Shaughnessy (1984) says, the thought of the paper is 'not altogether resolved'. I think this is partly because Klein includes within the paper a number of different mental states, with sometimes very different qualities, all of which she calls 'loneliness'. Some are clearly more related to depressive and others to paranoid situations but she does not always distinguish these clearly.

I want just to clarify this distinction myself for colleagues who use different theoretical paradigms. In the more primitive states of mind that are primarily 'paranoid schizoid' the individual projects out into others bad, unwanted mental content, and thus feels surrounded by persecutors. He fears predominantly for his own safety. In the process of movement towards the depressive position (both a long-term developmental process and a to and fro movement in everyday life) the individual owns, that is, integrates, what has been projected and thus must face his own hatred alongside his love. The depressive position, encountered over and over again, involves guilt and despair over the damage done to loved and needed others. It involves mourning on a small or large scale. It also allows progressive strengthening of the internal good object which forms the core of the healthy ego.

In her paper Klein (1963) first describes loneliness as 'A ubiquitous yearning for an unattainable perfect internal state' (p. 300) and later 'an unsatisfied longing for an understanding without words' (p. 301). These feelings arise from 'the depressive feeling of an irretrievable loss', and represent a wish to return to the earliest relation to the mother, where there was understanding without words based on direct contact between the unconscious of mother and infant.

This perfect state is an idealization; it is never entirely met, or at least quickly disturbed by persecutory anxiety, linked with the infant's inevitable destructive feelings. Klein (1963) writes 'When paranoid anxiety is relatively strong . . . the relation to the internal good object is impaired. As a consequence, there is increased projection of paranoid feelings and suspicions on others, with a resulting sense of loneliness' (p. 303).

Integration, however, has its own problems: It helps loneliness by mitigating hate with love, giving more safety both to the ego and its good object. At the same time the bringing together of destructive and loving impulses and the good and bad aspects of the object gives rise to a fear that the good object and loving feelings may be overwhelmed and endangered. Klein (1963) comments: 'I have heard patients express the painfulness of integration in terms of feeling lonely and deserted, through being completely alone with what to them was a bad part of the self' (p. 302).

Full integration is never achieved because anxiety keeps parts of the self split off and projected. Thus one will never feel fully understood either by oneself or by another. These lost parts cause a 'conviction that there is no person or group to which one belongs' (Klein, 1963, p. 302). Evocatively, Klein writes: 'The lost parts too, are felt to be lonely' (p. 302). Klein describes a male adult patient 'D' who always felt at peace in the countryside but had felt lonely in the town, and in the presence of mother, during childhood. This loneliness had never entirely left him, and Klein shows how in his analysis they were able to understand how he had always carried a lonely and persecuting internal object linked to the mother.

With a growing sense of reality omnipotence lessens, meaning in Klein's view 'a diminished capacity for hope' (p. 304). A patient of Klein's who comes to idealize less says 'the glamour has gone' (p. 305). This painful loss of the idea of the ideal self and ideal object contributes to loneliness.

Klein looks at loneliness in schizophrenia. Excessive projection and fragmentation leave the sufferer 'hopelessly in bits', and unable to internalize his primal object. He feels alone with his misery, often confused, and surrounded by a hostile world. He withdraws from people in a vicious circle of loneliness and isolation.

The manic depressive patient is less fragmented but still cannot keep 'an inner and external companionship with a good object' (p. 305), because hatred and thus paranoia continue to intrude. Loneliness here is characterized by a hopeless longing to restore things, and in severe cases Klein comments that this can lead to suicide.

Giving clinical material from two male patients, Klein spends some time on the difficulties caused by conflicting male and female elements in the personality and conflicting allegiances to the parents. Integration inevitably leads to guilt caused by the jealous and envious oedipal wish to attack the rival parent.

Lastly the paper describes factors which mitigate loneliness. Secure internalization of the first good object and a happy relation with it is vital for the ability to give and to receive love and understanding. These capacities stimulate gratitude, which in turn includes the wish generously to return goodness received. Generosity, Klein feels, is necessary for creativity, and all this counteracts loneliness. The capacity for enjoyment helps toleration of imperfection. The individual can identify with the pleasures of others without too much envy and jealousy. This helps both in the child who has to wait to be adult and in the older person who has lost some capacities and pleasures but can bear to identify with the pleasures of youth without too much resentment.

Loneliness can never be eliminated, Klein says. Identification with others and over-dependence on them may be excessively and defensively employed to try to rid oneself of lonely feelings. She suggests that older people, to avoid and deny loneliness and current frustrations, may get lost in, and idealize, the past, just as young people may idealize the future for similar reasons.

New material

I will go on to discuss additional material on the subject of loneliness that Klein was collecting for her book.

Of great interest are two letters from Wilfred Bion and one from Elliott Jaques [PP/KLE/C.29 images 1–7].

Letter from Elliott Jaques (on which Klein has handwritten at the top 'for book')

Dr Elliott Jaques
Knightsbridge 2273
35, Ennismore Gardens Mews,
London S.W.7

1st June, 1959

Mrs. M. Klein,
20 Bracknell Gardens,
N.W.3

Dear Mrs Klein,

The point I wanted to make about your Congress paper is that in it you dealt not only with the problem of loneliness but also with the allied problem of the sense of belonging.

a) The greater the integration, the greater the capacity for a feeling of belonging to oneself as well as to one's internal parents, family, etc.

b) At the same time, the sense of belonging is not inconsistent with the feeling of loneliness; for, as you point out, greater integration implies acceptance of loss and hence toleration of a certain amount of loneliness; I think you will find, however, that what you have written also includes the notion that the capacity for greater toleration of loneliness in itself reinforces feelings of belonging and the capacity to allow oneself to belong, that is to say, to commit oneself to good objects.

I think you will find, if you look through your paper that just as the theme of gratitude was in fact already in your previous paper, so here is the theme of the sense of belonging.

The working title that came into my mind on reading your paper was 'Loneliness and the Sense of Belonging'.

Yours sincerely
Elliott Jaques

The letters from Bion are handwritten, and dated 'Feb 14th' and 'Mar 29th'. I think it was almost certainly 1960, as Bion in the first letter regrets the fact that illness will prevent him from attending the reading of her loneliness paper to the Society on 17 February 1960. The second letter from Bion, I think one can assume is also from 1960. If so, Klein's paper has already been given to the Society, but she was still to talk in Philadelphia, and Bion is also clearly aware of Klein's aim to write a book on loneliness.

First letter from Wilfred Bion (on which Klein has handwritten at the top 'to book on loneliness')

Redcourt,
Feb 14th

Dear Mrs Klein
Many thanks for letting me see a copy of your paper: I have sent it on as you asked, after reading it. I found it very interesting and I think improved by its greater scope.

There is one aspect of loneliness which I think I would have liked to speak to – unfortunately I shall not be coming as I am trying to keep a bronchial cough at bay – and that is related to the change from paranoid-schizoid to depressive position which is involved in each new learning experience of any importance, or so it seems to me.

I think that there is a tendency for a personality to become increasingly unwilling to face this change and in those who do become increasingly unwilling to do so an attack is made on the ego with a view to destroying contact with reality rather in the way the psychotic patient does. This is especially so in unwillingness to learn of increasing physical limitations which is reminiscent of very early juvenile physical limitations. This drastic attempt to avoid transition from p-s position to depressive position by cutting the patient off from the stimulations of reality contributes to a state usually assumed to be senility and, of course, a sense of loneliness. It would be good to discuss the paper at a group, but in the mean time I hope you will have a very successful evening.

With very best wishes
Wilfred.

Second letter from Wilfred Bion, written the day before Klein's birthday on 30 March

Redcourt
Stanhope Road
E. Croydon
Mar 29th

Dear Mrs Klein
First of all Francesca and I want to send our love and very best wishes for your birthday. We hope you will pass it happily and with the pleasant prospect of your Easter holiday to come.

With regard to your paper – I do not know if this is a birthday subject but maybe it is very appropriate – it occurred to me if you are going to make it into a book later you might care to expand the appreciation on page 4 second paragraph of integration and synthesis as something continuing through life [Author's note: These references to 'page 4 second paragraph' and 'at later the bottom of page 5′ do not correspond to any of the four versions of the paper in the archive]: to me it seems that something should be said of a sort of normal capacity for achieving the depressive position, but I think there may be a kind of 'normal' loneliness which is an accompaniment of a capacity for integration and synthesis. Unfortunately there is no real word for it. I think of isolation, loneliness, but all carry something of a pathological meaning which is misleading. The idea that there is 'no friendships at the top' also comes near to it, but again fails because the phrase has been used to describe what essentially a grievance. It seems to me there may be a 'loneliness' which is essential to the really creative person which is not simply secondary to the envy to which they are subjected, but is, partly and in extreme cases, due simply to the fact that there are not any more – the outstanding person is alone. I am aware of course that this is not what is meant ordinarily by a feeling of loneliness but nor is it described by calling it independence. However you may feel that this is not the exploration you were intending and anyhow I find it difficult to say what I myself am trying to grope for. It is a kind of hunch that loneliness of a particular kind may not be painful or misplaced but springs from the fact that some people of outstanding ability to tolerate the painful concomitants of a capacity for synthesis live in a mental environment, partly described at the bottom of page 5, but chiefly dependent on their choice to live in contact with the un-synthesised and in coherent with a view to bringing synthesis and coherence. They always confront the paranoid schizoid position in its external form, namely the unknown which science has to make known.

With very good wishes from us all, yours very sincerely
Wilfred Bion

Klein also notes ideas and corrections from Herbert Rosenfeld and Hanna Segal, and makes notes to herself about Winnicott's (1958) paper 'On the capacity to be alone'. The Rosenfeld note is obscure, as it is refers to small corrections on untraceable numbered pages. However the notes related to Segal and Winnicott are more substantial.

Hanna Segal

On C.29 image 41, in Klein's handwriting, appears:

> **From Segal re Congress paper. P.4 difference between paranoid and depressive loneliness to come out more throughout and first on page 4. P 4 and 5 loneliness due to split off parts of self make more out; and stress the more paranoid the more feeling of lost parts.**

Donald Winnicott

On C.29 image 86, Klein notes as follows:

> **An infant who can experience repeated feelings of enjoyment and gratitude is also able at times to be quite happy by himself because he has enough trust in the internal object to be able to hope for the return of the external one. Winnicott, in his paper 'On the Capacity to be Alone' suggests that the infant learns to be alone by having his mother still near and also by internalization of her. I would add that at times when anxiety is not uppermost, even young infants are able to picture the presence of the mother. But this is much more the case in the second year, when the child's reality sense increases and he can interpret sounds in the house as the presence of the mother. This no doubt helps him to acquire a certain sense of independence because at the beginning his feeling of loneliness is mitigated by the knowledge that his mother is not far away.**

I will move on now to some of the further notes Klein made for her book. I have each time marked in bold, as with the two notes above, those ideas which do not appear, or at least are not fully elaborated, in the published paper.

C.29 consists of 129 sheets of paper. Many of these are isolated sheets; sometimes two or three sheets are consecutive. Occasionally a sheet consists simply of one underlined idea. Repeatedly in the C.29 notes Klein writes 'for book' or 'to book on loneliness', and lists *what she wants to bring out about loneliness.*

Klein seems full of ideas, and her language is often poetic, in what feels an upwelling of creativity in this final part of her life. Some ideas might have been very personal to her and her own lifetime of struggles. The need for, and the difficulty of, integration is clearly an important preoccupation for her, and we have seen how she was collecting and wishing to integrate ideas from colleagues. Klein comes back again and again to what she sees as the fundamental *source of loneliness* in the imperfect and lost experience of being understood by the mother in infancy. She links this with a *need for harmony, balance and inner peace in the personality*.

Klein devotes considerable space to Segal's suggestion that she *distinguishes more between paranoid and depressive loneliness*. Perhaps prompted by Bion, she develops the theme of *the loneliness of the creative person*. In relation to this she develops her own ideas about the *need for solitude*. Another new theme that appears is that of *the loneliness of the child*. Klein also comes back several times in her notes to her belief that *a degree of omnipotence is necessary for hope*, just touched on in the published paper. It is particularly striking how much Klein worries away at *the difficulties of integrating male and female parts of the personality*. There is considerable extra material about the dreamer of the 'lioness and snake' dream of the published paper, whose difficulty integrating male and female identifications in the personality was, Klein felt, a major source of the loneliness uncovered in his analysis. Also on this theme she collects some material from other patients.

Finally, Klein writes more than appears in the published paper on the themes of *ageing well or badly, of acceptance or denial of death*.

What follows are samples of Klein's further thoughts on loneliness, collected under the headings above. Where I quote Klein, the passages I have put in bold seem to me more or less new, or at least developing the thoughts in the published paper.

General aims of book on loneliness – what Klein 'wants to bring out' in the book

C.29 image 8 typed heading: **Note for book on Loneliness.**

> **I want to speak more about the loneliness of old people and link it with the attitudes of the infant, and enlarge on the integration between male and female.**
>
> **Also the loneliness of the creative person and the painful pleasure of that loneliness.**

The basis or source of loneliness – linked with the need for 'harmony', 'balance', 'wholeness' and 'inner peace' in the personality

The longing for 'wholeness' comes up on page 302 of the published paper and Klein accentuates this more in her notes, repeatedly using the words 'harmony', 'balance' and 'inner peace' and once 'the longing to find oneself'. Insofar as all this is not achieved, a feeling of loneliness remains.

Image 52

> **Loneliness – this has to do with inner peace or lack of inner peace, which not necessarily counteracted by external activities. It goes back to having sufficiently brought together oneself with the good object.**

Image 137

> **The mother's breast, which gives food, warmth and love, maybe be felt also to bring about the harmony between different parts of the self.** ... There is little doubt that some satisfaction of this primal need is found in external relations. But it never fully counteracts **the deep and excessive need for wholeness of the self**. This excessive need is also perhaps an explanation why external relations, however helpful and satisfactory, still leave the individual with a core of loneliness.

Image 140

> Danger to the self is bound up with danger to the good object; and **only if the trust in one's capacity for love is strong enough can relative harmony within the self and with the good object be achieved**.
>
> In spite of the difficulties which are in the way, **the longing to find oneself is never given up and is, as I suggested, the origin of the sense of loneliness**.

Distinctions between paranoid and depressive loneliness

Probably partly prompted by Segal, Klein makes extensive notes in C.29 more clearly distinguishing paranoid from depressive sorts of loneliness. Here are some examples:

Images 42–43

> When depressive anxiety culminates in the depressive position ... **If the sense of guilt and paranoid anxiety prevent synthesis and integration, the all important processes of making reparation are impeded and an overwhelming feeling of guilt which is among other factors due to a strong sense of destructive omnipotence, requires an equally strong constructive omnipotence of which the weakened ego is not capable. As a result there is a strong feeling of damaged internal and external objects which is a cause of loneliness ... One could therefore describe as the core of depressive loneliness the incapacity to keep the good object and the good part of the self alive**.

> **Paranoid and depressive loneliness have in common that integration of the ego, reliance and trust on the capacity for love, have not come about. But it is a difference in emphasis: with the paranoid it is the need to pacify persecutors; with depressives it is the need to preserve the object. Since integration is deficient in both cases, the first and main means of counteracting loneliness is inadequate.**

Image 60

> **The sense of loneliness takes somewhat different forms according to whether paranoid or depressive anxiety is prevalent. Paranoid loneliness leads to a greedy need for people and relations, for external values such as prestige and success at any price. None of this actually counteracts the core of loneliness. Loneliness in which depressive anxieties predominate is more centred on a failure of the capacity for reparation which centres primarily on the inner object whereas in paranoid loneliness projection is much stronger and therefore the external object is so much more important.**

The loneliness of the creative person/leader

Bion's letter probably played some part here:

> Image 20 [typed] **'to be added'** [and in handwriting] **'for the book'**
>
> **The loneliness of the leader, the loneliness of the creator, and the satisfaction of that loneliness.**

Image 121

> **In creating you find the companionship you have been looking for. Real creativeness can only be expressed if one is by oneself with one's good object and with one part of the self. One is creating ideal companions. The same feeling is transferred to include the creating of beauty and truth. It implies giving to the external world, and giving counteracts loneliness. Also it is restoring to the external world the longed for harmony and unity which cannot entirely be achieved internally. All this extends to humbler forms of creativeness. People who are capable of doing things for others or for a cause are also actuated by a similar drive. It is particularly great or fruitful in the creative artist or scientist. There is also a special loneliness in particularly creative people (expand this for book).**

The following passage is from another part of the archive, D17 Images 23–24. Interestingly it is dated 23 January 1958 (meaning well before Bion's letter).

> **There is another type** [of splitting and projective identification], **to which I have already referred, and that is a flight to the internal good object, away from everything external. This flight is based on the anxiety relating to internal and external persecutors. We find it often in artists, for whom the whole external world hardly exists, but who are craving to find inside what is good. 'Visionary' persons are often under the urge of this process. They may completely ignore external relations and their visions are an expression of what they are trying to find within themselves. They may not have a feeling of loneliness, but I believe that their states of mind are very closely linked with loneliness, for it is the interactions between a self sufficiently based on peace of mind and the relations to external people which are the foundations for not feeling lonely. Of course we have to consider that there are many ways of dealing with loneliness, which do obscure this fact. For example, certain capacities of an artistic kind, or love for nature, love for animals, are all expressions of a belief in good objects, which, however, may not have been able to develop in connection with people. There is no doubt, since I mentioned the love for artistic creation, that during this process the whole emphasis lies on inner processes, but the return to the external world at other times seems to me evidence that what I conceive as loneliness is not prevalent.**

The need for solitude

The published paper does not address solitude, and so this is a substantial addition.

> C.29 Image 18 [typed] **'to be added'** [and in handwriting] **'for the book'**
>
> **All of us at times need solitude. It is not only because we have to think about something or do something, but because we need time to be by ourselves. In these times of solitude which we need, there is that attempt to regain parts of oneself, as well as a close connection with the internal object, and at these times, external objects are intruders. If this is exaggerated, it turns people into recluses, but it would also show that the relation to the internal object is not secure enough, because if it is, the relation to external objects succeeds.**

Image 53

There is an urge to be by oneself in one's mind.

To develop a creative thought or phantasy.

One cannot follow out an idea of one's own without doing it by oneself.

But distrust of the internal object not understanding or disapproving or grudging it comes in, which means an element of depressive or persecutory anxiety is bound up with it, this need to be alone.

It is impossible to anyone to follow all one's thoughts and phantasies and one of the greatest satisfactions in life is the freedom to phantasy and think and this would be impeded by someone else even by a loved internal. Phantasies are very substantial and do not just fly, they are a very important part of trains of thought, of work, etc. One wants to be free to let them develop, but anxiety comes in because nobody can follow.

Image 55

Integration means bringing oneself together. But there is also the wish to be by oneself. One has to get oneself together. It cannot be done by not taking in the good object. But one even wants to get away from that good object. It is the self one longs for. There is the feeling that one cannot burden one's good object with decisions. There is also too much envy of it. One wants to do it all by oneself. It is the wish to get away from something which has become part of the self but is not the self.

The giving out of goodness gives great satisfaction, but you feel deprived. The feeling that you have taken in the good object and it is part of yourself still means that it is felt as an internal good object-it is never identical with the self. It is an essential part of one's inner life but it can at times turn into a persecutor if it becomes too demanding. There is a longing to be without it.

Image 122

The other reason for being by oneself is needed is due to a surfeit of projective and introjective identifications, after which the self is in need of reintegration. This has been expressed by Wordsworth in the famous lines:

> ***The world is too much with us; late and soon,***
> ***Getting and spending, we lay waste our powers.***
>
> ***Little we see in nature which is ours;***
>
> ***We have given our hearts away, a sordid boon!***
>
> **I have mentioned that to give out love and goodness, which implies giving out some of the gifts received from the good object, leads to enrichment. But there is another side of this process: in giving out parts of the self there is also a feeling that whatever is returned is not identical with the parts of the self which have been given out. So in spite of enrichment there is also a feeling of loss.**

Another new subject for the book is:

The loneliness of the infant/child

Image 104

> **The loneliness of the child includes idealizing adulthood and thinking that one will have real companionship then. Idealisation of adulthood is an important factor in the child and also links with omnipotence, for it means the hope to be able to do all the things as adults which children cannot do now. They expect to be happy as adults.**
>
> **Identification with an object exposed to suffering and far from omnipotent also leads to de-idealisation and lessening of omnipotence, and then life in front of one becomes hard without the companionship one so much longed for.**

And related to this latter point of Klein's:

Image 124

> **If the child is overwhelmed by his inability to make his parents or siblings happy, his feelings of guilt and his sense of loneliness are reinforced and he is driven to introject their unhappiness. As a result of such infantile anxieties, some depressive patients feel that their internalised figures are in urgent need or help and should be given that before the patient himself can experience relief.**

Image 133

> **For instance the patient D** [mentioned in the published paper as the man who had the lioness/snake dream]**, who was thought by himself**

and others to have been a contented child, has discovered that he actually was extremely lonely. He was not forthcoming in telling his thoughts as a child, but it appears that his desire was to have his unconscious approved and understood by a very beloved mother. This was partly fulfilled because in the earliest stages, and I have suggested, there is this unconscious understanding between a good mother and the baby and the relatively exclusive relation between them ... In the course of his analysis he had referred to a photo of himself as a baby not more than two, speaking into a toy telephone in which he looked preoccupied and, as he now realised, unhappy. At the time, and during the course of his analysis, it was understood that he was trying to speak to an internal object to establish a connection which was missing.

Omnipotence and hope

Image 102

<u>Note re Omnipotence</u>

Optimism and the feeling of being able to wait is supported by omnipotence. This need not be omnipotence to such a degree that it falls under the heading of megalomania – it can be much more moderate form and degree. But it is a part of that feeling 'never mind, I shall achieve what I want, I shall preserve my good object, etc'.

This feeling, like idealization, goes when integration is achieved.

The feeling of flatness is not only that the glamour is gone, but also what glamour consists of, and that is omnipotence.

One never loses omnipotence. Any optimism still derives from that original source. This element persists, and links with hope. There is a stimulus towards hope derived from omnipotence.

Image 127

<u>For book</u>

The importance of omnipotence: without it one cannot live. Hope is impossible without omnipotence. If you have not the feeling that you can carry something through, you cannot carry through anything.

There are other sources for the feeling of hope: trust in oneself and one's capacities and the good object.

The difficulties of integrating male and female parts of the personality

This topic takes up a lot of C.29; Klein seems to be worrying away at it in her notes. She expands upon the cases mentioned in the published paper, giving more clinical material from them and also from additional patients. This material would be a paper in itself and I will mention it only briefly here.

Image 12

Note to loneliness

Integration between male and female. Feelings of badness are split between them – sometimes they are put onto one part, sometimes on to the other. This increases the difficulty of integration.

Sometimes what we encounter is not integration but only bringing things more closely together. Full integration is impossible.

Image 20

For book on loneliness

It is to be enlarged why the superego demands identification with each of the parents. Guilt towards either of them prompts reparation towards them. This is a point worth going into in more detail, that identification is a way of making reparation. Since it is very difficult to identify with the father and mother in a way in which the masculine and feminine position is held, and competition and envy still enter into the process of reparation, there is a special point about integration between the masculine and feminine side in either case.

She adds in Image 28:

One has to be developed at the cost of the other. This is a great source of loneliness.

Image 32

One factor which makes for difficulty in experiencing the self as a whole is bisexuality. Both in male and female children the masculine and feminine aspects are fundamentally not entirely compatible. The biological factor in bisexuality is reinforced by the relation to and identification with both parents, which contain elements of admiration as well as the envious and greedy desire to

possess what both parents represent. In addition, the superego demands to identify with each of them are prompted by the need to make reparation for early desires to rob them. We know the difficulties women have over their penis envy and men over their longing for femininity. In the infant's development there is a polarity between these two parts of the self which in successful development finds some solution.

Ageing and death; resignation

Image 37

It is well known that some people become more and more bitter the older they get. The resentment about the futility of their lives, about unfulfilled wishes and disappointments – going back to the earliest ones – takes hold of them. On the other hand there are people who become more mellow as they age, which implies greater tolerance and resignation. This tolerance and resignation is, as I found, linked with a longing for reconciliation – reconciliation with all the figures in their lives by whom they felt hurt or to whom they bore grievances. As always this applies to the earliest experiences as well. In the current situation it also means reconciliation with the fate of becoming old, with all the frustrations and disadvantages of age.

Image 38 headed 'to Loneliness'

Reconciliation before death. The superego has become more mitigated. The terrifying figures are not only more split off, but become less terrifying. These are the people who can die peacefully.

Image 120

Their [old people] identification with youth, especially children and grandchildren, makes up for the fact that youth and all its pleasures have gone. **This implies also gratitude for irretrievably lost situations and pleasures, either related to the people who contributed to them or to the causes of pleasure, such as that art and beauty exist and go on existing.** [This is a poetic extension to what is said on 311 of the published paper.]

If early development has been successful, resignation – which always implies some painful elements but means that envy, greed and hate are not predominant – is bound up with hope and tolerance and a sense of proportion in which the course of nature and the fact that

death is not only inevitable but is up to a point accepted plays an important part. It means an acceptance of reality.

Image 128

The fear of death is particularly strong where persecutory anxiety is in the ascendant; death is then felt as persecution by bad internal objects that would destroy the good parts of the self and the good object. The stronger persecutory anxiety is – and here we are touching on illness – the less is enjoyment in life and the greater is the sense of loneliness.

Particularly in childhood the actual death of a sibling or parent leaves deep marks, and the fear of death which is stirred up by such losses increases loneliness. [NB of course Klein lost a much loved older sister as a child] . . . **but the feeling that these loved persons could not live their lives increases by introjective processes guilt and loneliness . . . The desire to enter into and share the lives of children or grandchildren in the future, as well as the wish to know that their lives will develop happily, can never be fulfilled; and in a wider sense this applies to the future of humanity. Such unfulfilled desires add to the feeling of loneliness and loss.**

Conclusion

In this chapter my aim has been to bring to light some archival material which I have not attempted to analyse. However it is striking that many of these notes appear to have been written only months before Melanie Klein's death. They feel to me moving and intense, at times possibly expressing something personal. I feel this particularly in her notes about the need to achieve inner harmony, balance and peace. While talking of the need for, and the pain of, integration it can be seen how Klein is at the same time herself striving to collect and integrate the ideas of her close colleagues. In this archive she keeps coming back to the difficulty of integrating male and female parts of the personality in a way that may suggest that it was of particular significance to her in her work. This subject alone would repay much further study. Klein's writing about the need for solitude feels poignant, as do her reflections on preparedness for old age and death.

Note

1 An earlier version of this chapter was presented to the British Psychoanalytical Society on 6 June 2018. It was then published as Milton, J. (2018). 'From the Melanie Klein archive: Klein's further thoughts on loneliness'. *International Journal of Psychoanalysis*, 99, 929–946.

References

Klein, M. (1963). On the sense of loneliness. In *Envy and gratitude and other works 1946–1963*. London: Hogarth Press 1984.
O'Shaughnessy, E. (1984). Explanatory notes to Klein M. In *Envy and gratitude and other works 1946–1963*. London: Hogarth Press.
Winnicott, D.W. (1958). The capacity to be alone. *Int. J. Psychoanal.*, *39*, 416–420.

13

NOTES ON 'DICK' IN THE MELANIE KLEIN ARCHIVES

Maria Rhode

Introduction

In 1930, Melanie Klein published her seminal paper 'The importance of symbol-formation for the development of the ego' (Klein, 1930), in which she discussed the processes by which the developing child invests the outside world with emotional meaning and becomes able to engage in reality testing. Symbolism, she wrote, 'is the foundation of all sublimation and of every talent, since it is by way of symbolic equation that things, activities and interests become the subject of libidinal phantasies' (Klein, 1930, p. 220). Her clinical illustration used material from the earliest sessions of a 4-year-old boy she called Dick, who functioned at the level of a child of 15–18 months, had virtually no words or interests, showed no attachment to adults and treated her like a piece of furniture. His behaviour as described would today lead to a diagnosis of autism; in the absence of this diagnosis, Klein considered him to be schizophrenic. She shows how she managed to get in touch with him and, by analysing his latent anxiety, to mobilize his manifest anxiety and, with it, his attachment to his family and to her.

Extensive detailed process notes from Dick's analysis have been discovered in the Klein Archives (PP/KLE/B.31–34 and B.48–49) held at the Wellcome Library. These cover 5 months at the beginning of his analysis, and also later periods of his life when he was 8–9 years old, 16–17 years old, and 20. Because there is some identifying material in these files, general access is restricted until 2031. However, in view of the important scientific nature of the material, I have been given permission by the Melanie Klein Trust to use it for this chapter, with careful attention to confidentiality. In what follows, I will consider some of the main themes from these various periods of Dick's analysis. I will give illustrations of Klein's technical approach and of her conceptualizations. I will focus on Klein's understanding of Dick in relation to later psychoanalytic work on autism; both on ideas that she did not publish and that anticipate later theories, such as the construction of the body image. Finally, I will discuss aspects of the relation between autism and schizophrenia in the light of Klein's reflections on Dick and of work by later authors.

Klein's published 1930 paper on 'The importance of symbol-formation in the development of the ego'

'The clinical material of this paper,' as the editors of *The Writings of Melanie Klein* say in their Notes, 'opens a new era' (in Klein, 1975, p. 428). In the first published analytic account of psychotic states in a child, Klein showed that it was possible to make contact with 'Dick', a 4-year-old boy who had only a few words, no interests except trains, stations and doorknobs, and no reciprocal relationships. The paper built on her previous explorations of psychotic processes in children, and she suggested that research into these processes must be a central task of child analysis. In her view, there was great therapeutic potential in treating children's psychotic features, and the new knowledge gained would allow more refined differential diagnosis and illuminate such questions as the part played by psychosis in failures of cognitive development.

Theoretical formulations

Kanner's delineation of the syndrome of childhood autism (Kanner, 1943) did not appear until 13 years after Klein's paper. Her description of Dick makes clear that today he would be diagnosed with autism. Before Kanner, children who were not neurotic were seen as 'feebleminded' or as suffering from childhood schizophrenia, and Klein devoted a long discussion to the question of whether Dick could properly be described as schizophrenic. In favour of such a diagnosis were his mutism, his withdrawal and his almost total absence of involvement with other people. Against it was the fact that schizophrenia generally involved regression from a more advanced developmental level, which Dick had failed to reach in the first place. In the end, Klein decided that schizophrenia was an appropriate diagnosis, but her reservations are clear.

The paper develops a number of ideas that were central to Klein's thinking at the time. These include the fundamental role of anxiety in development and inhibited development; early manifestations of the Oedipus complex; the ramifications of hostile and sadistic impulses towards the parents; the child's phantasy relation to the mother's body and the people it was felt to contain; and the internalization of important figures leading to the construction of the child's internal world. The paper also introduces new theoretical formulations. Klein points out that repression, the defence mechanism *par excellence* of neurosis, did not apply to Dick's early material. Instead, he resorted to the more primitive mechanism of expulsion in order to rid himself both of his aggressive impulses and of the bad internal figures by whom he felt threatened. Expulsion was Klein's first attempt at outlining projective identification, as she was to call it 16 years later in 'Notes on some schizoid mechanisms' (Klein, 1946). A further theoretical innovation was her description of the emotional basis for cognitive functioning. She had touched on this earlier (Klein, 1921, 1923), and it was in Bion's (1962a, 1962b) work that this line of thought later became central. But Klein's 1930 paper demonstrates the connection between the child's ability to tolerate various kinds of anxiety and his ability to engage with reality testing and so to differentiate between external figures and the inhabitants of his own internal world. This in turn underpins an increasingly realistic view of other people as well as of inanimate objects.

Technical considerations

In her published paper, Klein quotes material from Dick's very first sessions only, and follows this with a summary of some of the improvements he had made after 6 months. She documents the impressive changes that took place in treatment, illustrates how her knowledge of other children allowed her to establish contact with him, and describes how, once she had done so, she could begin to rely on Dick's own material rather than on previous knowledge. Crucially, she assumed that the interests he did have – in trains, stations, doors and doorknobs, interests that are all typical of children with autism – meant the same thing to him as they might to a neurotic child and reflected a preoccupation with the father's penis inside the mother. This in itself implies that he had already developed some capacity for symbolic representation.

Accordingly, she adopted an active technique: she presented him with two trains, large and small, and told him they were a Daddy train and a Dick train. Dick immediately responded by driving the Dick train towards the window, explaining, 'station'. When Klein commented that the station was Mummy and Dick was driving into Mummy, he ran to the dark space between the double doors to the consulting room and said, 'Dark'. Klein said that Dick was inside dark mummy. Later he picked up a railway truck containing coal, and said, 'Cut'. He was too inhibited to cut it himself – Klein noted that he was unable to hold a knife or a pair of scissors, though he had no difficulty in holding a spoon. She cut the coal for him, interpreting that Dick wanted to cut faeces out of mummy's tummy – material that was familiar to her from her early child patients in Berlin. Her understanding was that the analysis and alleviation of unconscious anxiety allowed conscious anxiety to become manifest, and with it Dick's attachment to his parents and his nurse, whom he now for the first time missed and was pleased to see. His interest in the toys and his capacity to play increased. Klein theorized this as being at least partly because of the search for new symbolic representations of the mother's body once the familiar ones had, as it were, become saturated with anxiety. She was later to elaborate in many places this central idea that an optimal level of anxiety was necessary for development: enough to encourage the child's exploration of different forms of symbolization, but not so much as to lead to the shut-down of reality testing and the paralysis of the epistemophilic instinct.

'Dick' in the Klein Archives

Dick was the first child of a couple with an interest in psychoanalysis. Detailed notes exist for the first 5 months of work (January to May 1929); Klein also retained some useful information provided by the parents. In the second main section of notes Dick was about 9. In the third main section (in 1941 and 1942) Dick was 16 and 17. The last notes, from 1945 when Dick was 20, cover a few sessions when he was extremely anxious about having to go into hospital to have teeth extracted under a general anaesthetic. Further short passages are difficult to place.

The first tranche of notes (PP/KLE/B.32) highlights central areas of Klein's technique, including her handling of the transference and her evolving views on reassurance. They illustrate her emphasis on Dick's persecutory anxiety, in contrast to later work on the existential bodily fears of children with autism. They also show his unusual sensitivity to adults' state of mind, which anticipates later observations on autistic children. Finally, they provide evidence for her assertion that Dick had made more developmental progress than was immediately visible.

The notes from the two main later periods (B.33/34 and B.48/49) show us Dick when he was fully verbal and apparently doing fairly well academically and musically (he was largely home schooled). However, he still had major social difficulties, and his tutor or governess informed Klein when he was 9 just how shockingly unusual his behaviour in public places could be. When he was 16, too, external circumstances that made him anxious could easily trigger meltdowns that had a psychotic quality, and Klein discusses various factors contributing to his confusional states.

Inevitably, these notes contain far more important material than there is room to discuss. I will emphasize those aspects that are most relevant to conceptualizations of autism, rather than the general theoretical points that are familiar from Klein's published papers.

Dick at 4: The first 5 months of treatment

Dick's early history: Environmental factors

Klein describes Dick at 4 as being at the general developmental level of a child of 15 or 18 months. He had a few words, which he had begun to use at the age of 2 after producing his first word (which was 'No!') at 18 months. As Klein wrote in the published paper, Dick's mother was desperate to continue feeding him in spite of having little milk, so that he went virtually without food for his first 2 or 3 weeks. Indeed, the paper contains enough facts about this very difficult beginning to show how mistaken is the view that Klein paid no attention to external circumstances.

The notes provide further detail. Because of his mother's small nipples, the parents said, Dick did not latch on; instead he bit and chewed. After 2–3 weeks he was finally given a bottle, but he still did not suck properly. Although a wet-nurse kept him alive (the parents' view was that he hardly needed to suck as she had so much milk), he appears not to have taken to that feeding experience either. What is not explicitly stated is just how invalidated his mother must have felt. It is recorded that she apparently tried to restrain herself from loving and cuddling him, as this might lead to problems. She must have been left feeling that she had nothing of value to give him. Information that she provided to Mrs Klein shows her capacity for careful observation of Dick and her detailed knowledge of his likes and dislikes.

A new nurse who joined the family when Dick was 2 was much more affectionate than the first, and at that point he also spent time with his very loving grandmother (Klein, 1930). Under their influence, Klein notes, he managed to become clean and dry, but not to accept emotional contact with them. He did not play and his interests were seriously restricted, but he did engage in peep-bo when he was in a good mood. This implies the beginning representation of losing and re-finding an emotionally significant person, and is therefore prognostically encouraging. But Dick's mother also reported that, when he was asked to repeat words, he might deliberately repeat the opposite of what was expected. This suggests a greater level of understanding than one might have assumed from his general behaviour, but it also raises the question of how far he might come to be able or willing to cooperate with adults.

These recorded details of Dick's history reinforce the impression that Klein paid full attention to the importance of early experience, though therapeutically she focused on the child's internal world. She acknowledged the trauma Dick suffered through nearly starving, but emphasized even more the absence of love although he 'had every care'.

Klein's conceptual framework

When Klein began working with Dick, she had not yet formulated her concept of the paranoid-schizoid and depressive positions, though in her notes she frequently refers to his fears concerning persecutory or damaged people or part-objects. Equally, this was some 40 years before Bick (1968) and Meltzer (1975a) described the adhesive mode of relating, which was central to Tustin's work with children on the spectrum (Tustin, 1980, p. 80; Tustin, 1994, p. 15) as well as to Meltzer's (1975b). In line with her experience with previous patients, Klein's interpretations to Dick emphasize his phantasies about his mother's body and its desirable contents (babies, faeces and father's penis) as well as his sadistic impulses towards these, since she believed at this point (Klein, 1928, 1932) that the early Oedipus complex arose at the time of what she called the 'phase of maximal sadism'.

In fact, Dick soon showed unmistakeable signs of being frightened of the consequences of his aggression. For example, in the third session:

> 'When finds wagon with "coals" cut it'. I give him some scissors he takes them tries to jab at coals, but cannot hold scissors. At a look from him I scrape & cut out with scissors the coal inside & for the first time I get an expressive look (gratitude). He throws pieces into drawer, likewise damages wagon & says 'gone'. – Likewise had repeatedly said about wagon & engine that was looking at & had then thrown away like that. – I interpreted: [Dick] cuts etete [faeces] out of Mummytummy. – He then runs away from drawer & to door space & scrapes something with nail on glass of doors. I make same interpretation. – Afterwards repeats this a few times running out of door space & corner behind chest from there looking anxiously at door space .... – Has also discovered cupboard & now does the same things there as with door space. Asking for Nurse more and more often running out of room into hall. Anxiety much clearer.
>
> *(B.32)*

'Gone', like 'broken', is often among the first words spoken by children with autism (though not by Dick), but lengthy work is often necessary before this fear can be linked to any action on the part of the child. In this extract, Dick had already reached a level of being able to understand the consequences of aggression: an example of his hidden developmental achievements that Klein referred to in the published paper. Klein focused on Dick's impulse to cut 'etete' (faeces) out of Mummy, rather than on his fear of the consequences, though in the published paper she stressed that his inhibition made him unable to hold scissors or a knife.

Expulsion as a defence

Somewhat later, Klein described the bodily expulsion of damaged objects as well as of Dick's own aggressive impulses:

> Looks at wagon in drawer takes out a brown-striped one loaded with small logs & says: 'cut it, – knife' I give him scissors, then at his wish knife that can hardly hold (all aggression/paralysed) demands I cut it. When I have broken the logs out looks at them & partly broken wagon puts it back in the drawer. Finds a hairpin on the ground, wants it alternately fixed in his & my hair, takes knife again & begins to scrape table. Suddenly puts it on fireplace says: 'Naughty knife.' Then runs to dark door space stands in there, opens door into passage runs out, – fearfully comes back takes a wagon & puts it first in door-space then in hall says 'good by'. (Running out partly running away in front of me partly projecting outward the cutting Dick as well as putting away naughty knife &

> putting out object also putting back into mother.) . . .. He avoids cupboard today (/change of anxiety object/between cupboard & door-space./
>
> *(B.32)*

This passage illustrates how Dick's fear of aggression leads to an inhibition in grasping; it also illustrates how he tries to expel his 'naughty', cutting self, though Klein comments that he is 'also putting back into mother'. The very interesting material concerning the hairpin anticipates later work: Tustin (1972a) was to describe how her patient David built up his own bodily identity by 'snipping bits off his father as though he were a lifeless thing'. This constellation is often met with in autistic children, leading to a fear that any growth is at the adult's expense. This can be associated with impaired introjection and with the kind of feeding difficulties that Dick experienced.

Levels of interpretation: Dick's hidden developmental achievements

Klein's early notes contain various examples of Dick's hidden developmental achievements. Unlike many children with autism, he played peep-bo and could point to share attention. He frequently looked at Klein to gauge her reaction, particularly after doing something aggressive. This implies that Dick possessed a so-called 'Theory of Mind' (a realization that others have a mind similar to one's own), which is frequently absent in children with autism.

Klein's early child cases often focused on early oedipal rivalries. In *The Psycho-analysis of Children* (Klein, 1932), she described the oral precursors of these although, in contrast to some currents of contemporary Kleinian work with children (for example, Meltzer, 1967), the masculine part-object she referred to was the penis rather than the nipple. When interpreting Dick's material, she generally talked about the 'Daddy wiwi in Mummytummy', though towards the end of this first block of notes she also mentioned babies. When Dick put objects into his mouth, she addressed this in terms of phantasies of eating or drinking the Daddy wiwi.

Dick's response did in fact appear to confirm her interpretations. In the second week of work (B.32 sheets 42–43), he sat anxiously in the cupboard with the door open. Klein brought over the drawer with his toys, in which he found a broken wagon. He pushed it away, commenting, 'Naughty'. He then:

> took out a stall with little man looks at it closely from all sides says: tea (I: Daddy drinks tea etete weewee in Mummytum Dick wants etc.) Lies down on ground on his back looks at stall and hits his feet on ground. Then asks for (after interp. that wants in mother tea weewee etc. kicks to go in there) knife and runs it along table just like yesterday when said 'walk & train'. Interpret. – Grabs (through his trousers) at his genitals.

> Later in treatment, when Klein had talked about a cutting and burning Daddywiwi, he picked up a sharp toy tree and said, 'Daddy go away.' (B. 32). Though this focus on the genital level was characteristic of Klein's work at this time, it is also one of the indications that Dick had achieved a greater degree of development than many children with autism, whose material for a long time typically centres on the mouth or on primitive anxieties concerning the body
>
> *(Tustin, 1972b).*

Later in the second week Klein records material in which the fear of robbing the mother of the father appears both on the genital and on the oral level:

> Says repeatedly: poor nurse ... Asks for scissors & box of matches – throws matches out (but very fearful & hesitant & then back again (I interpret Dick takes Daddyweewees, etete out of Mummytummy puts them in Dicktummy. [Previously/he had looked at little signal box, shown me, said: Soldier gone – I interpreted Dick cuts, Daddy, daddyweewee out of mummy tummy)] Repeats: poor nurse. Cuts a sliver off matchbox lid, puts it in his mouth. 'Poor nurse' Then wants to put it in my mouth.

This links with the material of the hairpin, which Dick had passed back and forth between himself and Klein. Klein convincingly interprets that Dick is competing with the mother for her contents, which he wishes to incorporate orally himself.

In some respects, this material foreshadows Tustin's (1972b) later description of her patient John, who was convinced that the nipple that produced sensations in his mouth was part of his own body. Even in his second week of treatment Dick was functioning on a more developed level: he was concerned with separate and separable objects such as the matches that could move between his mouth and Klein's, in contrast to John's focus on the more primitive, adhesively based level of sensation and damage to his body. Similarly, when Dick pointed out the plugholes in a basin and said 'water', Klein interpreted that there was 'much water in mummy tummy/much wiwi, much etete in Mummy tummy' (B.32 sheet 3). This is clearly far more sophisticated than a characteristic fear met with in autistic children, namely that water spilling away through plugholes implies that their own body contents could spill away through holes in their skin (Tustin, 1986). This more primitive level was to re-surface when Dick was 9 (see pp 239–240).

The location of the 'black hole'

Tustin's John felt that his mouth, in the absence of the sensation-giving nipple, contained instead a 'black hole with a nasty prick' (Tustin, 1972b). In spite of functioning on a less primitive level, Dick shared with John (and with other children with autism) the fear of a black hole in the form of a dark place. This began as the dark space between the doors that he ran into in his first session, and was later sometimes represented by the dark waiting room or a dark, empty cupboard. While Klein suggests at one point later on that Dick is seeking refuge in the dark empty space in order to be safe from a dangerous 'Daddy weewee', it is clear that in far more instances he felt that, by driving the 'Dick train' into Mummy, he ended up in a dark place that he was often frightened of getting stuck in. This foreshadows Meltzer's (1992) notion of the Claustrum, in which he outlines the child's intrusive identification with various compartments of the maternal body. According to such a conceptualization, Dick's mind and glance might have been dark and empty because he was intrusively identified with a dark and empty womb. Again, this illustrates that, despite his typically autistic behaviour, Dick was operating at a surprisingly sophisticated level of development, availing himself of projective mechanisms instead of the adhesive ones that usually characterize children with autism at the beginning of treatment. Most importantly, he experienced his 'black hole' as being located in the mother's womb and mind, rather than in his own mouth: he could sustain a greater level of separateness from the Other than is typical of children on the spectrum, who often relate to their own body as though it were the mother's body, for example in episodes of self-mutilation. In two later instances, when he was 9 (B. 34 and B. 49), Dick was overwhelmed by anxiety about losing a part of his mouth (teeth); but he was terrified of hostile figures rather than focused on bodily sensation.

Achievement of the good-bad split: Meaning and sensation

Many children with autism come to treatment without having achieved the fundamental split between good and bad that Klein outlined in 1946. Emilio Rodrigué, for example, described in 1955 how his 3-year-old patient Raoul was able to take this fundamental step in the course of his analysis (Rodrigué, 1955). In contrast, Dick's very early weeks provide evidence that he had made this split: for example, he used words such as 'naughty'. Interestingly, the opposite of 'naughty' at the beginning seems to have been 'soft' rather than 'good' or 'nice'. This anticipates later findings on the importance of softness to children with autism: Tustin (1980, pp. 83–85) describes the integration of 'hard' and 'soft', which she saw as the forerunners of male and female, as one of the earliest developmental tasks, which fits with autistic children's typical reliance on sensation rather than meaning (Tustin, 1972b; Meltzer, 1975c).

In line with this, Dick was particularly focused on the softness of the velvet collar on his coat. In his sixth session (B.32 sheets 9–10) he was frightened of the dark space between the two doors and in the cupboard. Klein interpreted this as 'naughty, strict Mummy', which, together with her saying, 'soft coat' and 'nice mummy says soft coat', seems to have helped him over the fear.

Klein's handling of the transference and other technical issues

Klein wrote of this example, 'I nurture positive transference/to me' (B.32). This seems to go against her later conviction that the right way to proceed was to analyse the positive and negative transference as they arose. In the present example, she appears to have been encouraging the split between the 'naughty, strict Mummy' and herself as the 'nice' one associated with the soft coat: she spoke to both aspects of Dick's experience, even if she did not link the 'naughty, strict Mummy' to herself. The following week, she attempted again to calm Dick down by referring to the soft coat after noting (though not interpreting), 'clearly also afraid of me'. This time, Dick failed to be reassured, and she wrote: 'it did nothing to reassure (takeover positive transference only achievable by dissolving anxiety') (B.32 sheet 36). Dick had moved to the realm of meaning, and sensation no longer worked as a refuge. In later instances of his turning to the soft coat, Klein describes his eyes taking on the vacant look typical of autism, which she refers to as 'dreamy' or 'introverted'.

As she continued to do for many years, Klein focused on delineating her patient's experience at any moment in terms of a variety of internal constellations involving family members in relation to one another – good and bad mother, father and babies. (Even in the *Narrative of a Child Analysis* (Klein, 1961), where transference work is central, she might interpret 10-year-old Richard's suspicions of her as following from the idea of her getting together with 'the Hitler Daddy'.) In an amusing vignette (B.32) in fact, after she had helped Dick to enact his aggressive impulses, she talked about his worries concerning Mummy's breast, and he corrected her: 'Mrs. Klein's breast.'

Klein enacted Dick's aggressive impulses in a number of instances, particularly at the very beginning when he was still extremely inhibited. She saw this as doing for him what he could not yet do for himself, whether because of extreme anxiety or inhibition leading to physical incapacity. She wrote, 'I represent the id' and emphasized his 'asking' her by means of a glance to do this, and his look of gratitude afterwards. Clearly he was able to differentiate between her standing in for his id in this way, and her colluding with him or becoming the hostile, dangerous mummy. This was so even in a very striking instance when together they attacked the table with a knife, particularly places where there were screws. Klein asked him where Mummy's breast was on the table: he pointed it out, and seems to have added that the screws were Daddy's eyes.

In general, Klein appears to have been quite relaxed about the limits she imposed on Dick. He was allowed to damage the furniture, not just his own toys. He ran in and out of the consulting room and waiting room, generally in response to anxiety; she followed him and interpreted rather than insisting that he should remain in the room. Even when his excursions were motivated by curiosity rather than anxiety, as when he explored her dining room, she interpreted instead of preventing this. Possibly she was encouraged by the development of his impulse to investigate and did not feel it was necessary to curtail it.

The development of symbolism and language

Klein's theoretical focus in the published paper was the centrality of symbolism, and comments on this are interspersed throughout this section of the notes, particularly at the beginning. The only instance of didactic behaviour on her part involves her seemingly encouraging his symbolic capacities by playing out with the toys what he had expressed by means of his body: when he went to sit in the cupboard, which she interpreted in terms of his wanting to be in mummy's tummy, she accompanied this by putting a woman doll in a box (to show that the box was part of her) and then having a Dick doll enter it. This occurred only at the very beginning, as Dick's symbolic capacities increased very quickly.

A particularly interesting passage in B.32 seems to imply that this increase was directly connected to Dick's experience of Klein's attention. She describes how

> a few days ago when leant with him over drawer for a moment thought about something else, he lifts my head at chin & looks into my eyes. Doubtless an element of positive transference not only by interpretation in this instance but also there uncons. so much closer by my identifying with his uncons. allowing him aggression etc.

We see just how in tune Dick was with Klein's state of mind, and that he was able to check what was going on in her mind/in her head behind her eyes and at the same time to take steps to bring her back into contact. Many writers, beginning with Tustin and Meltzer, have remarked on how sensitive children with autism are to the analyst's feelings. Klein gave full weight to Dick's inability to tolerate anxiety as well as to the emotional atmosphere of his early life, but she did not extrapolate from this vignette that he might have been exceptionally aware of the darkness of his mother's mood in his early weeks. The evidence of his acute sensitivity suggests why he might have found depressive anxiety so hard to bear.[1]

Very interestingly, this vignette is immediately followed in the notes by a new sequence of play about losing and re-finding a gate: Klein mentions the *fort-da* game (Freud, 1920). While Dick had already been capable of playing peep-bo at 18 months, this passage implies that the Fort-Da play may have rested on the capacity to reclaim the analyst's attention after destructiveness had been expressed.

Klein also provides two striking examples of the link between the analysis of Dick's phantasies and his language development. The first concerns his vocabulary. At the beginning of the second week (B.32 sheet 24), he came into the room and looked at everything much more intensely and with greater comprehension.

> In drawer asks for 'etete'. I give him pencil case where I had shown him the pencils like that. He satisfied: etete pencil (*keeps the word because the right symbolic connection was made*) [italics added].

The second (considerably later) example concerns the beginnings of Dick's use of complete sentences with proper syntax. Very interestingly, the context involved his greater acknowledgement of the father's existence and rightful place (B.32 sheet 94). This is a topic that was not subsequently touched upon for decades: It calls to mind Segal's (1997) suggestion that there may exist an inborn knowledge of structured object relationships that parallels the inborn knowledge of grammatical structure.

A different aspect of symbolism concerns Klein's reading of the symbols in Dick's fast developing play. It is well known that she likened children's play to adults' dreams. Some of Dick's play constellations, for instance the various times when he pushed a brick under another one that was shaped like a bridge, which Klein took as a representation of parental intercourse, might indeed be encountered in a Freudian account of dream material; in one instance she interprets a toy rooster as a penis symbol. Elsewhere, however, her symbolic interpretations are convincingly based on context. For example, she interprets the flowers on the curtain fabric as representing babies inside the mother, but this is immediately preceded by material about attacking babies in Mummy's tummy and about animals in the drawer as representing children.

In this context, Klein noted that, after some months of work, Dick's parents reported improvements in all aspects of his behaviour. It is tantalizing that no write-ups of sessions are available for this *precise* time. However, she also noted that the parents were expecting another child. It seems reasonable to link Dick's improvement to this fact: his mother's mood may well have lightened, and he would have been reassured that his attacks on her babies had not succeeded. (Anecdotally, some children with autism react to a pregnancy by improving, while in others it may trigger further withdrawal.)

Bodily anxieties

Later work with autistic children and psychotic adults has made fundamental contributions to our understanding of the body image. Themes include primitive fears of losing body parts and body contents (Bick, 1986; Rey, 1979; Tustin, 1972b, 1986; Winnicott, 1949, 1963), as well as the relational aspects of constructing the body image (Haag, 1985, 1991). As in her other cases, Klein discusses Dick's phantasies concerning his body, particularly in connection with the aggressive use of urine and faeces: another example of addressing a more sophisticated level than later workers. The more primitive level came into focus in the second tranche of notes (see below).

A particularly striking sequence in B.32 anticipates later work (Haag, 1991) on bodily identifications: Klein describes Dick's internalization of the parents, one into each shoulder. Equally, she sees Dick's unsteady gait as being to do with his relation to an internalized penis, though this is a hostile penis that attacks him rather than a link (Haag, 1991) that has not been securely internalized.

Dick at 9 years old

Dick's material at 4 was striking for the way Klein managed to make contact with him; in view of his developmental delay, one might imagine him continuing to catch up. In fact, at 9, in material to be found in B.33 and B. 34, he was speaking fluently and playing expressively, but was clearly struggling with strong psychotic anxieties and often behaving in bizarre ways, though functioning quite well academically. At times he seemed to be hallucinating. Numerous sessions describe his pre-occupation with bogies: he personified them as babies or children of his own age; they were sometimes said to be damaged, or associated with the presence of a monster who spoke in a deep voice: 'Hi, Ho, Hu'. These phantasies about bogies modulated into an extreme fear of germs and poison, which Dick later tried to deal with by obsessional means. Klein documents many instances of his fear of these fantastical sibling figures: Dick frequently wanted to bar them from the therapy room, but sometimes asked Klein to bring them in and include them. This is an instance of his struggle to deal with frightening internalized figures who at the same time felt essential to the construction of his internal family and therefore of himself. For example, Klein records how Dick tore out and scrambled boards lining a cupboard, and then lay down on them; he later restored the cupboard by making sure that each board was returned to its proper place (see Rosenfeld, 1950). Klein interpreted this in terms of his bodily identification with a mother containing the father's penis and babies. She describes Dick's conflict between wishing to eliminate dangerous, attacked and attacking paternal part objects from the mother cupboard, and needing them to ensure the health and survival of the mother: if the father was killed, Dick's internalized mother was dead too, and so was he, as he could not restore her on his own. Similarly, the rival babies needed to survive as they were a means of restoring the mother. Dick often lay on his back on the couch, dirtying the wall with his shoes. He would say that the wall was full of crying babies and that the marks left by his shoes were their tears. On one occasion, saliva escaped from his mouth as he said this, as though it were the same as the babies' tears.[2]

In these examples, Dick's body is felt to be damaged in identification with internal figures. Klein repeatedly points out that evacuating these frightening figures leads to emptiness and to a dead internal mother, whereas not doing so spells persecution. From babyhood, Dick had retained his stool for days on end and shown distress when he finally passed it, although it was soft. Klein takes this as an example of his need to be in control of an enormous, frightening penis, and two months' work on this led to the symptom clearing up. Her theoretical focus throughout is on the effect of frightening internalized objects, and she made frequent notes about melancholic anxieties and Dick's ways of dealing with them.

However, a more primitive level now also appeared, as when Dick watched water flowing out of holes in the sink and told Klein that he had holes all over his body. He then grabbed at his anus, and Klein interpreted that holding back faeces also proved that he had no holes. In his sixth session Klein had taken Dick's interest in the water and drainage holes in terms of water in Mummy's tummy, in line with her early cases. Here, however, without the benefit of later work on fears of losing the body contents (Bick, 1986; Tustin, 1986; Rosenfeld, 1984) she followed Dick's material to formulate this more primitive dimension to his anxieties concerning defaecation. He was also pre-occupied with skin and wanted Klein to measure him for a coat, as though making his skin and putting his body together.

Dick was often unreachable and manic, and manifested strong psychotic anxiety that spilled over into the outside world. For instance, his nurse or governess reported when he was nearly 9 that he provoked a group of schoolboys by calling them 'damn fools', persisting until they hit him. He clearly envied them for going to school and wanted their attention, but was also terrified of their attacks. These 'Marylebone boys' came up often in sessions as representatives of the 'bogies' – human representatives rather than germs or 'bumfleas'.[3] Klein noted that interpreting his fears of his internal situation led to greatly improved reality testing, academic performance and general functioning, along with a better functioning of projective mechanisms and a recognition that animals and inanimate objects had their own nature, and were not merely stand-ins for internal figures of phantasy. She frequently comments, 'quite normal at this point'. Dick was obviously extremely attached to her, and recognized her role in helping him to deal with his fantastic terrors. As he improved, he focused more on the state of internalized people, whereas earlier he had talked about inanimate objects as though they were alive, and had compulsively checked Klein's clock, couch, and so on to see whether they were 'alive' and working.

Dick at this age comes over as an imaginative child, not just as one tormented by psychotic anxiety, and Klein's imagination was obviously in tune with his. The material and interpretations are often startling and poetic. For example, he switches the light off so as not to see shadows, which he says are dead. In response to her question, he explains the dead person is Captain Hook (one of his representations of a bad father figure). The dark place between two doors evolves into Captain Hook's grave, and Dick shows his identification with this dead father, and his experience of Klein as representing life, when he switches the light on while she speaks and off when he answers. In a sequence that prefigures her first paper on mourning (Klein, 1935, pp. 276–277), he says that he is fed up with being alive and wants 'nice flowers on top' of the grave with a tombstone that Klein must dig for him before throwing the balls at him with which he killed Captain Hook. Klein interprets that he wants to die to kill the bad father inside him and allow the flower-babies to grow. Dick then says that the couch is a bed, not a grave: the two cushions at either end are the parents, and other children share the bed with him.

Dick at 16–17 years old

This section of the notes covers a period from the autumn of 1941 to the early summer of 1942 and is to be found in B.48 and B. 49. Dick is greatly affected by his father's serious illness, which he takes as confirmation of his destructive attacks; Klein goes so far as to interpret that his father is the most important person in his life, since he relies completely on him to restore the mother and give her babies. Dick himself feels unable to do this on a symbolic level, as he has no belief in his own constructive capacities: this keeps him unhelpfully dependent on his good objects and inhibits his initiative in all areas. While we repeatedly hear about his phantasies of marrying Klein one day, we also hear that he will arrange for his mother to divorce his father and go with Dick to Germany to marry Hitler. Hitler would also come to Britain where Dick would 'make love' to him.

Dick was very pre-occupied with the progress of the war, which Klein interpreted in terms of his inner world constellations. Under their overwhelming influence he often completely misunderstood newspaper articles, and Klein outlined the origin of various kinds of confusion – of good and bad, of himself with other people, and of internal and external – distinctions later developed by Rosenfeld (1950). There are many instances – which diminish as time goes on – of Dick having a psychotically tinged meltdown in which he urgently and unreachably ascribes his own disturbed behaviour to other people and insists on completely unrealistic ways of controlling them, At other times he urgently and unreachably insists on something Klein must believe, or on a completely unrealistic course of action. Klein deals with these outbursts both by interpreting in terms of Dick's inner world and by drawing his attention to reality. In one fascinating late example, Dick is so oppressed by the fear that a bad internal father is winning that he completely misunderstands the newspaper account of a battle, believes that the war is lost and produces a frenzied outpouring of talk that Klein cannot get through. When he notices that she is frustrated and tired, he asks whether she will give up the work: she mustn't, she has to keep going, and if Dr Winnicott knew that she was tired he would come and stay for the whole 50 minutes to make sure she carried on. After he has allowed Klein to interpret, he seems transformed and is amazed to realize that the newspaper article was in fact quite optimistic.

Dick's bodily anxieties during this time focus on castration, in a way that Klein suggests is both developmentally appropriate and unusually charged. She describes the panic that tinges his experience of his adolescent body, in which Hitler's genital is felt to be growing through his own. However, he could also be affectionate, humorous and good company: this was confirmed even by his landlady, who said that he could behave like a normal, helpful adult or focus for an hour on practising a Mozart sonata, although at other times he had 'commotions' during which he insulted her and produced anxiety-driven streams of mad talk. He was placed with her so that he could attend analysis, but also because his behaviour at home was intolerable, something he was painfully aware of. He hoped to become an analyst and to have ideas that his father and Freud had not thought of. Klein responded very gently to this (and to his statement that she herself had had no new ideas), suggesting that he wanted to be an analyst to revive his father and make babies together. At the same time she noted that his total dependence on good internal objects to counteract bad ones left him no scope for his own initiative, which would have required greater assimilation of his good objects. She reacted with similar gentleness when he reproached her for analysing his aggression in a way that Dr Fairbairn, Dr Glover and Dr Schmideberg would never have done: this a few months before the Controversial Discussions!

Klein stresses the appearance of depressive anxieties towards the end of this period, which is otherwise largely characterized by persecution and manic behaviour. There is however a striking vignette towards the end of B.49, where Dick had the vacant look characteristic of autism and said that there was nothing in his mind. Klein reminded him of his frustration with a school administrator and suggested that, in killing him off, Dick had lost his good internal object as well. He seemed transformed by the interpretation, lost his vacant look and re-engaged with the analysis. I will return to this in connection with conceptualizations of autistic blankness.

Technically, Klein's work in this period follows on from the notes when Dick was 9. Though she emphasizes the transference slightly more, this is still within the context of elucidating internal object relationships, which she always prioritises in her interpretations. She continues to be relaxed about the boundaries of the sessions, which take place sometimes in central London and sometimes at her home in Pinner. Dick accompanies her to the train while continuing to discuss material, and she answers factually when he asks whether she has seen a certain film or what she thinks of a speech by Churchill.

Concluding remarks

Klein's notes on Dick show her developing and working with concepts that are familiar from her other works: the prime importance of good and bad internal objects, the ramifications of the early Oedipus complex, persecutory and depressive anxiety, the assimilation of internal objects. We get a close-up view of her technique – and of her warmth – comparable to that afforded by the *Narrative of a Child Analysis* (Klein, 1961) and see her anticipating later Kleinian and post-Kleinian formulations: most strikingly perhaps in her interpretations concerning Dick's experience of a body full of holes and of the way his relationship to an internal family underpins the construction of his body image as well as his psychological make-up.

The notes also raise questions central to a psychoanalytic conceptualization of autism, without providing definitive answers. In the absence of the concept of adhesive identification, Klein addressed Dick's material on the level of internal objects, which tend to be incompletely developed in children with autism given their difficulties with internalization. Indeed, while Tustin (1983) suggests on the basis of his history and behaviour that Dick's presentation was typical of Kanner's syndrome, she also sees Klein's interpretations as being more appropriate to a schizophrenic child. Dick's striking response to them may well have been a function of his having achieved a greater degree of development than is true of many autistic children beginning treatment. This includes the acquisition of some words and of a rudimentary ability to play; the attainment of some degree of separateness from the other and of a good–bad split; and the beginnings of projection. He had less recourse to sensation than many children with autism, and even this diminished very quickly during the first period of treatment.

Both Tustin and Meltzer contrasted the adhesive, sensuous, two-dimensional world of the autistic child with the three-dimensional functioning of schizophrenia, where a greater degree of separateness has been achieved and projection and projective identification predominate. Tustin (1990), however, also described children who made use of an 'autistic straitjacket' to hold psychotic anxieties in check: these emerged once the autistic protections had been modified. While the schizoid phenomena can sometimes be seen to have been present from the beginning of treatment (Rhode, 2011), other cases document the varying presentations that may appear once autistic features have been ameliorated – schizophrenic, manic-depressive or obsessional (Haag, 1997). Finally, Durban (2018) has proposed the existence of an 'autistic-psychotic' spectrum, where the child oscillates between anxieties and defences typical of autism and of psychosis.

Klein's notes on Dick do not resolve these debates, but Dick's episode of 'autistic' blankness at the age of 17 makes it plausible that he may have similarly been blanking out frightening constellations from early on, which would be consistent with the speed of his response in analysis. Reading the details of his development is not just fascinating in itself, but provides insights that remain fundamental after decades of developments in the field.

Notes

1 Meltzer (1975c) was later to suggest that children with autism were assailed by 'premature' depressive concerns at a time when their mothers were suffering from depression, whereas Klein, in her published paper, writes in terms of premature genital tendencies.
2 This anticipates Meltzer's later view that the child cannot repair the mother himself: he can only allow the father to carry out his function of doing so.
3 These permutations of fantastical sibling figures anticipate Tustin's (1972: 177–178) description of the 'nest of babies' that is a recurrent constellation in children with autism.

References

Bick, E. (1968). The experience of the skin in early object relations. *International Journal of Psycho-Analysis*, *49*, 484–486.

Bick, E. (1986). Further considerations on the importance of the skin in early object relations: Findings from infant observation integrated into child and adult analysis. *British Journal of Psychotherapy*, *2*, 2992–2999.

Bion, W.R. (1962a). A theory of thinking. In *Second thoughts*, London: Heinemann, 1967.
Bion, W.R. (1962b). *Learning from experience*. London: Heinemann.
Durban, J. (2018). 'Making a person' – Clinical considerations regarding the interpreting of anxieties in the analyses of children on the autisto-psychotic spectrum. *International Journal of Psycho-Analysis*. Open vol. *5*.
Freud, S. (1920). Beyond the pleasure principle. *Standard edition of the complete works of Sigmund Freud*. Vol *18*. London: Hogarth.
Haag, G. (1985). La mère et le bébé dans les deux moitiés du corps. *Neuropsychiatrie de l'Enfance*, *33*, 107–114.
Haag, G. (1991). Nature de quelques identifications dans l'image du corps (hypothèses). *Journal de la Psychanalyse de l'Enfant*, *4*, 73–92.
Haag, G. (1997). Psychosis and autism: Schizophrenic, perverse and manic-depressive states during psychotherapy. In M. Rustin, M. Rhode, A. Dubinsky and H. Dubinsky, *Psychotic states in children*. London: Karnac.
Kanner, L. (1943). Autistic disturbances of affective contact. *Nervous Child*, *2*, 217–250.
Klein, M. (1921). The development of a child. In *Love, guilt and reparation and other works 1921–1945: The writings of Melanie Klein vol. 1*. London: Hogarth Press, 1975, pp. 1–53.
Klein, M. (1923). Early analysis. In *Love, guilt and reparation and other works 1921–1945: The writings of Melanie Klein vol. 1*. London: Hogarth Press, 1975, pp. 77–105.
Klein, M. (1928). Early stages of the Oedipus conflict. In *Love, guilt and reparation and other works 1921–1945: The writings of Melanie Klein vol. 1*. London: Hogarth Press, 1975, pp. 186–198.
Klein, M. (1930). The importance of symbol-formation in the development of the ego. In *Love, guilt and reparation and other works 1921–1945: The writings of Melanie Klein, vol. 1*. London: Hogarth Press, 1975, pp. 219–232.
Klein, M. (1932). Early stages of the Oedipus conflict and of super-ego formation. In *The psycho-analysis of children: The writings of Melanie Klein vol. 2*. London: Hogarth Press, pp. 123–148.
Klein, M. (1935). A contribution to the psychogenesis of manic-depressive states. In *Love, guilt and reparation and other works 1921–1945: The writings of Melanie Klein vol. 1*. London: Hogarth Press, 1975, pp. 262–289.
Klein, M. (1946). Notes on some schizoid mechanisms. In *Envy and gratitude and other works: The writings of Melanie Klein vol. 3*. London: Hogarth Press, 1975, pp. 1–24.
Klein, M. (1961). *Narrative of a child analysis*: *The writings of Melanie Klein vol. 4*, London: Hogarth Press, 1975.
Klein, M. (1975). *Love, guilt and reparation and other works 1921–1945: The writings of Melanie Klein*. London: Hogarth Press.
Meltzer, D. (1967). *The psychoanalytic process*. London: Heinemann.
Meltzer, D. (1975a). Adhesive identification. *Contemporary Psychoanalysis*, *11*, 289–310.
Meltzer, D. (1975b). Dimensionality in mental functioning. In D. Meltzer, J. Bremner, S. Hoxter, D. Weddell, and I. Wittenberg (eds), *Explorations in autism*. Strath Tay: Clunie Press, pp. 223–238.
Meltzer, D. (1975c). The psychology of autistic states and of post-autistic mentality. In D. Meltzer, J. Bremner, S. Hoxter, D. Weddell, and I. Wittenberg (eds), *Explorations in autism*. Strath Tay: Clunie Press, pp. 6–32.
Meltzer, D. (1992). *The claustrum*. Strath Tay: Clunie Press.
Rey, H. (1979). Schizoid phenomena in the borderline. Reprinted in E. Spillius (ed.), *Melanie Klein today, Vol. 2. Mainly Theory*. London: Routledge, 1988.

Rhode, M. (2011). Asperger's syndrome: A mixed picture. *Psychoanalytic Inquiry, 31*, 288–302.

Rodrigué, E. (1955). The analysis of a three-year-old mute schizophrenic. In M. Klein, P. Heimann and R.E. Money-Kyrle (eds), *New directions in psycho-analysis*. London: Tavistock Publications.

Rosenfeld, D. (1984). Hypochondrias, somatic delusion and body scheme in psychoanalytic practice. *International Journal of Psycho-Analysis, 65*, 377–387.

Rosenfeld, H. (1950). Note on the psychopathology of confusional states in chronic schizophrenias. *International Journal of Psycho-Analysis, 31*, 132–137.

Segal, H. (1997). Phantasy and reality. In *Psychoanalysis, literature and war: Papers 1972–1995*. The New Library of Psychoanalysis. London: Routledge, p. 28.

Tustin, F. (1972) *Autism and childhood psychosis*. London: Hogarth Press.

Tustin, F. (1972a). Autistic processes in action. In *Autism and childhood psychosis*. London: Hogarth Press, pp. 32–50.

Tustin, F. (1972b). Psychotic depression. In *Autism and childhood psychosis*. London: Hogarth Press, pp. 4–31.

Tustin, F. (1980). Psychological birth and psychological catastrophe. In *Autistic states in children*. London: Routledge. Second revised edition, 1992, pp. 78–94.

Tustin, F. (1983). Thoughts on autism with special reference to a paper by Melanie Klein. *Journal of Child Psychotherapy, 9*, 119–131.

Tustin, F. (1986). Spilling and dissolving. In *Autistic barriers in neurotic patients*. London: Karnac. Second revised edition, 1994, pp. 197–214.

Tustin, F. (1990). *The protective shell in children and adults*. London: Karnac.

Tustin, F. (1994). The perpetuation of an error. *Journal of Child Psychotherapy, 20*, 3–23.

Winnicott, D.W. (1949). Birth memories, birth trauma and anxiety. In *Through paediatrics to psycho-analysis*. London: Tavistock Publications.

Winnicott, D.W. (1963). The mentally ill in your caseload. In *The maturational process and the facilitating environment*. London: Hogarth Press, pp. 217–229.

INDEX

References to endnotes consist of the page number followed by the letter 'n' followed by the number of the note.

For Product Safety Concerns and Information please contact our EU
representative GPSR@taylorandfrancis.com
Taylor & Francis Verlag GmbH, Kaufingerstraße 24, 80331 München, Germany

www.ingramcontent.com/pod-product-compliance
Ingram Content Group UK Ltd.
Pitfield, Milton Keynes, MK11 3LW, UK
UKHW022030061126
477531UK00003B/140
9780367337896